SURGICAL ANATOMY
OF THE HUMAN BODY

DEAVER

GENERAL ARRANGEMENT OF CONTENTS

SURGICAL ANATOMY
OF THE HUMAN BODY

BY

JOHN B. DEAVER, M.D., SC.D., LL.D., F.A.C.S.

SURGEON-IN-CHIEF TO THE LANKENAU HOSPITAL, PHILADELPHIA, EMERITUS
JOHN REA BARTON PROFESSOR OF SURGERY, UNIVERSITY OF PENNSYLVANIA

SECOND EDITION. IN THREE VOLUMES
THOROUGHLY REVISED AND REARRANGED

PROFUSELY ILLUSTRATED WITH DRAWINGS FROM ORIGINAL DISSECTIONS
MADE ESPECIALLY FOR THIS WORK

VOLUME I
SCALP, CRANIUM, BRAIN, FACE, MOUTH, THROAT, ORGANS
OF SPECIAL SENSES

PHILADELPHIA
P. BLAKISTON'S SON & CO.
1012 WALNUT STREET

PRINTED IN U. S. A.
BY THE MAPLE PRESS COMPANY, YORK, PA.

TO

Surgeons and to Students of Surgery and Anatomy,

WHOSE LABORS IT IS INTENDED TO LIGHTEN IN A FIELD WHERE
LABOR ALONE IS THE PRICE OF ATTAINMENT,

THIS WORK

IS RESPECTFULLY DEDICATED
BY THEIR FRIEND AND FELLOW-STUDENT

THE AUTHOR.

PREFACE TO THE SECOND EDITION

It is now twenty-five years since the appearance of the original edition of this book. While gross human anatomy undergoes no change, the passing of time has seen a closer correlation of anatomy and physiology, and a greater emphasis placed upon the surgical anatomy of the brain, neck, thorax and abdomen. Therefore it has been necessary to largely rewrite sections of the book, this being especially true of the brain.

Time, experience, and improvement in operative technic have enabled the surgeon to explore certain fields that were but rarely entered when this work was first published, so that those surgical procedures which have a definite anatomical bearing have also had to be rewritten and brought in conformity with modern methods.

Twenty-five years ago there had been little attempt made to obtain a uniform nomenclature, but since then the Basle nomenclature has come into more or less general use, and although it is not ideal, it marks the beginning of a uniform, international, anatomical terminology. In revising the work the English equivalent of the B.N.A., has been used (Jamieson's Basle Anatomical Nomenclature serving as a guide) so that those who are more familiar with it may use the text without confusion. At the same time, since the book will probably be used by the older surgeons as well as by students, the old terminology has been retained in the text, followed by the English equivalent of the B.N.A. in parenthesis.

It is hoped that the present rearrangement of the text, will do much to enhance its value from the point of view of accessibility. The first volume now consists of the surgical anatomy of the head and the brain, the face, mouth, nasopharynx, eye, and ear, so that the surgeon who confines himself to one of the surgical specialities of this region will not have to turn from this volume to find the material he desires. The second volume contains the anatomy of the upper extremities, neck, shoulders, back, and lower extremities; the third volume that of the chest, abdomen, pelvis, and perineum.

The demands of a busy surgical practice have retarded the preparation of this edition of the work for a period of years. Even now publication would have been much prolonged had it not been for the valuable assistance I have been fortunate in obtaining. Dr. Temple Fay, formerly associated with the

neurological department of the University of Pennsylvania, has assisted in bringing the work on the brain and spinal cord, up to date, and I here acknowledge my
indebtedness to him.   In the revision of the work as a whole, I have been
assisted by my former pupil and friend, Dr. I. S. Ravdin, Assistant Surgeon to
the University Hospital and Associate in Surgery in the Graduate School of
the University of Pennsylvania, where he has had charge of Surgical Anatomy
in the Surgical Section for the past six years.   He has devoted much time and
thought to this revision which I deeply appreciate and this appreciation expressed
in words gives only a faint idea of my gratitude to him.   To Dr. Elizabeth G.
Ravdin was entrusted the insertion of the B.N.A. nomenclature and also the
reading of the proof.   It gives me pleasure to express my sincere thanks for her
valuable services.   Throughout the years during which the revision has been in
progress I have had the constant help of Miss A. M. Jastrow.   Without her
assistance the work would yet remain unfinished.   I owe her an everlasting
debt.   My thanks are also due to Miss Eleanor Paxson for the new drawings
that appear; and to Dr. A. D. Whiting for the preparation of the index.   Special
acknowledgement is due to the publishers, Messrs. P. Blakiston's Son & Co. for
their patience and consideration.   In this connection mention must be made
of the valuable advice of Mr. C. V. Brownlow and particularly of the painstaking
co-operation and helpful suggestions of Mr. E. B. Barnes, to whom I herewith
express my warmest thanks.

I have always maintained that the road to efficient surgery leads to and
from the dissecting room, and if in these volumes I have succeeded in inculcating
this principle in the minds of the surgeon and the student, I shall feel satisfied
that the labor expended has not been in vain.

JOHN B. DEAVER.

PHILADELPHIA,
April, 1926.

PREFACE TO FIRST EDITION

This book has been twelve years in preparation. During this time, while no change has been made in its plan, its scope has been much enlarged, to meet a wider field than for which it was first intended. My original purpose was to furnish for students a text-book of Surgical Anatomy, then much needed and not obtainable by them. I have made a book which will be serviceable, I hope, not alone to them, but to practising physicians and surgeons. While, I regret to say, this subject is much neglected in our American institutions, there came to be nevertheless, during the progress of this work, an increasing and encouraging recognition of its importance. In some schools the course was much enlarged; in others new courses were established. In my own classes the work has constantly grown, until it has become not alone an adjunct to, and application of descriptive anatomy, but rather the bridge between the study and practice of surgery itself. To meet these requirements it has not been sufficient for me to emphasize and clarify the facts of descriptive anatomy as required of undergraduates. I have been compelled to bring to them the knowledge of anatomy which I have used and as I have used it in surgical practice.

My book has kept pace with this change and growth. I have in no case cut down descriptions nor the teaching devoted to surgical anatomy, nor directions for and procedure in dissection, but I have added much relating to surgical work. I have endeavored to regard fully the necessities of undergraduates, and at the same time have had in mind constantly the requirements which they will meet as surgeons in their chosen field, and have tried to make for them a sufficient work of reference for use in actual practice.

I am aware that much of the ground, particularly that portion relating to regional anatomy, has been covered by other books. The valuable works of Cunningham, McLaughlin, Holden, Treves, Heath, Owen, and others, the companions and guides of many years, have been at my hand for constant reference. I welcome this opportunity to acknowledge my great indebtedness to them.

I have hoped, gathering freely from every source, adding much from surgical experience, and arranging the whole as systematically as possible, to make for the student and practical doctor a work of reference which is, comparatively speaking, complete.

The illustrations have been for the most part made from dissections, and are, therefore, original and accurate. Too much praise can not be given the artists and engravers who have expended in their production infinite care and an interest which has been most conscientious. I believe that use will lead to appreciation of the great value of their labors.

I take this opportunity to thank, and acknowledge the services of, Dr. Carl Hamann, my old student and house surgeon, now Professor of Anatomy in the Western Reserve University, Cleveland, Ohio, for reading the manuscript; Dr. J. Rex Hobensack, formerly my prosector in the University of Pennsylvania, for the excellent dissections from which the illustrations were made and for other valuable services in the preparation of this book, and Dr. A. D. Whiting, for making the index.

1634 WALNUT STREET,
    PHILADELPHIA.

CONTENTS OF VOLUME I

LIST OF ILLUSTRATIONS

SURGICAL ANATOMY

SURFACE ANATOMY OF THE CRANIUM (Plate I)

The **cranium** is the bony enclosure of the brain, and is that portion of the head which extends from the lower margin of the forehead in front to the upper extremity of the neck behind, from ear to ear laterally, and along the base of the brain-case below. The base of the brain-case is represented by a line which extends from the median line about one centimeter (one-half inch) above the naso-frontal suture, along the upper part of the orbit, one centimeter from its edge, to the external angular process of the frontal bone; thence to the middle of the zygoma, and posteriorly, along its upper border above the external auditory meatus, following the superior curved (*superior nuchal*) line to the external occipital protuberance. This corresponds roughly to a line from the eyebrows, through the external auditory meatus, to the nape of the neck. The covering of the cranium, with the exception of that of the forehead and part of the temporal regions, constitutes the scalp.

The **scalp** is covered by a more or less abundant amount of hair. At the junction of the middle and posterior thirds of the sagittal suture can be seen a dividing point of the hair, from which it falls radially in all directions. It is at this point that baldness usually begins. The density of the scalp is well marked. The integument is closely connected with the cranial, or occipito-frontalis (*epi-cranial*) aponeurosis, this attachment in many persons permitting mobility of the scalp by the alternate contractions of the occipital and frontal divisions of the muscle. The scalp, especially its posterior part, is much less elastic than the skin in other parts of the body, so that in peeling it back during postmortem examinations it sometimes tears, and in the subsequent suturing stitches, if drawn very tight will pull through.

The **arteries** supplying the frontal region of the scalp are derived from the internal carotid, while the remainder are from the external carotid. There is free anastomosis between the two sets of arteries. The arteries of the scalp are the *frontal*, which ascends near the median line; the *supra-orbital*, which is found above the supra-orbital notch and for some distance up the forehead; the *anterior branch of the temporal artery* (often very tortuous), found about three centimeters (one and one-quarter inches) behind the external angular (*zygomatic*) process of the frontal bone; the *posterior branch of the temporal*, which runs above and in front of the ear; the *posterior auricular*, above and behind the ear, and the *occipital*, distinguishable about midway between the mastoid process and the external occipital protuberance. These arteries communicate freely with each other, both laterally and across the top of the scalp.

In examining the head as a whole, it will be noticed that the two sides are not always symmetrical—the left half usually being the larger.

The **cranial bones** forming the brain-case are: the *frontal*, two *parietal*, two *temporal*, the *occipital*, the *sphenoidal*, and the *ethmoidal*. In the adult they are immovably connected with one another, their lines of junction being termed sutures. In infancy the frontal bone consists of two portions, which coalesce very early in life, the line of union being known as the **frontal suture.** The two parietal bones are joined at their superior margins by the **sagittal suture.** The course of the frontal and sagittal sutures corresponds to a line drawn from the root of the nose, directly backward over the median line of the vault of the skull, to the external occipital protuberance. In this line, within the skull, are the superior longitudinal (*superior sagittal*) sinus and the longitudinal fissure of the cerebrum. The parietal bones are joined to the frontal bone by the **coronal suture,** and to the occipital bone by the **lambdoid suture.** The **bregma,** which is the situation of the anterior fontanelle of the infant, is the location of the junction of the coronal and sagittal sutures, and lies on the mid-point of a line connecting the pre-auricular points of the zygomatic arches. The **coronal suture** corresponds to a line drawn from the bregma to the middle of the zygomatic arch. The **lambdoid suture** is represented by a line drawn from the posterior border of the base of the mastoid process to a point six centimeters (two and a half inches) above the external occipital protuberance. The **lambda** is the point of junction of the sagittal and lambdoid sutures, and is the site of the posterior fontanelle in infants. The **pterion**—the junction of the antero-inferior angle of the parietal, the frontal, the temporal, and the greater wing of the sphenoidal bone—is found about three centimeters (one and one-quarter inches) behind the external angular (*zygomatic*) process of the frontal bone, and about the same distance above the zygoma. Davis states that Broca named the pterion as the point where the frontal, parietal, and sphenoidal bones meet. He distinguished this from the Sylvian point which in some skulls is about sixteen millimeters (five-eighths of an inch) farther back, and marks the junction of the temporal, parietal, and sphenoidal bones.

The **superciliary ridges,** or arches, commence on each side of the **glabella,** which is the smooth elevation above the root of the nose, and extend lateralward in a gentle curve, gradually becoming less prominent. The superciliary ridges

PLATE 1.

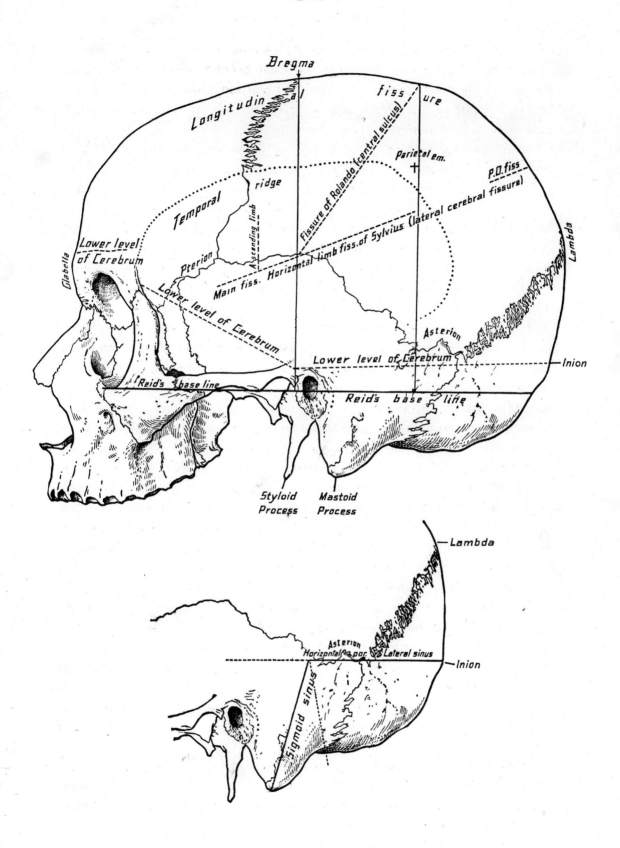

CRANIAL LANDMARKS AND LINES OF CEREBRAL FISSURES.

mark the location of the sinuses of the frontal bone, but may vary greatly, generally because of the difference in size of the frontal sinuses. They are small in females and absent in children. Although the size of the ridge may be an indication of the size of the frontal sinus, yet this does not always hold good, as a large ridge may be associated with slight development of the sinus, and vice versa. Some of the Australian aborigines have very small sinuses, but large ridges, due to great thickness of the bone.

Above the superciliary ridges are found the **frontal eminences,** slightly convex elevations which mark the original centers of ossification in the two frontal bones. The increase in the development of the skull as a whole causes the frontal bones to become upright, and thus makes the frontal eminences more prominent.

Immediately behind the external ear is the **mastoid process** of the temporal bone, which during infancy is rudimentary, developing, as a rule at about puberty, the typical mastoid cells. It extends downward for about two and a half centimeters below the external auditory meatus, and projects forward slightly under it. Medial to, and under cover of the mastoid-process is the **digastric fossa (mastoid notch).** The body of the mastoid process is honeycombed with air-cells, which are connected with the middle ear. The incision for mastoiditis should be made in the hairless space behind the ear (Wilde's incision). A line connecting the tips of the two mastoid processes would pass through, or immediately under the condyles of the occipital bone.

About one centimeter (one-half inch) above, and one and a half centimeters (three-quarters of an inch) behind the posterior border of the mastoid process is the **asterion**—the junction of the lambdoid and squamous sutures.

The **external occipital protuberance, or inion,** is distinctly felt in the median line at the posterior part of the head, at the junction of the skin of the neck with that of the head. It is the thickest part of the vault of the skull. From it the superior curved (*superior nuchal*) lines of the occipital bone extend laterally and give attachment to some of the muscles which support the head. The external occipital protuberance marks the position of the torcular Herophili (*confluens sinuum*), or the confluence of the superior longitudinal (*superior sagittal*), the two lateral (*transverse*), the straight, and the occipital sinuses. Above the superior curved (*superior nuchal*) lines the general contour of the skull can be readily seen, as the covering is composed of thin structures. Below these lines, however, the skull recedes to a considerable extent, the space being filled in with the strong muscles and fasciæ of the neck. It is in the region of the occiput that a bulging of the membranes of the brain (meningocele) or of the brain itself (encephalocele) sometimes occurs, and is due to defective ossification of the occipital bone, the tumor being always located in the median line.

The **parietal eminences** which mark the position of the centers of ossification in the parietal bones are readily distinguishable on the sides of the skull above the ears.   They are much more marked in infancy, gradually becoming rounded and less prominent.   Anterior to the parietal eminences, and running along the sides of the head, are the two **temporal ridges** which limit the temporal fossæ above, and give attachment to the temporal fascia.   They commence at the external angular (*zygomatic*) process of the frontal bone and arch upward, backward, and then downward, to become lost on the posterior roots of the zygomatic process of the temporal bone.   The point where the coronal suture is crossed by the temporal ridge is known as the **stephanion**.   It is about three centimeters (one and one-quarter inches) above the pterion.

The **middle meningeal artery** passes upward on the antero-inferior angle of the parietal bone, and is found by trephining three centimeters (one and a quarter inches) behind, and about three centimeters above the external angular (*zygomatic*) process of the frontal bone, which corresponds to the pterion.

The **course of the superior longitudinal (superior sagittal) sinus** is indicated by a line drawn over the median line of the top of the head, or from the root of the nose to the external occipital protuberance.

The **course of the horizontal portion of the lateral (transverse) sinus** is shown by the posterior part of a line drawn from the external occipital protuberance to a point two and a half centimeters (one inch) above the external auditory meatus.   The sinus turns downward and becomes the *sigmoid sinus* at the point where a vertical line drawn through the posterior border of the base of the mastoid process crosses the line for the horizontal portion.

SURFACE ANATOMY OF THE FACE

The appearance of the face differs at different periods of life, as well as in health and disease.   In infancy, owing to the greater abundance of subcutaneous fat and the lack of development of the muscles of expression, the face is full and round; the relatively greater development of the brain and sense organs causes the upper portion of the face to be broader than the lower; the nasal fossæ are shallow, and the maxillary bones are small.   In old age, the subcutaneous fat largely disappears, and the integument becomes wrinkled and thinner.   Not infrequently there are observed areas of thickened, brownish epidermis (*keratosis senilis*), particularly in persons much exposed to the weather.

The **supra-orbital** ridges are readily recognized as the dividing line between the forehead and the face.   They are strong arches which form the superior boundary of the circumference of the orbit, and are covered by the eyebrows. Medially, the arch ends in the internal angular process of the frontal bone, which articulates with the lacrimal bone and the nasal process of the superior maxilla (*maxilla*). It is between the two internal angular processes, at the fronto-nasal suture, that a meningocele or an encephalocele sometimes appears. Laterally, the supra-orbital arch terminates in the external angular (*zygomatic*) process which articulates with the malar (*zygomatic*) bone. Immediately below the supra-orbital arches are the orbital fossæ.

In size the eyes do not vary much in different individuals, the apparent difference being due to the variations in the length of the palpebral fissure, which thus permits a larger or smaller portion of the ocular surface to come into view. The **palpebral fissure** is the aperture between the edges of the two lids, and extends from the medial to the lateral canthus, or commissure. The fissure is not, as a rule, exactly horizontal, the lateral canthus being generally a little higher than the medial. By everting the eyelids, the **tarsal cartilage** may be felt as a thickened portion of the lid. The vertical arrangement of the *Meibomian (tarsal) glands* in the tarsal cartilage can also be made out. The skin of the eyelids, especially of the upper lid, is very thin, and is connected to the orbicularis oculi muscle by lax subcutaneous tissue destitute of fat, which accounts for the marked swelling in the so-called "black eye."

The lacrimal gland which is situated behind the lateral portion of the supra-orbital margin is not palpable unless enlarged. The **puncta lacrimalia**, which are situated on the lacrimal papillæ, are readily discernible near the medial canthus, the lower being the larger and more lateral, and mark the beginning of the lacrimal ducts. Before introducing a probe into the lacrimal canaliculus the lid should be drawn lateralward, thus straightening the canal.

The **tendo oculi** (**median palpebral ligament**) can be felt after drawing the eyelids lateralward, or forcibly closing the eye. Immediately behind this is the **lacrimal sac.** A knife pushed backward just below the tendo oculi (*median palpebral ligament*) would enter the sac, with the angular artery and vein on the medial side of the puncture. A probe passing through this opening into the sac, and then downward, slightly lateralward, and backward, would enter the naso-lacrimal duct and appear in the inferior meatus of the nose. Tension upon the tendon, as in closure of the eyelids, compresses the sac, with which it is closely connected, thus emptying the sac and forcing the tears which have collected at the medial angle of the eye down the naso-lacrimal duct.

The **naso-lacrimal duct,** about two centimeters (three-quarters of an inch) in length, and constricted in its middle, extends from the lacrimal sac to the inferior nasal meatus, just under the inferior turbinated bone (*inferior concha*). The opening in the nasal mucous membrane is a slit, but there is a comparatively large opening in the dry bone. When the inferior end of the duct lies in the lateral wall of the meatus instead of in its roof, greater difficulty is experienced in passing a probe into the duct.

The **infra-orbital margin,** the inferior border of the orbit, lies immediately below the eyeball and is formed by the superior maxillary (*maxillary*) and malar (*zygomatic*) bones. It can be readily felt throughout its entire extent.

The **glabella** is a flat, triangular eminence situated between the two medial extremities of the superciliary ridges. Immediately below the apex of the glabella is found the prominence of the nose formed by the nasal bones.

The form of the nose and much of the general expression of the face are due to the size and form of the nasal bones. The difference in these bones accounts for the variations in the nose in the different races.

The nose is rigid at its root and base as far as its middle, beyond which it is cartilaginous and flexible. The lack of cutaneous elasticity due to the intimate adherence of the skin to the nasal cartilages, which are attached to the lower ends of the nasal bones, makes furuncles or erysipelas in this region exceedingly yainful.

The inferior end of the nose is open and is divided into the two **anterior nares** by the nasal septum and the *columella* (*septum nasi mobile*). Since the nose is attached lower than the floor of its cavity, it must be elevated when the interior is to be inspected.

Below the nose are the lips, which bound the aperture of the mouth which is the upper opening of the gastro-intestinal tract, and which extends backward to be continuous with the pharynx. The lips contain muscles and vessels, and play a large part in the general expression of the face. The pulsations of the superior and inferior coronary (*labial*) arteries can be easily felt by holding the lips between the finger and the thumb. In the operation for harelip these arteries are divided, the ensuing hemorrhage being easily controlled by pressure with the finger and thumb. This vascularity accounts for the relative infrequency of infection after operation or injury. Carbuncle or malignant furuncle of the upper lip is exceedingly serious since the superior coronary (*labial*) vessels anastomose with the ophthalmic vessels, and sinus thrombosis or meningitis may result.

Below the lips is the prominence of the symphysis of the mandible, or lower jaw which can easily be felt from the symphysis to the condyle where it articulates with the temporal bone. By slight pressure along the bone the alveolar border, in which the teeth are set, can readily be distinguished. In passing the finger backward along the inferior border of its body the angle of the mandible, at the junction of the body with the ramus, can be distinguished. In front of the angle at the anterior border of the masseter muscle is a depression through which passes the *facial* (*external maxillary*) *artery*, and at this point its pulsation can be detected.   The condyle of the mandible is felt in front of the tragus of the external ear and below the zygomatic arch.   When the mouth of a living person is opened, the condyle can be felt leaving the glenoid (*mandibular*) fossa and advancing upon the eminentia articularis.   This forward motion of the condyle affords a freer access to the external ear; it can be demonstrated by passing the little finger into the external auditory (*external acoustic*) meatus and opening and closing the mouth.

In the supra-orbital margin, at the junction of its medial with its intermediate third, is the **supra-orbital notch, or foramen,** which gives passage to the supra-orbital vessels and nerve.   The **mental foramen,** which gives passage to the mental vessels and nerve, is normally found in the mandible, opposite the second bicuspid tooth.   It varies in its vertical location according to age, being low in the infant, and gradually becoming higher as life advances.   In a line drawn between the supra-orbital notch and the mental foramen, and just below the infra-orbital margin, is the infra-orbital foramen, which gives passage to the infra-orbital vessels and nerve.   These nerves are derived from the fifth cranial (*trigeminal*) nerve.   Frequently accessory foramina are found lateral to the constant ones, and usually transmit a portion of the nerve which commonly passes through the normal foramen.   These anomalies, being rather common, are of considerable significance in the treatment of neuralgias by nerve section.   The anomalous openings occur most frequently in connection with the supra-orbital, the infra-orbital, and the mental foramina, in the order named, and upon the right side.   At times a deep groove extends for several centimeters upward from the accessory supraorbital foramen and about one centimeter medial to the temporal ridge.

Continuing lateralward from the external angular process is the **zygomatic arch,** formed by the temporal process of the malar (*zygomatic*), and the zygomatic process of the temporal bone.   The anterior part of the arch is flat and broad, and forms the prominence of the cheek, or the "cheek bone."   Posteriorly, the zygomatic arch terminates just anterior and superior to the external auditory meatus.   On account of the attachment of the dense temporal fascia to the superior border of this arch, the inferior border is more easily distinguished. The zygomatic arch forms a dividing line between two depressions, which, in the healthy individual, are generally filled with fat and, therefore, are not very marked.   But in a wasting disease the fat above the zygoma is absorbed, and the bony arch becomes much more prominent; as the disease progresses, the masseteric depressions can be plainly seen and, at the same time, the fat in front of the anterior margin of the masseter muscle and below the anterior half of the malar (*zygomatic*) bone disappears, with resultant sinking of the cheeks.

The **arteries of the face** are the *temporal*, between the ear and the zygoma, and the *facial (external maxillary)*, which runs from a point on the body of the mandible just anterior to the masseter muscle, to the angle of the mouth, and passes along the naso-labial fold and the side of the nose to the median canthus of the eye. The *facial (anterior facial) vein* runs straight across the face from the medial canthus of the eye to the anterior inferior angle of the masseter muscle at the inferior border of the mandible. The anterior temporal and facial (*external maxillary*) arteries are useful to the anesthetizer in studying the pulse, and also to the physician when the patient is sleeping.

Expression is due to muscular traction upon the facial integument. In facial hemiplegia, when the muscles of the affected side have lost their power, expression is gone, and the wrinkles of the face disappear. The "expression of the eye" is due to wrinkling of the lids and the peri-ocular integument.

The **external ear** (**auricle**) is placed at the junction of the face, the neck, and the cranial vault, and in general conformation and direction is designed for the collection and partial condensation of sound. During inspection of the tympanic membrane and of the whole length of the external auditory canal (*external acoustic meatus*), the direction of the latter is of practical importance. The canal is about three centimeters (one and a quarter inches) long. When removing foreign bodies, which frequently lodge in this canal, it is important to note that it sags at its outer end, and can be straightened by pulling the ear upward. The upper and posterior portions of the tympanic membrane incline outward. The external opening of the canal is oval, while further in the canal is more nearly circular.

THE SCALP

DISSECTION.—(Plate II). The dissection of the scalp should be made before that of the face and neck. The body should be placed on its back, the head being well elevated by means of a large block placed under the nape of the neck. The head having been shaved, an incision should be carried from the root of the nose over the middle line of the vertex to the external occipital protuberance; a second incision, at a right angle to the first, commencing at the nasal eminence, should extend on each side as far back as the ear. Beginning at the junction of the two incisions, reflect the skin backward and lateralward, forming two flaps. When dissecting these flaps great care must be taken to remove only the skin, the best guide being the bulbs of the hair, which are in the superficial fascia.

The scalp is that portion of the cranial covering which lies in front of the superior curved (*superior nuchal*) ridges of the occipital bone and above the two

PLATE II.

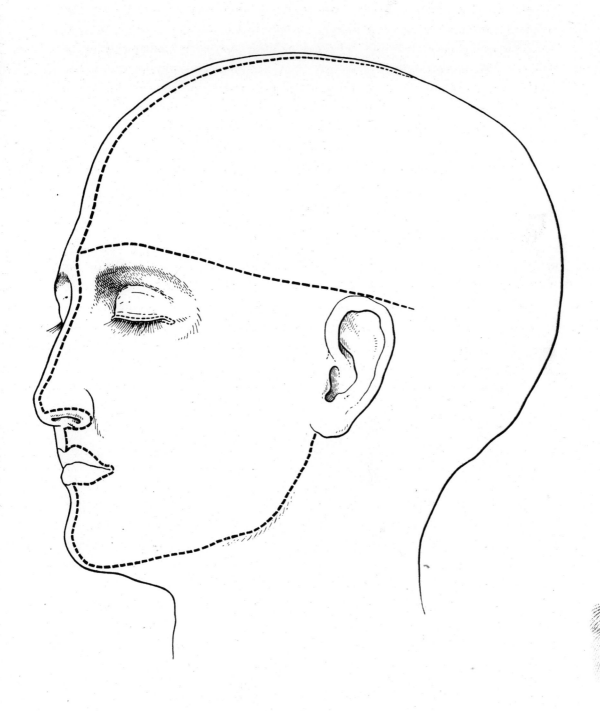

INCISIONS FOR DISSECTION.

II

PLATE III.

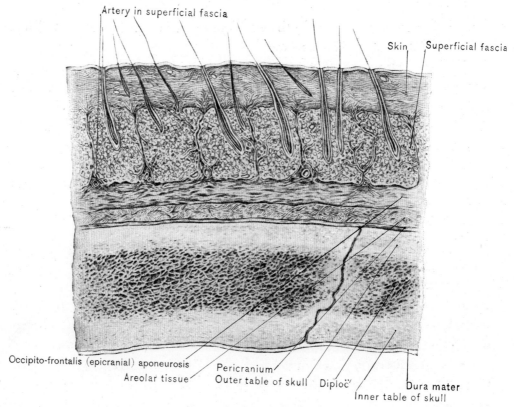

Artery in superficial fascia

Skin   Superficial fascia

Occipito-frontalis (epicranial) aponeurosis

Areolar tissue

Pericranium

Outer table of skull

Diploë

Inner table of skull

Dura mater

FIG. 1.—LAYERS OF SCALP.

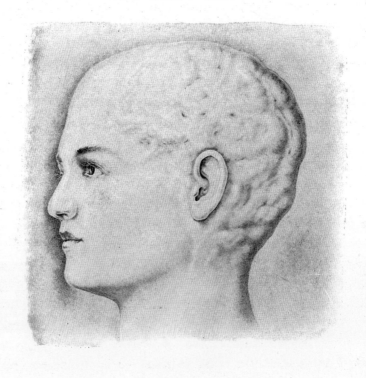

FIG. 2.—CIRSOID ANEURYSM.

14

temporal ridges, although in the dissection of the scalp the tissues in the temporal region are included for convenience.

Layers.—(Plate III, Fig. 1). The scalp above the temporal ridges is made up of five layers: skin, superficial fascia, occipito-frontalis (*epicranial*) aponeurosis, laose areolar tissue, and pericranium, or external periosteum. The first three layers are so closely connected that from a practical standpoint they may be considered as one layer, and they are the layers commonly meant by the term scalp. In the frontal and occipital regions, in place of the aponeurosis, are the muscular bellies of the occipito-frontalis (*epicranius*) muscle. Below the temporal ridges (in the temporal regions) the scalp is composed of eight layers: skin, superficial fascia, attolens aurem (*auricularis superior*) and attrahens aurem (*auricularis anterior*) muscles, occipito-frontalis (*epicranial*) aponeurosis (*galea aponeurotica*), areolar tissue, temporal fascia, the temporal muscle, and the periosteum.

The **skin of the scalp** is thicker than that of any other part of the body. By means of the dense, inelastic, superficial fascia it is closely adherent to the occipito-frontalis (*epicranius*) muscle and aponeurosis, which accounts for the movement of the skin with the muscle and its aponeurosis. It is rich in sebaceous glands which, when enlarged on account of occlusion of their ducts, constitute sebaceous cysts, or wens, so common in this region. These growths, even when large, are superficial to the occipito-frontalis (*epicranial*) aponeurosis, and, by carefully dissecting close to the sac, can be removed without risk of opening the subaponeurotic layer, thus minimizing infection should it occur. The skin is well nourished by the vessels of the superficial fascia.

The **superficial fascia of the scalp** consists of a single layer, which presents a granular appearance, due to the nodulated fat and dense fibrous septa. Its septa firmly connect the skin to the occipito-frontalis (*epicranial*) aponeurosis. In its density and resistance to pressure it resembles the superficial fascia of the palm of the hand and the sole of the foot. Posteriorly, it is continuous with the superficial fascia of the back of the neck; laterally and anteriorly, with the superficial fascia of the face. It contains the principal blood-vessels and nerves of the scalp, in this respect differing from the superficial fascia elsewhere, with the exception of that of the face and the ischio-rectal fossæ, of the muscles of the auricle, and of the hair-bulbs. The arteries of the scalp lie in compartments within the fascia, to the walls of which they are attached by loose fibrous tissue; when divided, they have only a slight tendency to retract or to contract within these channels, and, on account of the density of the fascia, it may be difficult to seize them with the artery forceps, so that some form of pressure is often required to check the bleeding which may be abundant and persistent. Suppuration in this layer is very limited because of this dense inelastic tissue, which also accounts for the

slight swelling accompanying superficial infections, such as erysipelas. Hematomata after contusions, like the deeper hematomata, may simulate a fracture
of the skull. The presence of the hair-bulbs in this dense fascia and
their firm attachment to the scalp enable a strong person, by securely
grasping the hair, to lift the entire weight of the body without tearing out
the hair-roots. (Plate IV.)

DISSECTION.—Upon one side of the head the superficial fascia with the
vessels and nerves should be removed as one common layer, bringing into view
the corresponding half of the occipito-frontalis (*epicranius*) muscle and its
aponeurosis; while upon the other side only the superficial fascia in the immediate
neighborhood of the vessels and nerves should be removed, in this way exposing
and giving a clear idea of the blood and nerve supply of the scalp. In reflecting
the superficial fascia preserve the attolens aurem (*auricularis superior*) and
attrahens aurem (*auricularis anterior*) muscles which lie between it and the
aponeurosis.

The **Extrinsic Muscles of the Ear** are very feeble and rudimentary, the
auricle in man being practically immovable They are three in number: the
attolens aurem (*auricularis superior*), attrahens aurem (*auricularis anterior*),
and retrahens aurem (*auricularis posterior*); they require considerable care in
dissection to avoid being overlooked and destroyed.

DISSECTION.—Draw the auricle downward and fasten it with hooks, thus
putting the attolens aurem (*auricularis superior*) and attrahens aurem (*auricularis anterior*) muscles on tension.

The **attolens aurem (auricularis superior)**, the largest of the three muscles,
is broad and fan-shaped, converging to a narrow tendon below. It *arises* from
the superficial surface of the occipito-frontalis (*epicranial*) aponeurosis (*galea
aponeurotica*) below the temporal ridge, and is *inserted* into the cranial aspect of
the upper part of the root of the auricle.

NERVE SUPPLY.—From the temporal branch of the facial nerve.

ACTION.—It draws the auricle upward.

The **attrahens aurem (auricularis anterior)** is the smallest muscle of the
three, and *arises* from the occipito-frontalis (*epicranial*) aponeurosis (*galea
aponeurotica*) in front of the attolens aurem (*auricularis superior*) muscle, and
is *inserted* into the top of the root of the auricle.

NERVE SUPPLY.—From the temporal branch of the facial nerve.

ACTION.—It draws the auricle forward and upward.

DISSECTION.—Release the auricle from its position and draw it forward;
fasten it with hooks, and divide the integument over the tense band behind the
auricle to expose the retrahens aurem (*auricularis posterior*) muscle.

PLATE IV.

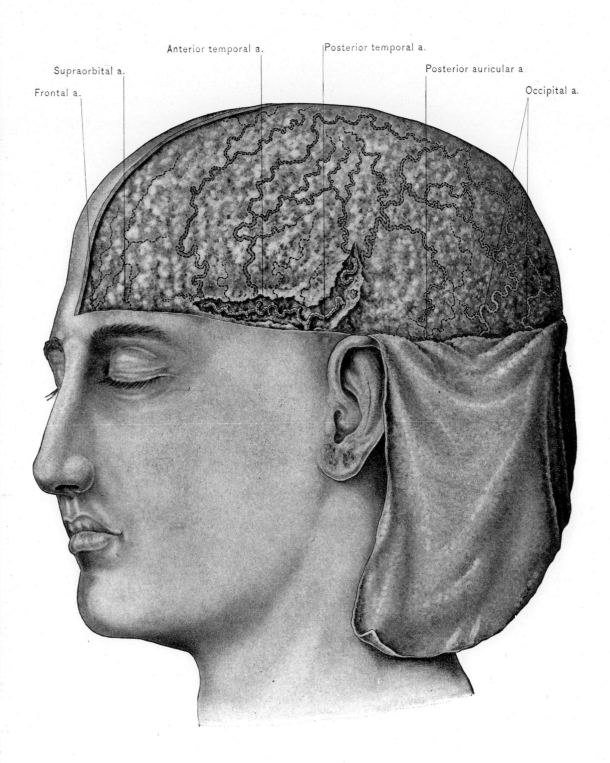

Frontal a.

Supraorbital a.

Anterior temporal a.

Posterior temporal a.

Posterior auricular a.

Occipital a.

SUPERFICIAL FASCIA AND ARTERIES OF SCALP.

PLATE V.

PLATE V.

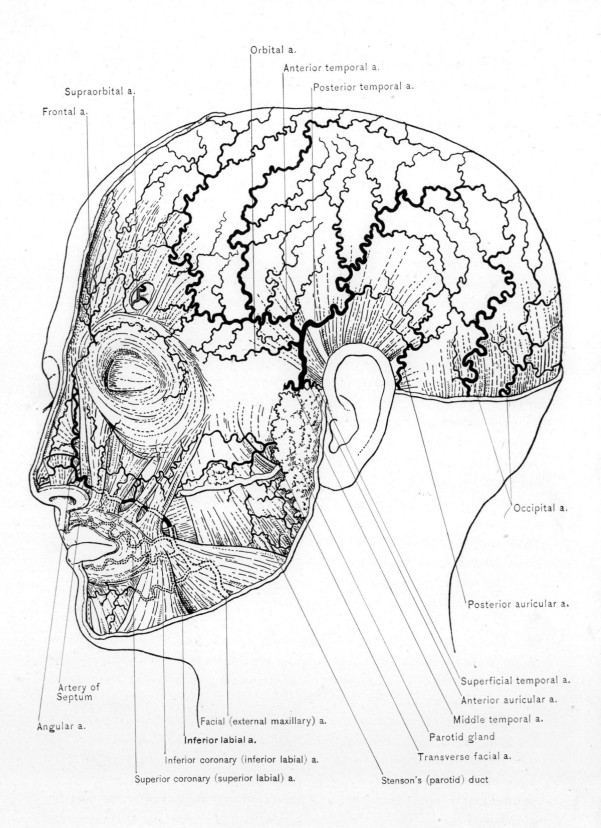

Orbital a.

Anterior temporal a.

Posterior temporal a.

Supraorbital a.

Frontal a.

Occipital a.

Posterior auricular a.

Superficial temporal a.

Anterior auricular a.

Middle temporal a.

Parotid gland

Transverse facial a.

Stenson's (parotid) duct

Artery of
Septum

Angular a.

Facial (external maxillary) a.

Inferior labial a.

Inferior coronary (inferior labial) a.

Superior coronary (superior labial) a.

ARTERIES OF SCALP AND FACE.

The **retrahens aurem (auricularis posterior)** muscle consists of two or three short muscle bundles, which *arise* from the mastoid process of the temporal bone and are *inserted* into the posterior part of the concha.

NERVE SUPPLY.—From the posterior auricular branch of the facial nerve.

ACTION.—It draws the auricle backward.

The **Arteries of the Scalp** (Plate V), which are five on each side, are derived anteriorly from the frontal and the supra-orbital, which are from the ophthalmic branch of the internal carotid; laterally, from the superficial temporal; posteriorly, from the posterior auricular and occipital arteries, which are from the external carotid.

The **frontal artery,** a small branch of the ophthalmic, leaves the orbit at its medial angle in company with the supratrochlear nerve, and is distributed to the skin over the glabella and to the pyramidalis (*procerus*) and frontalis muscles.

The **supra-orbital artery,** a branch of the ophthalmic, leaves the orbit, accompanied by the supra-orbital nerve, through the supra-orbital notch, and divides into a superficial and a deep branch, which ascend toward the vertex, anastomosing with the temporal and frontal arteries and with the supra-orbital artery of the opposite side. It supplies the tissues of the forehead.

The **superficial temporal artery,** the smaller of the two terminal divisions of the external carotid, arises in the substance of the parotid gland posterior to the neck of the mandible, and ascends over the posterior root of the zygoma at about one centimeter (one-half inch) in front of the ear. It lies on the temporal fascia, and at about two and a half centimeters (one inch) above the zygoma it divides into the *anterior* and *posterior temporal.* It is accompanied by branches of the facial and auriculo-temporal nerves. It is covered by the attrahens aurem (*auricularis anterior*) muscle and is crossed by one or two small veins.

The *anterior temporal (frontal branch of superficial temporal) artery* is tortuous, and can be seen pulsating. It anastomoses with the supra-orbital and frontal arteries and with the anterior temporal artery of the opposite side.

The *posterior temporal (parietal branch of superficial temporal) artery,* the larger of the two, passes upward and backward above the auricle and anastomoses with the posterior temporal artery of the opposite side and with the occipital and posterior auricular arteries.

The transverse facial, anterior auricular, and middle temporal branches of the temporal artery will be described with the dissection of the face.

The *posterior auricular artery* arises from the external carotid after it has passed beneath the posterior belly of the digastric muscle. It passes under the parotid gland which it supplies, and thence upward and backward between the auricle and the mastoid process, and divides into two branches: an anterior and a posterior. The *anterior branch* passes forward and anastomoses with the posterior temporal artery; *the posterior branch* passes backward and anastomoses with the occipital artery. It is accompanied by the posterior auricular nerve, a branch of the facial nerve.

The **occipital artery** pierces the trapezius muscle at its attachment to the superior curved (*superior nuchal*) line of the occipital bone, about midway between the mastoid process and the external occipital protuberance. Thence it ascends in a tortuous course over the back of the head to the vertex, dividing into numerous branches, which anastomose with the occipital artery of the opposite side and with the posterior temporal (*parietal branch of superficial temporal*) and posterior auricular arteries. It is accompanied by the greater occipital nerve. When ligating the occipital artery near the mastoid process, care must be taken not to injure the mastoid venous branches of the occipital vein, which connect the vein with the lateral sinus.

The arteries of the scalp sometimes become elongated and dilated, producing what is known as **cirsoid aneurysm** (Plate III, Fig. 2). The participation of the capillaries in the process gives rise to **racemose aneurysm**; the anterior temporal artery is the one most commonly affected.

The **Veins of the Scalp** accompany the corresponding arteries, with the exception of the supra-orbital and frontal veins, which unite to form the angular, the beginning of the facial vein. The veins of the scalp communicate with the intra-cranial venous sinuses by anastomoses with the ophthalmic; through the veins of the diploë; through small veins which pass through the bones and sutures to the dura, and through anastomoses with the large emissary veins.

It is through these channels that pyogenic infection is carried from the scalp and cranial bones to the dura mater and the venous sinuses, and thence to the brain. Infection rarely spreads from the cranial cavity through the emissary veins to the scalp.

The **lymph vessels of the scalp** form a rich net work. The lymphatic drainage from the occipital region is into the occipital nodes, from the postparietal and temporal areas into the postauricular nodes, from the anterior parietal and temporal areas into the pre-auricular, or parotid, nodes, and from the frontal region into the submaxillary glands. The anterior cervical chain of glands is involved in infections of the lateral portion of the scalp.

The **Nerves of the Scalp** (Plate VI) are *branches* of the trigeminal, facial, and greater occipital nerves, and of the cervical plexus.

The **supra-orbital nerve,** the larger of the two terminal branches of the frontal branch of the ophthalmic division of the trigeminal nerve, leaves the orbit with the supra-orbital artery through the supra-orbital notch, or foramen, which is

PLATE VI.

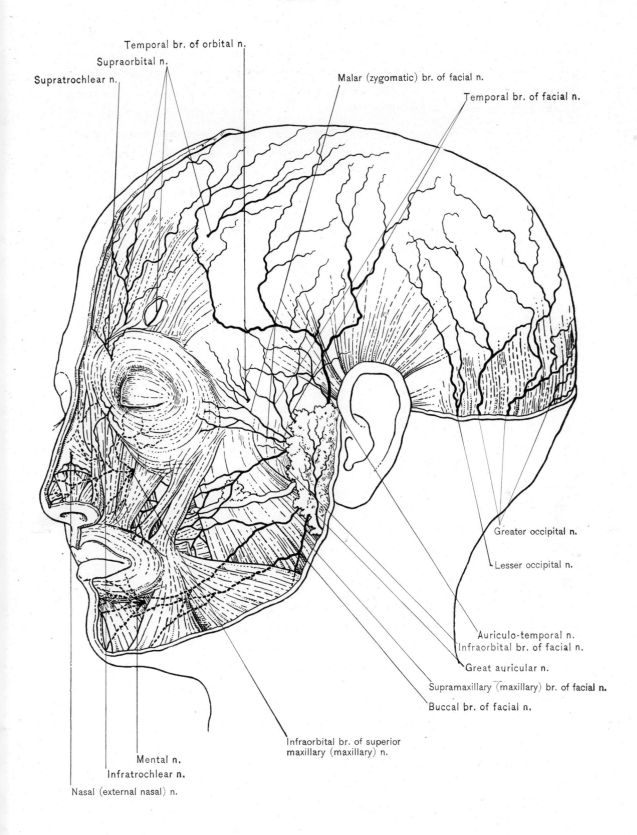

Temporal br. of orbital n.

Supraorbital n.

Supratrochlear n.

Malar (zygomatic) br. of facial n.

Temporal br. of facial n.

Greater occipital n.

Lesser occipital n.

Auriculo-temporal n.

Infraorbital br. of facial n.

Great auricular n.

Supramaxillary (maxillary) br. of facial n.

Buccal br. of facial n.

Infraorbital br. of superior maxillary (maxillary) n.

Mental n.

Infratrochlear n.

Nasal (external nasal) n.

NERVES OF SCALP AND FACIAL NERVE.

located in the superior margin of the orbit at the junction of its medial and intermediate thirds, and ascends upon the forehead beneath the orbicularis palpebrarum (*orbicularis oculi*) and the frontal belly of the occipito-frontalis (*epicranius*) muscle. It divides into two branches, and becomes subcutaneous: the *medial branch* pierces the frontal belly of the occipito-frontalis (*epicranius*) muscle, and ascends as high as the parietal bone; the *lateral branch*, the larger of the two, pierces the occipito-frontalis (*epicranial*) aponeurosis (*galea aponeurotica*), and ascends over the vertex as far as the occipital bone.

The **supratrochlear nerve,** the smaller of the two terminal branches of the frontal branch of the ophthalmic nerve, appears at the medial angle of the orbit above the pulley of the superior oblique muscle, and ascends upon the forehead. It is covered by the orbicularis palpebrarum (*orbicularis oculi*) and the frontalis muscles, piercing the latter to end in the integument. It supplies the medial portion of the skin of the forehead, the upper eyelid, and the root of the nose.

The **temporal (zygomatico-temporal) branch of the orbital (zygomatic) nerve.**— About two and a half centimeters (one inch) above the zygoma the temporal fascia is pierced by the temporal (*zygomatico-temporal*) branch of the orbital (*zygomatic*) branch of the superior maxillary (*maxillary*) nerve, which is distributed to the integument of the temple and communicates with the temporal branch of the facial nerve.

The **auriculo-temporal nerve,** a branch of the inferior maxillary (*posterior division of the mandibular*) nerve, accompanies the temporal vessels, lying posterior to them. The auriculo-temporal nerve emerges from beneath the upper part of the parotid gland, and divides into auricular and temporal terminal branches which supply the upper half of the auricle, the mandibular joint, and the skin of the temple and scalp, reaching almost to the vertex.

The **temporal branches of the facial nerve** extend upward over the zygoma upon the temple to supply the attrahens aurem (*auricularis anterior*) and attolens aurem (*auricularis superior*), the orbicularis palpebrarum (*orbicularis oculi*), the frontalis, and the corrugator supercilii muscles. They communicate with the temporo-malar (*zygomatic*), auriculo-temporal, lacrimal, and supra-orbital nerves.

The **posterior auricular nerve,** a branch of the facial, accompanies the posterior auricular artery, and divides into an *occipital* (posterior) branch which supplies the occipitalis muscle, and an *auricular* (anterior) branch which supplies the posterior auricular and the intrinsic muscles of the auricle. This nerve is joined by filaments from the auricular branch of the vagus nerve and from the greater auricular and small occipital (*lesser occipital*) nerves.

The **small occipital (lesser occipital) nerve,** a branch of the anterior divisions of the second and third cervical nerves, supplies the scalp behind the ear and over the lateral surface of the occiput. It communicates with the great auricular and the greater occipital nerve, and with the posterior auricular branch of the facial nerve. It can be seen in the neck running along the posterior border of the sterno-mastoid muscle.

The **greater occipital nerve** is the largest cutaneous nerve of the posterior part of the scalp. It accompanies the occipital artery over the occiput. It is the medial branch of the posterior division of the second cervical nerve. It pierces the complexus (*semispinalis capitis*) and trapezius muscles near their attachment to the occipital bone, enters the superficial fascia with the occipital artery, and breaks up into a number of large branches which spread over the back of the head, supplying the integument as far forward as the vertex. It communicates on the scalp with the great auricular, the small (*lesser*) occipital, the posterior auricular, the third occipital, and the first cervical, or suboccipital, nerves, and receives a lateral branch from the third cervical nerve.

The occipito-frontalis (*epicranius*) muscle and aponeurosis, exposed upon the side from which the superficial fascia has been removed, will now be studied.

The **occipito-frontalis** (**epicranius**) is a broad, musculo-aponeurotic layer stretching over the median plane of the skull from the occiput to the brow. It consists of two pairs of flattened muscular bellies, an occipital and a frontal, with an intervening epicranial aponeurosis.

The *occipitalis muscle* (*occipital belly*), thin and quadrangular, *arises* from the lateral two-thirds of the superior curved (*superior nuchal*) ridge of the occipital bone and the adjoining mastoid process, thus leaving a triangular interval between the two occipital muscles as their fibers eventually meet higher up in the median line. The fibers are about three centimeters (one inch and a quarter) in length and ascend to blend with the aponeurosis.

BLOOD SUPPLY.—From the occipital and posterior auricular arteries.

NERVE SUPPLY.—From the posterior auricular branch of the facial.

The *frontalis muscle* (*frontal belly*), a thin, muscular layer with intimate cutaneous connections, *arises* from the aponeurosis at about the level of the coronal suture. It descends over the forehead and blends with the orbicularis palpebrarum (*orbicularis oculi*), the corrugator supercilii, and, in the median plane, with the muscle of the opposite side.

BLOOD SUPPLY.—From the frontal, supra-orbital, and anterior temporal arteries.

NERVE SUPPLY.—From the temporal branch of the temporo-facial division of the facial nerve.

The *aponeurosis* (*galea aponeurotica*) extends over the entire vertex. It is continuous across the middle line with the aponeurosis of the opposite side; later-

PLATE VII.

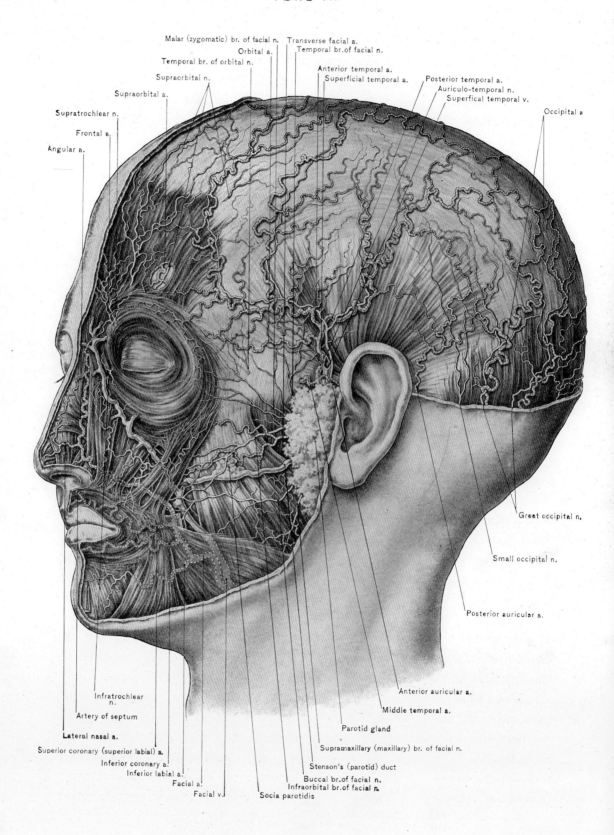

Malar (zygomatic) br. of facial n.
Transverse facial a.
Orbital a.
Temporal br. of facial n.
Temporal br. of orbital n.
Anterior temporal a.
Supraorbital n.
Superficial temporal a.
Posterior temporal a.
Auriculo-temporal n.
Supraorbital a.
Superfical temporal v.
Supratrochlear n.
Occipital a
Frontal a.
Angular a.

Great occipital n.

Small occipital n.

Posterior auricular a.

Infratrochlear n.
Artery of septum
Anterior auricular a.
Middle temporal a.
Lateral nasal a.
Parotid gland
Superior coronary (superior labial) a.
Supramaxillary (maxillary) br. of facial n.
Inferior coronary a.
Inferior labial a.
Stenson's (parotid) duct
Facial a.
Buccal br. of facial n.
Infraorbital br. of facial n.
Facial v.
Socia parotidis

ARTERIES, NERVES, AND MUSCLES OF SCALP AND FACE.
28

ally, it is prolonged over the temporal fascia to the zygoma, just above which it is attached to that fascia. Connected with the lateral portion of the aponeurosis are the attolens aurem (*auricularis superior*) and attrahens aurem (*auricularis anterior*) muscles. It is intimately connected with the skin through the attachment of the superficial fascia, and has a loose connection with the pericranium by the connective tissue which intervenes; this accounts for the movement of the integument when the occipito-frontalis (*epicranius*) muscle is in action.

ACTION.—Contraction of the frontal belly of the muscle elevates the eyebrow and produces horizontal folds in the forehead. Contraction of the occipital belly draws the scalp backward, and alternate contraction of the two bellies moves the scalp backward and forward. (Plate VII.)

DISSECTION.—Divide the aponeurosis in the median line, and make another incision at its junction with the frontalis muscle. Reflect the aponeurosis lateralward and backward, and the frontalis muscle downward.

Areolar tissue layer.—The mobility of the scalp depends entirely upon the laxity of the subaponeurotic, or subjacent areolar tissue layer; it is this layer which permits extensive flaps of the scalp to be torn loose. When the hair is caught in moving machinery the entire scalp may be torn off, laying this tissue bare. It was due to the laxity of this layer that the American Indian, with no knowledge of anatomy or surgery, was able to peel off the scalp with so much ease. Exposure of the skull in a postmortem examination is effected with remarkable ease by peeling off the scalp along this layer of tissue.

Tumors.—A careful examination will show that a tumor situated above or within the occipito-frontalis (*epicranial*) aponeurosis (*galea aponeurotica*) is freely movable. An immovable growth of the scalp should be very carefully examined before extirpation, for it is probably located beneath the aponeurosis. A tumor originating within the cranium may force its way outward and form a prominence on the scalp. Dermoids of the scalp are common at the anterior fontanelle and the external occipital protuberance, being formed by an inclusion of some of the ectodermal tissue of the bones as they grow in to unite in the median line. Encephalocele, meningocele, and cephalhydrocele all protrude through bony defects of the skull, pushing the aponeurosis before them.

Wounds involving only the skin and superficial fascia of the scalp do not gape, provided the occipito-frontalis (*epicranius*) muscle or its aponeurosis has not been divided, because of the close adherence of the skin to the superficial fascia and of the latter to the aponeurosis. The areolar tissue layer permits of wide separation of the edges of a wound which divides the occipito-frontalis (*epicranial*) aponeurosis (*galea aponeurotica*). Anteroposterior wounds which involve the aponeurosis gape but little, but the edges of transverse wounds are widely separated by the contraction of the occipito-frontalis (*epicranius*) muscle. The great vascularity of the scalp lessens the likelihood of sloughing and gangrene. A large flap of the scalp if attached by even a small pedicle is much less likely to undergo necrosis than a flap of skin torn from another part of the body, as the vessels of the scalp run immediately beneath the skin and are included in the flap. In phlegmonous erysipelas and in deep inflammation of the scalp the areolar tissue layer becomes infiltrated with pus and consequently sloughs. As the vessels are superficial to this layer, the skin does not necrose or ulcerate and allow pointing; for this reason early incision is important.

The **pericranium** (external periosteum) is loosely attached to the bone, except at the sutures, where the union is firm. In lacerated wounds of the scalp the pericranium is frequently stripped from the skull to the extent of exposing large areas of bone. Necrosis of the cranial bones rarely results from such an accident because these bones receive their blood supply chiefly through the endosteum—the outer layer of the dura mater—and not through their periosteal covering, as is the case with other bones which therefore necrose when deprived to any extent of their periosteum. The pericranium at the sutures, is continuous with the external layer of the dura mater, constituting the so-called intersutural membrane. It is also continuous with the dura at the foramina. Inflammation of the pericranium may thus extend by continuity and involve the dura mater, producing pachymeningitis.

Collections of blood or pus in the scalp may be situated superficial to the occipito-frontalis (*epicranial*) aponeurosis (*galea aponeurotica*), between the aponeurosis and the pericranium, or beneath the pericranium. A collection superficial to the aponeurosis is of little moment, since the density of the superficial fascia causes it to be circumscribed, but in the areolar tissue layer, between the aponeurosis and the pericranium, it is limited only by the attachments of the occipito-frontalis (*epicranius*) muscle and its aponeurosis, and may undermine the entire scalp and prove serious if not evacuated early. Collections beneath the pericranium are limited to a single bone, on account of the sutural attachments of the membrane. Hematomata in the areolar tissue layer are uncommon, except as a result of fissured fracture of the skull with rupture of one of the branches of the middle meningeal artery, or of the superior longitudinal or lateral sinus, as the areolar tissue between the aponeurosis and the pericranium contains very few vessels. Collections of blood beneath the pericranium, cephalhematomata, are limited to one bone, since the membrane dips into the sutures and becomes continuous with the dura mater; they are usually congenital, due to pressure upon the head at birth (caput succedaneum). These collections of

PLATE VIII.

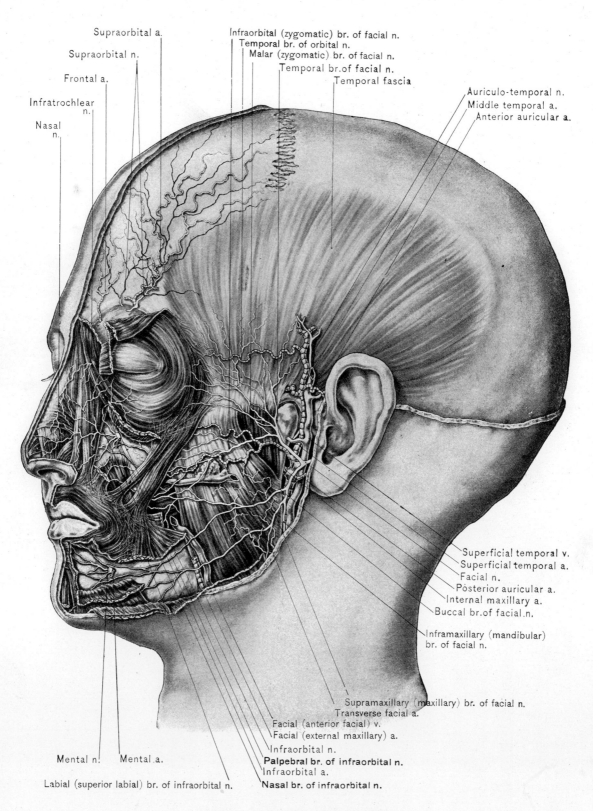

Supraorbital a.

Supraorbital n.

Frontal a.

Infratrochlear n.

Nasal n.

Infraorbital (zygomatic) br. of facial n.
Temporal br. of orbital n.
Malar (zygomatic) br. of facial n.
Temporal br. of facial n.
Temporal fascia

Auriculo-temporal n.
Middle temporal a.
Anterior auricular a.

Superficial temporal v.
Superficial temporal a.
Facial n.
Posterior auricular a.
Internal maxillary a.
Buccal br. of facial n.

Inframaxillary (mandibular) br. of facial n.

Supramaxillary (maxillary) br. of facial n.
Transverse facial a.
Facial (anterior facial) v.
Facial (external maxillary) a.
Infraorbital n.
Palpebral br. of infraorbital n.
Infraorbital a.
Nasal br. of infraorbital n.

Mental n.   Mental a.

Labial (superior labial) br. of infraorbital n.

TEMPORAL FASCIA AND NERVES OF FACE.

32

PLATE IX.

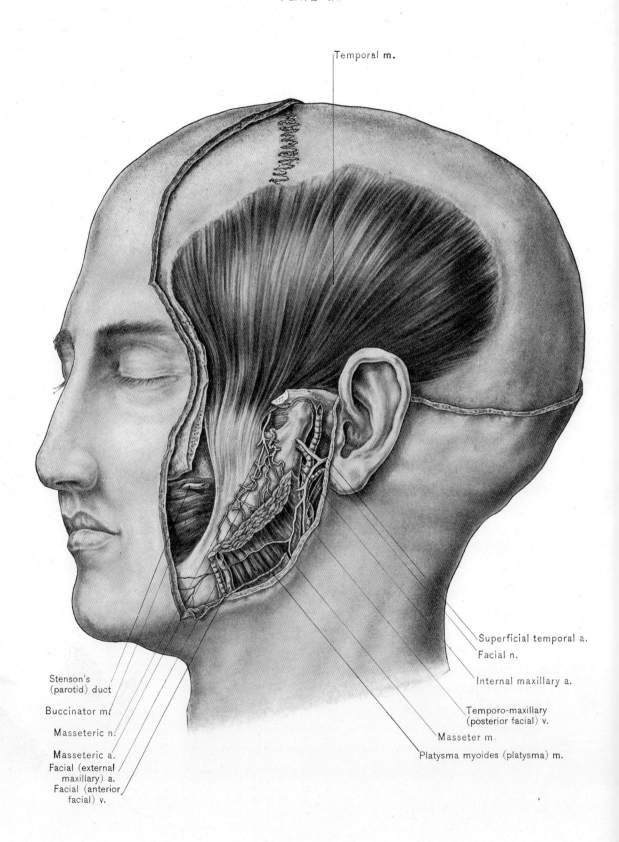

Temporal **m.**

Stenson's
(parotid) duct

Buccinator m.

Masseteric n.

Masseteric a.
Facial (external
maxillary) a.
Facial (anterior
facial) v.

Superficial temporal a.

Facial n.

Internal maxillary a.

Temporo-maxillary
(posterior facial) v.

Masseter m

Platysma myoides (platysma) m.

TEMPORAL MUSCLE.

blood, because of their sharp edges and softer centers, may be mistaken for a fractured skull.

Temporal fascia. (Plate VIII).—The temporal fascia is a white, shining membrane, which is stronger than the occipito-frontalis (*epicranial*) aponeurosis (*galea aponeurotica*) in this location, and which gives attachment by its under surface to the superficial fibers of the temporal muscle. Above, it is attached to the entire extent of the temporal ridge as a single layer, while below, it divides into two layers, the lateral of which is attached to the lateral, and the medial to the medial border of the superior margin of the zygomatic arch and the zygomatic process of the malar (*zygomatic*) bone. The structures between these two layers are: a small quantity of fat, the orbital branch of the middle temporal artery, and the temporal branch of the temporo-malar (*zygomatic*), or orbital (*zygomatic*) branch of the superior maxillary (*maxillary*) nerve. In relation with the outer surface of the fascia are: the extension of the occipito-frontalis (*epicranial*) aponeurosis (*galea aponeurotica*), the orbicularis palpebrarum (*orbicularis oculi*), the attolens aurem (*auricularis superior*) and attrahens aurem (*auricularis anterior*) muscles, the temporal vessels, the auriculo-temporal nerve, and the temporal branches of the orbital (*zygomatic*) and facial nerves. Immediately above the zygoma, it is pierced by the middle temporal artery, a branch of the temporal.

Owing to the density of this fascia abscesses beneath it very rarely point upon the surface, the pus passing in the direction of least resistance namely, through the pterygo-maxillary region into the mouth or neck.

DISSECTION.—The temporal fascia should now be detached from the zygomatic arch and reflected upward, when the greater portion of the temporal muscle and a quantity of fat overlying the muscle above the zygoma will be exposed. The tendon of insertion of the muscle will be seen in dissecting the face.

The **temporal muscle** (Plate IX), broad, flat, and triangular, is situated on the side of the head, and occupies the temporal fossa. It *arises* from the under surface of the temporal fascia and from the whole of the temporal fossa, whence its fibers descend and converge to a tendon which passes under the zygomatic arch to be *inserted* into the apex, the medial surface, and the fore part of the coronoid process of the mandible down to the last molar tooth.

BLOOD SUPPLY.—From the middle and deep temporal arteries.

NERVE SUPPLY.—From the temporal branches of the inferior maxillary (*anterior portion of the mandibular division of the trigeminal*) nerve.

ACTION.—The action of the temporal muscle is to elevate the mandible; its posterior fibers also assist in drawing the mandible backward after other muscles have carried it forward.

THE BRAIN
THE MEMBRANES AND VESSELS

DISSECTION.—Before entirely removing the calvaria, or skull cap, its outer compact table should be removed on one side, so as to expose the diploë, or middle table, with its bony channels for the accommodation of the diploic veins. This is most readily done by sawing through the outer table in the horizontal line described in the removal of the calvaria as a whole, and in the sagittal line of the skull, when it can be lifted off piecemeal with a chisel; the portion below the line of the horizontal section can be removed with a Hey's saw.

The **Diploic Veins** (Plate X) form a rich plexus in the spaces of the diploë. They vary in size in different subjects and at different periods of life, being small in young persons and increasing in size with advancing age. They are distinct before union of the cranial bones takes place, after which they anastomose freely with each other by numerous irregular channels. The veins when injured bleed actively, and it is frequently necessary to resort to the use of bone wax to plug their openings in order to control hemorrhage from them during intracranial operations. The veins are characterized by the absence of valves and the thinness of their walls. They terminate in four or five main channels which descend and open, either into the veins of the scalp, or the meningeal veins, or the cranial sinuses. These main branches are known as: the frontal, anterior temporal, posterior temporal, and occipital diploic veins.

Where increased intracranial pressure exists, incisions through the scalp may frequently encounter communicating branches between the diploic veins and those of the scalp. There may result profuse bleeding which can be controlled in one of two ways: immediate ventricular tap with relief of pressure by removal of fluid, or nicking of the outer table of the skull by means of the chisel at the bleeding point to allow the opening to be plugged with bone wax.

The **frontal diploic** vein is situated in the anterior part of the frontal bone; it usually passes through the supra-orbital foramen and empties into the supra-orbital vein. Varicosity of this vein, even to the extent of causing absorption of the outer table of the bone, sometimes occurs. This vein is found to be greatly enlarged and may become huge in size in the condition known as Leontiasis Ossium.

The **anterior temporal diploic vein** is situated in the posterior part of the frontal and in the anterior part of the parietal bone; it terminates either externally in the deep temporal veins, or internally in the superior petrosal (*sphenoparietal*) sinus or in a meningeal vein.

The **posterior temporal diploic vein** is situated in the parietal bone; it passes either through a foramen in the postero-inferior angle of this bone, or through

PLATE X.

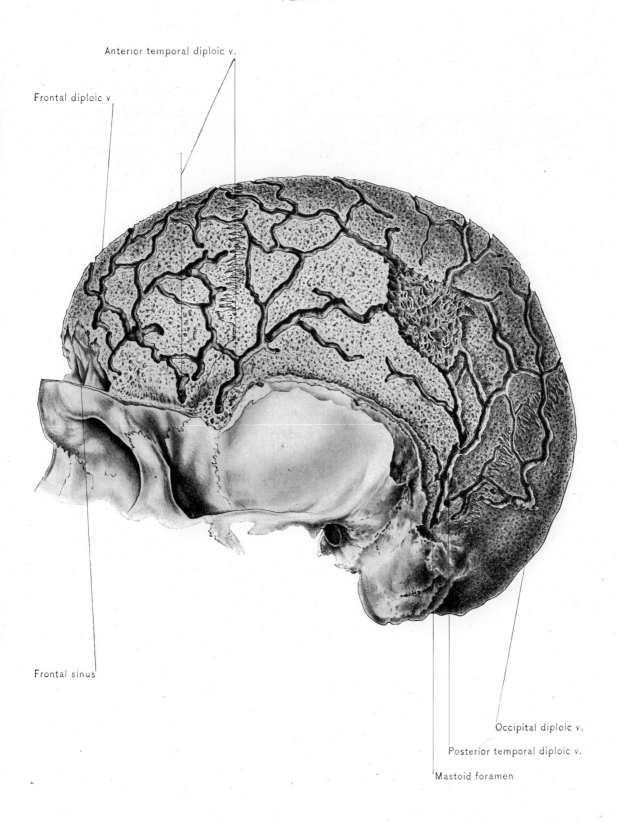

Anterior temporal diploic v.

Frontal diploic v

Frontal sinus

Occipital diploic v.

Posterior temporal diploic v.

Mastoid foramen

DIPLOIC VEINS.

the mastoid foramen, after emptying into the mastoid emissary vein, to empty into the lateral sinus. It also communicates with the posterior auricular vein.

The **occipital diploic,** the largest of the diploic veins, is confined to the occipital bone; it empties either externally into the occipital vein, or internally into the torcular Herophili (*confluens sinuum*) or the lateral sinus by joining the occipital emissary vein.

In **compound fractures of the skull** the diploic veins, through their communications with the extracranial and intracranial veins and sinuses, may give rise to osteomyelitis, septicemia, meningitis, or sinus thrombosis. Pyemia with necrosis may result from septic phlebitis; hepatic abscesses have also been known to result from this cause. Because of the extensive anastomosis, diploic infection has a tendency to spread rapidly.

The *emissary veins* are those branches which connect the intracranial venous channels with the veins external to the cranial cavity.

DISSECTION.—Remove the calvaria (*skull cap*) by sawing through the outer and middle tables along a line carried horizontally around the skull, connecting a point one centimeter (one-half inch) above the supra-orbital margin with a point the same distance above the external occipital protuberance; then, with a chisel and mallet, cut through the inner table, prying the calvaria from the underlying dura mater. In breaking through the inner table the mallet and chisel are better than the saw, because there is less danger of cutting the dura mater; even when closely adherent to the calvaria, the dura mater should be divided only as a last resort. In dividing the bone in the temporal region its thinness must be borne in mind, otherwise the brain, as well as the dura mater, may be injured.

Pacchionian Bodies (Arachnoid Granulations). The outer surface of the dura mater, exposed by removal of the calvaria, appears rough, especially along the lines of the sutures and in the neighborhood of the foramina, where it is most closely attached to the bone. The anterior and posterior branches of the middle meningeal artery, with the corresponding veins, will be seen to ramify upon the dura mater over each hemisphere; in most instances granular masses, *Pacchionian bodies*, will be seen upon the surface on each side of the middle line. These are numerous cauliflower-like projections of the arachnoid. They occur along the dural venous sinuses, chiefly on the sides of the superior longitudinal (*superior sagittal*) sinus, although they may be found along the cavernous, straight, and lateral (*transverse*) sinuses. They consist entirely of arachnoidal tissue and contain no blood vessels in themselves but project into the lacunæ (blood lakes), or sinuses, and allow the cerebro-spinal fluid to enter the venous circulation. The position of these bodies should be carefully noted, since they are apt to be regarded as pathologic when seen on the operating or postmortem table. In some cases they are quite large. The author has known an instance in which one of these bodies was so large as to cause sufficient pressure to give rise to focal (Jacksonian) epilepsy. These bodies are always impressed upon the calvaria after the period of adolescence, so that depressions, corresponding in size to the bulk of the bodies causing them, may be seen upon each side of the median line of the skull. At times they almost perforate the bone, and as a rule, they hollow the bone out sufficiently to render it translucent. They vary greatly in size in different persons, and in children are small and rudimentary.

The **dura mater** (Plate XI), the most external of the three membranes of the brain, forms the internal periosteum of the skull, and affords an excellent protection to the brain. Through the medium of this internal periosteum the bones of the skull receive the greater part of their nourishment; this explains why they seldom necrose in scalp wounds in which the pericranium or external periosteum is torn away. The dura mater is a dense, tough, inelastic, fibrous membrane sending portions in between the hemispheres and between the brain and cerebellum. It is composed of an endosteal and a meningeal portion. These are for the most part closely united so that they appear as only a single membrane. However, in certain localities the layers separate. On the sides of the sphenoidal bones they form the cavernous sinus, and in the interpeduncular region they enclose the pituitary gland (*hypophysis*). At the apex of the petrous portion of the temporal bone they enclose the Gasserian (*semilunar*) ganglion and over the aqueductus vestibuli they enclose the dilated end of the endolymphatic duct. The layers also enclose the venous spaces known as the dural sinuses. The dura mater is intimately adherent to the base of the skull, owing partly to the numerous foramina present there; so that extradural extravasations or collections of blood or pus between the dura and skull rarely occur at the base of the skull. At the sides and roof of the cranial cavity, however, where the membrane is comparatively loosely attached (except along the sutures and around the foramina), purulent collections and extravasations from rupture of one or both branches of the middle meningeal artery are not uncommon. These conditions may cause *compression of the brain*, symptoms of which, coming on immediately after an injury to the head, indicate depressed fracture; their appearance somewhat later would indicate hemorrhage, and after a few days, pus. The dura mater is less firmly attached to the temporal fossa, the most frequent site of extradural hemorrhage, than to any other portion of the interior of the skull. It is most closely adherent to the bone in infancy and old age. It may be separated from the vault and sides of the skull by striking the head of a cadaver a hard blow with a heavy mallet.

PLATE XI.

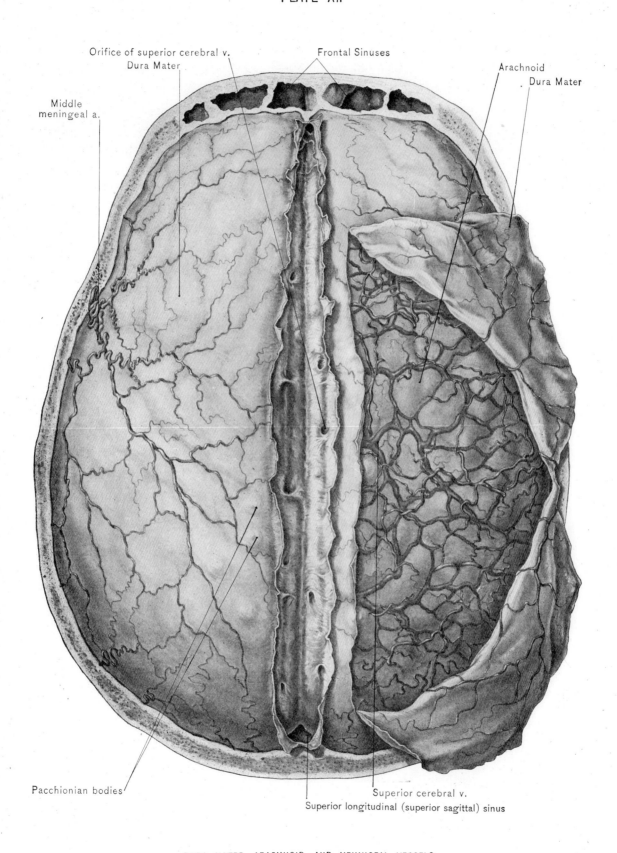

Orifice of superior cerebral v.
Dura Mater

Frontal Sinuses

Arachnoid
Dura Mater

Middle
meningeal a.

Pacchionian bodies

Superior cerebral v.
Superior longitudinal (superior sagittal) sinus

DURA MATER, ARACHNOID, AND MENINGEAL VESSELS.

Extradural hemorrhage.—The most common cause of extradural hemorrhage is rupture of the **middle meningeal artery** or one of its branches. This lesion may or may not be associated with a demonstrable fracture. If the hemorrhage is large and occurs rapidly, compression symptoms are manifested early, while if it is small and slow the symptoms are delayed. In many instances the patient reacts from the shock of the initial trauma and later again becomes unconscious as the compression symptoms develop. This is very characteristic of the lesion. Focal signs often indicate clearly the exact location of the lesion: usually weakness of the face on the opposite side, increasing weakness of the hand and arm, and later, paresis of the leg. If the lesion is on the left side of the brain, increasing motor and sensory aphasia and stupor may be of value in determining the presence and location of the lesion. Babinski's and Oppenheim's signs may show dorsal extension of the big toe on the opposite side.

Injuries to the parietal and occipital regions may give rise to middle meningeal hemorrhage on the opposite side by *contra coup* expenditure of the force of the blow. In fact, wherever severe injury to the head has occurred it will be found that usually the greatest damage to the brain lies *contra coup* to the site of injury.

Attachments of the dura mater.—Besides being closely adherent to the base of the skull, the dura mater is continuous, through the optic foramen, with the periosteum of the orbit; through the foramen magnum, with the dura mater of the spinal canal; through the fissures and the various foramina through which the vessels and nerves enter and leave the cranial cavity, clothed by prolongations of this membrane, and through the ununited sutures with the pericranium. As the dura mater is directly continuous with these various structures, it can be readily understood how inflammation may extend by continuity into the cranial cavity and cause secondary meningitis.

Pulsations of the dura mater.—The dura mater, when exposed in the living subject, may present two distinct pulsations, communicated from the underlying brain: one synchronous with the pulsation of the arteries, the other with respiration, rising in expiration and sinking in inspiration.

Tumors of the dura mater, if sarcomatous, may protrude through the bones of the cranium and cause a swelling in the scalp, or they may cause osseous erosion. If endotheliomatous they are called meningiomas, and frequently give rise to bony thickening directly over the tumor. X-ray evidence of this thickening with signs of intracranial pressure is diagnostic. Tumors with calcification along the falx are known as psammoma bodies, and may become quite large.

DISSECTION.—Preliminary to removing the brain, and in order to obtain the most correct idea of the normal relations of the two larger partitions formed by the inner layer, the falx cerebri and the tentorium cerebelli, divide the dura mater in the following manner: carry two incisions through it from before backward, one centimeter (one-half inch) on each side of the median line, thus avoiding the superior longitudinal (*superior sagittal*) sinus. From the center of these incisions carry a transverse incision upon each side as far as the divided margin of the bone. Reflect the flaps thus made, and with the fingers gently separate the hemispheres of the cerebrum. This exposes the falx cerebri with the veins from the surface of the cerebrum which empty into the superior longitudinal (*superior sagittal*) sinus. The tentorium cerebelli can now readily be exposed by lifting up the posterior extremities of the hemispheres of the cerebrum (occipital lobes). Next lay open the superior longitudinal (*superior sagittal*) sinus and inspect its interior. The small openings of the veins from the top of the hemispheres (superior cerebral veins), the diploë, and the dura mater will be seen along its entire course; they generally enter from behind forward. Divide the anterior uncut portion of the dura mater, and sever the falx cerebri from its attachment to the crista galli, along with the veins which empty into the superior longitudinal (*superior sagittal*) sinus; together with the falx cerebri turn back the strip of dura mater in which is contained the superior longitudinal (*superior sagittal*) sinus.

Removal of the brain.—The brain should now be removed in the following manner:

Draw the subject well up so that the head will hang over the edge of the table. With the fingers of the left hand lift the frontal lobes of the cerebrum from the anterior cranial fossa and raise the olfactory bulbs from the cribriform plate (*lamina cribrosa*) of the ethmoidal bone, thus severing the olfactory nerves. The optic nerves with the ophthalmic arteries beneath will now be seen, and both should be cut across with scissors, a short distance from the brain. By gently lifting and displacing the hemispheres backward, the internal carotid arteries and the infundibulum (*infundibulum hypothalami*), a process of gray matter which connects the pituitary body (*hypophysis*) with the tuber cinereum, will be seen. These should be divided or the arteries should be severed and the pituitary body removed from the pituitary (*hypophyseal*) fossa after incising the diaphragma sellæ. The third pair of cranial nerves, the oculomotor, will be seen lying behind the anterior clinoid processes on their way to reach the cavernous sinuses. Divide these nerves and then, turning the head to the right, lift the temporal lobes from the middle cranial fossa; the tentorium cerebelli will now be brought into view. This should be cut through close to its attachment to the posterior clinoid process and to the petrous portion of the temporal bone. The trochlear, or fourth, and the trigeminal, or fifth, pairs of cranial nerves should be severed on the left side; turn the head to the left, and divide the corresponding

PLATE XII.

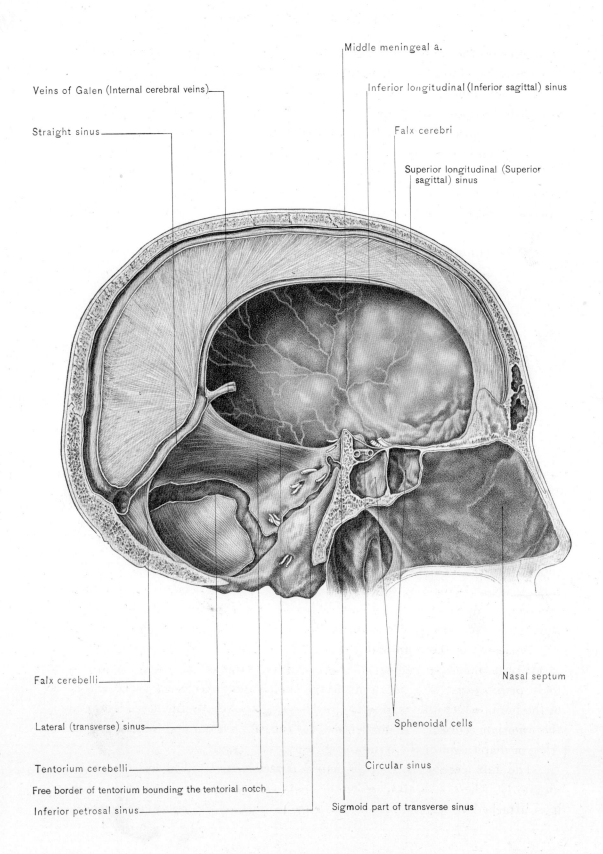

Middle meningeal a.

Inferior longitudinal (Inferior sagittal) sinus

Falx cerebri

Superior longitudinal (Superior sagittal) sinus

Veins of Galen (Internal cerebral veins)

Straight sinus

Falx cerebelli

Lateral (transverse) sinus

Tentorium cerebelli

Free border of tentorium bounding the tentorial notch

Inferior petrosal sinus

Nasal septum

Sphenoidal cells

Circular sinus

Sigmoid part of transverse sinus

SINUSES AND PROCESSES OF DURA MATER.

structures on the right side. Bring the face back to the middle line, draw the brain well backward, and divide the following structures from within outward in the order named: the abducens, or sixth, the facial, or seventh, the auditory, or eighth, the glosso-pharyngeal, or ninth, the vagus, or tenth, the spinal accessory, or eleventh, and the hypoglossal, or twelfth, pairs of cranial nerves. The next and final step consists in carrying a scalpel down into the spinal canal as far as possible and cutting through the spinal cord, the two vertebral arteries, and the spinal portions of the spinal accessory nerves. The fingers of the right hand should then be slipped beneath the cerebellum and the pons, and the brain removed.

Preservation of the brain.—If the brain is not to be dissected at once, it should be placed in a solution of chlorid of zinc or in alcohol and formaldehyd or in Müller's fluid. If placed in a zinc solution, the pia mater should be removed later, when it can be more easily separated than in the fresh condition. To preserve the brain in alcohol alone, the pia mater must first be removed, preferably under water; but if alcohol and formaldehyd are used, the membrane may be removed at leisure. Brains hardened in chloride of zinc should afterward be kept in alcohol. When the brain has been removed from a subject injected (embalmed) with chlorid of zinc, the pia mater can at once be separated and the brain placed in alcohol. If a fresh brain is immediately placed in alcohol, subsequent removal of the pia mater will be found almost impossible on account of its firm adherence. If the pia mater is not removed, the study of the convolutions is much less satisfactory. A brain which has been hardened in chloride of zinc and afterward kept in alcohol is much easier to handle than when kept in zinc alone as the latter, by its action on the skin makes, the fingers sticky. Brains preserved in alcohol and formaldehyd are preferable to those preserved in a solution of zinc chlorid and alcohol, because they are less shrunken than the latter. A brain taken from a subject embalmed with zinc chlorid should be hardened in a solution of the same; only fresh brains should be hardened and preserved in alcohol and a four per cent solution of formaldehyd.

Processes of the dura mater (Plate XII).—The dura mater, through duplication of its inner, or meningeal, layer, sends two large and two small partitions, folds, or processes, into the cavity of the skull and between certain subdivisions of the brain, which they support. The larger processes are the *falx cerebri* and the *tentorium cerebelli;* the smaller ones are the *falx cerebelli* and the *diaphragma sellæ,* or diaphragm of the pituitary (*hypophyseal*) fossa.

The **falx cerebri** is a sickle-shaped process, narrowed almost to a point anteriorly, where it is attached to the crista galli, and broad posteriorly, where it is attached to the middle of the upper surface of the tentorium cerebelli,

as far back as the internal occipital protuberance. The base of the falx
is oblique and is attached to the tentorium along the line of the straight
sinus. It projects into the great longitudinal (*longitudinal*) fissure of the brain
and separates the hemispheres of the cerebrum. Its convex upper border is
attached upon the inner surface of the calvaria to the edges of the groove which
accommodates the superior longitudinal (*superior sagittal*) sinus. The free
concave lower border arches over the corpus callosum, and contains in its
posterior half the inferior longitudinal (*inferior sagittal*) sinus.

The **tentorium cerebelli** is a somewhat triangular-shaped, tent-like process,
having its base attached upon the inner surface of the occipital bone to the edges
of the groove for the lateral (*transverse*) sinus; the sides are attached to the line
of junction of the upper and posterior surfaces of the petrous portion of the
temporal bone, from the apex of which they are continued to the posterior and
anterior clinoid processes. The apex corresponds to the free edge, which forms
the lateral and posterior boundaries of the triangular opening known as the
incisura tentorii, or *superior occipital foramen*. This foramen gives passage to
the crura cerebri (*cerebral peduncles*), the superior peduncles of the cerebellum,
the oculomotor and trochlear nerves, and the basilar artery. The tentorium
cerebelli projects into the great transverse fissure of the brain and separates the
posterior lobes of the cerebrum from the cerebellum. The convex border of
the base of the tentorium cerebelli contains the horizontal portions of the lateral
(*transverse*) sinuses; the sides contain the superior petrosal sinuses, and the
median portion, at its union with the falx cerebri, contains the straight sinus.
The base of the falx cerebri is attached along the entire median line of the upper
surface of the tentorium cerebelli, and the falx cerebelli to the median line of
the lower surface. The tentorium serves to support the posterior lobes of the
cerebrum, thus protecting the cerebellum from pressure.

The **falx cerebelli** is a small, vertical fold attached posteriorly to the internal
occipital crest, or inferior vertical limb of the occipital cross, and above to the
under surface of the tentorium cerebelli; it is situated between the hemispheres
of the cerebellum. Its posterior border contains the occipital sinus. This
border at times splits into two parts, which are attached to the sides of the back
part of the foramen magnum.

The **diaphragma sellæ** is a small, oval fold of the dura which projects horizontally from the margins of the sella turcica, roofing over the pituitary (*hypophyseal*) fossa. It is continuous on either side with the inner wall of the cavernous
sinus. It contains a small aperture, the *foramen diaphragmatis*, through which
the infundibulum connects the pituitary (*hypophysis*) with the brain. This
membrane often varies in thickness, and the foramen diaphragmatis may vary

PLATE XIII.

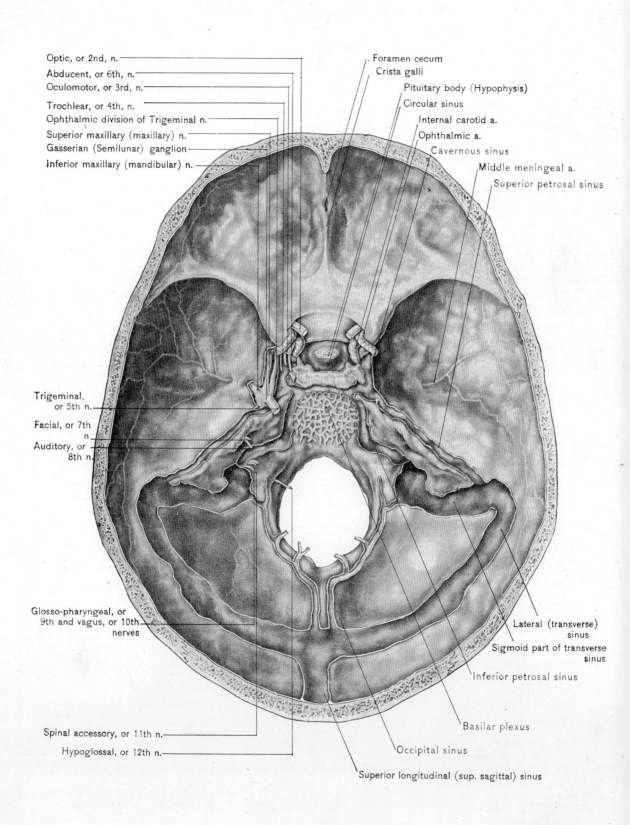

Optic, or 2nd, n.
Abducent, or 6th, n.
Oculomotor, or 3rd, n.
Trochlear, or 4th, n.
Ophthalmic division of Trigeminal n.
Superior maxillary (maxillary) n.
Gasserian (Semilunar) ganglion
Inferior maxillary (mandibular) n.

Foramen cecum
Crista galli
Pituitary body (Hypophysis)
Circular sinus
Internal carotid a.
Ophthalmic a.
Cavernous sinus
Middle meningeal a.
Superior petrosal sinus

Trigeminal, or 5th n.
Facial, or 7th n.
Auditory, or 8th n.

Glosso-pharyngeal, or 9th and vagus, or 10th nerves

Lateral (transverse) sinus
Sigmoid part of transverse sinus
Inferior petrosal sinus

Spinal accessory, or 11th n.
Hypoglossal, or 12th n.

Basilar plexus
Occipital sinus
Superior longitudinal (sup. sagittal) sinus

SINUSES AND CRANIAL NERVES.

from a small aperture to one almost the size of the sella. The thickness of this dural covering and the size of the infundibular opening often determine the direction of growth of pituitary tumors. Where the diaphragma sella is unyielding a pituitary growth will cause enlargement of the sella into the sphenoidal sinus below.

Sinuses of the dura mater (Plates XII; XIII).—The sinuses of the dura mater are venous channels formed by the separation of its endosteal and meningeal layers, and are lined with a prolongation of the lining membrane of the veins. They are rigid tubes which always remain patent, their function being to return the venous blood from the brain and its coverings, the diploë (with a few exceptions), and also the greater part of the blood from the orbit and the eyeball. They collect this blood and convey it to the jugular, or posterior lacerated foramina, where it is taken up by the internal jugular veins. There are sixteen sinuses in all, consisting of two groups, one situated at the superior and posterior part of the cranial cavity, and the other at the base of the skull. The first group includes the superior longitudinal (*superior sagittal*), the inferior longitudinal (*inferior sagittal*), the straight, the lateral (*transverse*), and the occipital sinuses. The other group includes the cavernous, the sinuses alæ parvæ (*spheno-parietal*), the circular (*intercavernous*), the superior and the inferior petrosal. They can also be divided into a median and a lateral group, the former including the single sinuses, situated in the middle line of the skull, and the latter, the paired sinuses, situated on both sides of the midline. Five are in pairs and six are single. The five pairs are the lateral (*transverse*), the superior petrosal, the inferior petrosal, the cavernous, and the sinuses alæ parvæ (*spheno-parietal*). The six single sinuses are the superior longitudinal (*superior sagittal*), the inferior longitudinal (*inferior sagittal*), the circular (*intercavernous*), the basilar, the straight, and the occipital. Some anatomists describes the sigmoid portions of the lateral (*transverse*) sinuses as an additional pair, thus making eighteen in all.

The **superior longitudinal (superior sagittal) sinus,** which has already been exposed, occupies the convex border of the falx cerebri. It passes from the foramen cecum at the root of the frontal crest through the mesial groove on the inner surface of the calvaria; deviating slightly to the right in the posterior part of its course, it runs to the internal occipital protuberance, to end in the torcular Herophili. The *torcular Herophili (confluens sinuum)* is the point of confluence of the superior longitudinal (*superior sagittal*), lateral, straight, and occipital sinuses, and is situated a little to the right of the internal occipital protuberance. The superior longitudinal (*superior sagittal*) sinus on section is triangular, its base being directed toward the calvaria; it is narrower in front, gradually increasing in width as it passes backward. Its lumen is crossed by a number of fibrous bands, the *chordæ Willisii*, and Pacchionian bodies (*arachnoid granulations*) are found projecting into it. It receives veins from the scalp through the parietal foramina, from the diploë, the dura mater, and the hemispheres of the cerebrum. These veins, particularly those from the cerebrum, the superior cerebral, run into the sinus anteroposteriorly, in the reverse direction to the blood stream, and pierce the wall of the sinus very obliquely. In the fetus the sinus communicates with the veins of the nose by a small emissary vein which passes through the foramen cecum, but this connection seldom occurs in the adult. The superior longitudinal (*superior sagittal*) sinus presents a variable number of lateral outgrowths or pouches, which have been named the *lacunæ laterales*. It is into these that the Pacchionian bodies (*arachnoid granulations*) project.

Wounds of, and line for the superior longitudinal (superior sagittal) sinus.—The relation of the sinus to the skull renders it liable to be wounded in fracture of the vertex and in trephining operations over the median line of the vertex. Hemorrhage from this or any of the sinuses is best controlled by the use of a small muscle graft taken from an accessible area. The graft should be large enough to cover the opening in the sinus and should be held in place by the finger for two or three minutes; the hemorrhage can thus be entirely controlled. Plugging with sterile gauze or, in case of a small wound, closure by sutures may be resorted to. The course of the sinus is represented on the scalp by a straight line drawn from the root of the nose over the median line of the vertex to the external occipital protuberance.

Septic or infective processes of the scalp may enter the superior longitudinal (*superior sagittal*) sinus through the parietal emissary veins, while septic infection of the nose may reach the sinus through the vein in which the sinus has its origin.

Superior longitudinal (superior sagittal) syndrome.—Attention has been called by Holmes, Sargent, and Wilensky to cases presenting a definite syndrome after injury to this sinus. Cushing has pointed out that the syndrome has its counterpart in the traumatic spastic paralysis of the newborn (Little's disease). Symptomatically, the cases present a spastic paraplegia of both lower extremities, symmetrical or asymmetrical.

The **lateral (transverse) sinus,** the largest of the paired cranial sinuses, extends from the internal occipital protuberance to the jugular foramen, terminating at the beginning of the internal jugular vein. The origin of the sinuses is at the point of junction of the two lateral (*transverse*), the superior longitudinal (*superior sagittal*), the straight, and the occipital sinuses. This meeting point is known as the torcular Herophili (*confluens sinuum*). The two lateral (*transverse*) sinuses may be entirely separate except for a small connecting branch which then represents the torcular Herophili (*confluens sinuum*). It then passes lateralward and forward, grooving the squamous portion of the occipital bone along the line of attachment of the tentorium cerebelli, the posterior inferior angle of the parietal, the mastoid portion of the temporal, and the jugular process of the occipital bone. Each sinus consists of two portions, a horizontal and a sigmoid. The *horizontal portion* is situated in the base of the tentorium cerebelli; it is triangular on section, with the base of the triangle directed toward the occipital bone and the posterior inferior angle of the parietal bone. The *sigmoid portion* is situated below the tentorium cerebelli, and grooves the mastoid portion of the temporal, and the jugular process of the occipital bone; it is semicylindrical on section, and is considered by some anatomists a separate sinus, the sigmoid. The superior petrosal sinus empties posteriorly into the sigmoid portion of the lateral (*transverse*) sinus at its origin. The lateral sinus varies somewhat in size and position, a fact to be remembered in trephining operations.

Tributaries of the lateral (transverse) sinus.—The right lateral (*transverse*) sinus is usually larger than the left; it begins at the torcular Herophili (*confluens sinuum*), and is the continuation of the superior longitudinal (*superior sagittal*) sinus. The left lateral (*transverse*) sinus is the continuation of the straight sinus, In addition to the superior petrosal sinuses, the lateral (*transverse*) sinuses receive emissary veins from the scalp, which pass through the mastoid and posterior condyloid foramina (*condyloid canals*), also veins from the diploë (the occipital and the anterior temporal), the lateral inferior cerebral, and some of the superior and inferior cerebellar veins.

Thrombosis of the lateral (transverse) sinus.—The sigmoid portion of the lateral (*transverse*) sinus, or the sigmoid sinus, is the part of the intracranial venous circulation which is most commonly the seat of sinus thrombosis. Macewen has shown that this may occur in one of six ways: (1) extension from acute or chronic purulent inflammations of the middle ear; (2) extension of acute inflammatory disease from the mouth, pharynx, and tonsils to the middle ear, mastoid antrum, and cells; (3) extension of thrombosis from other sinuses or emissary veins; (4) trauma, such as fracture of the base of the skull extending through the middle ear to the sinus; (5) pressure of tumors or discharge associated with them; (6) infection from septic wounds of the head, neck, or mastoid region. Thrombosis of this portion of the sinus and of the commencement of the internal jugular vein constitutes one of the most frequent complications of suppurative middle ear disease, and is due to the proximity of the sinus to the middle ear and mastoid cells, and to the fact that veins pass directly from the mastoid portion of the temporal bone to the lateral (*transverse*) sinus. This condition demands exposure of the sinus and removal of the clot, which should, if possible, be done before general systemic infection takes place. When sepsis is present and the mastoid antrum and cells have been drained without producing the desired effect, the sigmoid portion of the lateral (*transverse*) sinus should be exposed without delay. Frequently a perisinus abscess is found without thrombosis of the sinus itself. The presence of a clot can readily be determined by palpation; removal of the clot should immediately be followed by antiseptic packing of the sinus. In all exposures of the lateral (*transverse*) sinus for evacuation of a clot, the jugular vein should previously be ligated in the neck to prevent pulmonary infection. The four most serious complications of suppurative otitis media are septic thrombosis of the lateral (*transverse*) sinus, septic meningitis, abscess of the temporal lobe of the cerebrum, and cerebellar abscess.

Line for the lateral (transverse) sinus.—The relation of the lateral (*transverse*) sinus to the exterior of the skull is important when trephining for depressed fracture of the occipital bone, cerebellar tumor, or cerebellar abscess; when opening the mastoid cells or mastoid antrum, or when exposing the sinus itself in septic thrombosis. The sinus follows a line drawn from the external occipital protuberance to a point two and a half centimeters (one inch) above the external auditory meatus as far as the base of the mastoid process; it then runs downward parallel with the middle line of the mastoid. The right sigmoid groove is generally wider and deeper, projects farther lateralward, and reaches farther forward than the left sigmoid groove. The closer proximity of the sigmoid portion of the right lateral (*transverse*) sinus to the middle ear perhaps explains the greater frequency of intracranial lesions following right-sided otitis media.

Operations on the mastoid process.—In opening the mastoid cells or mastoid antrum it is better to expose the entire surface of the mastoid process than to expose a limited surface, particularly if the disease is advanced, and the overlying soft parts are so swollen as to render it impossible to outline the process with any degree of certainty. When the mastoid process is exposed, draw two lines: a horizontal one through the roof of the external auditory meatus, and a vertical one through its posterior wall. In adults apply the gouge at a point a little below the horizontal and behind the perpendicular line; in children apply the instrument at a point directly over the horizontal and behind the perpendicular line. With the gouge make an opening in an anteromedial direction. After removing the external table, the mastoid antrum can usually be entered with a small elevator or a stiff director; this is preferable to the gouge, as it lessens the risk of injuring the sigmoid portion of the lateral (*transverse*) sinus. Both the tympanum, or middle ear, and the mastoid cells can be drained through the mastoid antrum, although if extensive disease is found, the mastoid cells should also be opened. In the majority of cases the pus is primarily in the tympanum, but occasionally suppuration originates in the mastoid cells. It must be remembered that in children and in many adults there are no well-developed mastoid cells, so that opening directly into the mastoid antrum is the safest course to pursue in all cases.

The **inferior longitudinal** (**inferior sagittal**) **sinus** is a small sinus situated in the free concave margin of the falx cerebri. It is cylindrical on section, and terminates in the straight sinus at the junction of the falx cerebri with the anterior margin of the tentorium cerebelli and at the posterior boundary of the incisura tentorii, or superior accipital foramen. It receives veins from the falx cerebri, the median surface of the cerebral hemispheres, and the basilar surface of the frontal lobes.

The **straight sinus** which is an unpaired sinus, is formed by the union of the inferior longitudinal (*inferior sagittal*) sinus with the veins of Galen (*internal cerebral veins*). It is situated at the junction of the falx cerebri with the tentorium cerebelli, and terminates at the internal occipital protuberance, where it joins the torcular Herophili (*confluens sinuum*); it is continued as the left lateral (*transverse*) sinus. It is triangular on section, and increases in size as it passes backward. It receives veins from the tentorium cerebelli and the superior surface of the cerebellum. Its direction is downward and backward.

The **veins of Galen** (**internal cerebral veins**) drain the large subcortical area of the brain. Severe traumatic injuries to the head may result in rupture of these veins. The patient shows bilateral increase in reflexes, bloody spinal fluid, a loose and soft brain upon decompression with no evidence of pressure. Restlessness and stupor are marked throughout. The outcome is always fatal.

The **occipital sinus,** usually an unpaired, but sometimes a paired sinus, is formed by the union of two small veins (*marginal sinuses*) which pass around the lateral margins of the foramen magnum and communicate with the sigmoid portion of the lateral (*transverse*) sinus near the jugular foramen and with the posterior spinal veins. It passes along the attached margin of the falx cerebelli to the internal occipital protuberance, where it empties into the torcular Herophili (*confluens sinuum*); it may also empty into one of the lateral (*transverse*) sinuses or into the straight sinus. It receives veins from the tentorium cerebelli and cerebellum, and also communicates with the vertebral veins and the anterior spinal plexus.

The **spheno-parietal sinus,** or **sinus alæ parvæ,** one of the paired sinuses, occupies a groove on the inferior surface of the lesser wing of the sphenoidal bone, and runs through the *sphenoidal fold* of the dura mater. This fold is attached to the base of the lesser wing of the sphenoidal bone, and is continuous with the

dura mater at its attachment to the anterior clinoid process.   It empties into
the cavernous sinus, and receives dural, diploic, and anterior cerebral veins.

The **cavernous sinus,** a large paired sinus, is situated along the side of the
body of the sphenoidal bone, and extends from the sphenoidal (*superior
orbital*) fissure to the apex of the petrous portion of the temporal bone.   The
lateral wall of the sinus, the most distinct, contains the oculomotor and trochlear nerves and the ophthalmic division of the trigeminal; the medial wall is not
a distinct lamella, but is formed by the structures which it contains: the internal
carotid artery, the abducent nerve, and the cavernous plexus of the cervical
sympathetic.   Arterio-venous aneurysm between the sinus and the internal
carotid artery may occur.   The signs of such a lesion are dilatation of the
ophthamic vein, causing exophthalmos, and a pulsatory swelling behind the
medial angular process of the frontal bone.   The endothelial lining membrane
of the sinus prevents the blood from coming into contact with the nerves and
artery,   In addition to these symptoms of venous obstruction, the aneurysm
may lead to paralysis in the distribution of the nerves contained within the walls
of the sinus and which lie in close relation with the internal carotid artery.   Section of the sinus discloses numerous bands and fringes forming spaces on its
interior, hence its name.   The nerves which occupy the lateral wall of the sinus
observe the same order, both from above downward and from within outward,
in which they have been mentioned.   Of the structures occupying the medial
wall, the abducent nerve is the most lateral.   The sinus receives the ophthalmic
vein in front, and the spheno-parietal above the oculomotor nerve.   It communicates with its fellow by means of the circular sinus and the basilar plexus.
This communication between the two sinuses is important in providing a mechanism by which the pressure of venous blood within the cranium is equalized.
The sinus divides posteriorly at the apex of the petrous portion of the temporal
bone into the *superior* and *inferior petrosal sinuses.*   It receives the middle
cerebral veins and those from the basilar surface of the frontal lobe, and communicates with the pterygoid plexus of veins by means of the vein of Vesalius
which runs through the foramen of Vesalius in the greater wing of the sphenoidal
bone.   It also communicates with the internal jugular vein through the venous
plexus surrounding the petrous portion of the internal carotid artery, and with
the pterygoid and pharyngeal plexuses of veins by means of veins which run
through the foramen ovale and the foramen lacerum medium (*foramen lacerum*).

Infective material may reach the cavernous sinus from the scalp and face
through the supra-orbital or the frontal and the ophthalmic veins, and through
the anterior diploic vein and the spheno-parietal sinus; from the orbit, through the
ophthalmic vein, and from the pterygo-maxillary region, through the vein of

Vesalius and emissary veins which pass through the foramina at the base of the skull.

Relations of the cavernous sinus to the Gasserian (semilunar) ganglion.— Only one of the cavernous sinuses should be opened at this stage of the dissection, the opening of the other being deferred until the nerves which run in the walls of the sinus to enter the orbit have been traced. The cavernous sinus, like the other sinuses, will be seen to occupy an interval between the endosteal and meningeal layers of the dura mater. In the posterior portion of this interval is the cavity occupied by the Gasserian (*semilunar*) ganglion, known as Meckel's space. The comparatively intimate relation existing between the sinus and the ganglion is one of the reasons for avulsion of the sensory root in trigeminal neuralgia, rather than extirpation of the ganglion.

The **circular sinus,** through which the two cavernous sinuses communicate, surrounds the pituitary body (*hypophysis*). The anterior half is larger than the posterior, and enlarges still more in advanced life. It receives veins from the pituitary body (*hypophysis*) and the neighboring bone and the dura mater. Sometimes one-half of the sinus is wanting.

The **superior and inferior petrosal sinuses** are the terminal divisions of the cavernous sinus. The *superior petrosal sinus* runs in a small groove in the superior edge of the petrous portion of the temporal bone, in the margin of the tentorium cerebelli. It terminates in the lateral (*transverse*) sinus at the point where the sigmoid portion of the sinus begins. At its origin it is crossed by the trochlear nerve, and, in turn, crosses the trigeminal nerve. It receives some of the inferior cerebral and superior cerebellar veins, a vein from the middle ear which makes its exit through the petro-squamous suture, and some diploic veins.

The *inferior petrosal sinus,* which is shorter and wider than the superior, runs in the groove formed by the junction of the inferior border of the petrous portion of the temporal, with the basilar process of the occipital bone, and at the jugular foramen empties either into the superior bulb of the internal jugular vein, or into the vein below the bulb. The terminal portion of the inferior petrosal sinus separates the glosso-pharyngeal from the vagus and the spinal accessory nerves. It receives some of the inferior cerebellar veins and some veins from the medulla oblongata and the pons; veins from the internal ear which make their exit by way of the aqueductus vestibuli and aqueductus cochleæ also empty into it.

The **basilar plexus,** through which the inferior petrosal sinuses communicate with each other, passes across the basilar process of the occipital bone. It extends inferiorly as far as the anterior margin of the foramen magnum, where it communicates with the anterior spinal veins. The abducent nerve passes through it.

BLOOD SUPPLY.—The blood supply of the dura mater is derived from the meningeal arteries, though the chief function of these vessels is to supply the bones of the cranium. These arteries comprise practically three sets, an anterior, a middle, and a posterior, and in the dried skull their course can readily be traced by following the grooves in the bones which they occupy. The meningeal arteries are accompanied by relatively small veins.

NERVE SUPPLY.—The nerve supply of the dura mater is derived from the Gasserian (*semilunar*) ganglion through the first, second, and third divisions of the trigeminal nerve, from the vagus, the hypoglossal, and the cervical sympathetic nerves.

DISSECTION.—Before studying the courses of the meningeal arteries, which necessitates stripping the dura mater from the skull, examine the cranial nerves as they pass through the foramina at the base of the skull.

INTRACRANIAL COURSE AND MODE OF EXIT OF THE CRANIAL NERVES
(Plate XIII)

In tracing the cranial nerves to their exit through the foramina at the base of the skull, observe that each pair of nerves receives investments from all three membranes of the brain. The coverings derived from the dura mater and the pia mater are continuous with the sheaths of the nerves, while the covering from the arachnoid terminates as the nerves enter the dura mater.

The twelve pairs of nerves are designated by number, beginning anteriorly and passing posteriorly, in the order in which they pass from the dura, and by name according to their distribution and function. They are: the olfactory, the optic, the oculomotor, the trochlear, the trigeminal, the abducent, the facial, the auditory, the glosso-pharyngeal, the vagus, the spinal accessory, and the hypoglossal nerves. These nerves for the most part are distributed to, or come from the structures of the head. Conventionally, all the nerves are regarded as passing away from the brain, and the separation of motor and sensory nerves into centrifugal and centripetal nerves is frequently disregarded.

The **olfactory,** or first, **nerves** together with the olfactory tracts and bulbs have been removed with the brain and their branches divided. The olfactory nerve consists of some twenty filaments whose cells lie in the Schneiderian membrane (*mucous membrane of the nose*) which embraces, on the lateral nasal wall, less than the medial surface of the superior turbinate and a somewhat larger field on the adjacent portion of the septum. These fibers pass upward through the cribriform plate of the ethmoid and enter the inferior surface of the olfactory bulb. Here the axons make connection with the dendrites of the mitral cells. Some confusion is encountered in the study of this nerve, since formerly the olfactory bulb and tract together with the filaments were known as the olfactory nerve. These latter structures, however, are of an entirely different morphologic character, since the bulb and the tract are the rudimentary remains of the olfactory lobe found in animals, and strictly speaking, they should be regarded as a portion of the brain. Fractures of the anterior fossa involving the cribriform plate may damage the olfactory nerves and cause a loss of the sense of smell. An abscess in the frontal sinus frequently involves by extension the olfactory nerve on the same side giving unilateral anosmia. Frontal lobe tumors, by direct pressure, may cause a loss of smell on one side.

The **optic,** or second, **nerve** extends from the eyeball to the optic commissure. It leaves the apex of the orbit through the optic foramen of the sphenoidal bone in company with the ophthalmic artery which lies to its lateral and inferior side.

The **oculomotor,** or third, **nerve** pierces the dura mater behind and slightly lateral to the carotid artery and behind the anterior clinoid process, and enters the superolateral wall of the cavernous sinus. In this situation it lies above the trochlear nerve and the ophthalmic branch of the trigeminal. Entering the orbit through the sphenoidal (*superior orbital*) fissure, it then lies below the trochlear nerve and part of the ophthalmic. It next divides into a *superior* and an *inferior branch.* These branches pass between the heads of the external (*lateral*) recti muscles, in company with, but separated from each other by the nasal branches of the ophthalmic nerve. They supply all the extrinsic muscles of the eyeball, with the exception of the superior oblique and external (*lateral*) rectus, and also the circular muscular fibers of the iris and the ciliary muscle through sympathetic nerves which originate close to its nucleus.

The **trochlear,** or fourth, **nerve** pierces the dura mater near the free edge of the tentorium cerebelli, a little posterior and lateral to the posterior clinoid process and above the oval opening for the trigeminal nerve. It enters the lateral wall of the cavernous sinus, where it lies below the oculomotor and above the ophthalmic branch of the trigeminal nerve, passes through the sphenoidal (*superior orbital*) fissure, in which it lies above the oculomotor nerve and the ophthalmic division of the trigeminal, and enters the orbit above the heads of the external (*lateral*) rectus muscle, crosses above the levator palpebræ superioris and the rectus superioris to reach the superior oblique, or trochlearis, muscle, which it supplies.

The **trigeminal, trifacial,** or fifth, **nerve** arises from the mid-pons on its lateral aspect, and consists of a large sensory (*portio major*), and a small motor (*portio minor*) root. It passes through an oval opening in the dura mater beneath the attachment of the free border of the tentorium cerebelli to the posterior clinoid process. Strictly speaking, the sensory portion enters the dura here and the motor portion emerges. It lies below the trochlear nerve and above the apex of the petrous portion of the temporal bone and the internal auditory meatus. Upon the larger or sensory root is the Gasserian (*semilunar*) ganglion which, however, cannot be seen until the dura mater is raised from the base of the skull. (Its description will therefore be deferred until later.) The ophthalmic branch of the trigeminal nerve is exposed, and is seen running through the lateral wall of the cavernous sinus, where it lies beneath the trochlear nerve. It divides into three terminal branches, *lacrimal, frontal*, and *nasal*, after which it enters the orbit by way of the sphenoidal (*superior orbital*) fissure. In the wall of the sinus the ophthalmic branch is joined by filaments from the carotid plexus of the cervical sympathetic, communicating with the oculomotor, trochlear, and abducent nerves, and giving off a *recurrent branch* which passes backward between the layers of the tentorium cerebelli.

The **abducent,** or sixth, **nerve** pierces the dura mater behind the body of the sphenoidal bone immediately below the posterior clinoid process and slightly medial and posterior to the opening for the trigeminal nerve, and passes to the lateral side of the inferior petrosal sinus and over the apex of the petrous portion of the temporal bone. It then courses along the medial wall of the cavernous sinus to the lateral side of the internal carotid artery, and enters the orbit by way of the sphenoidal (*superior orbital*) fissure, lying between the ophthalmic vein and the inferior branch of the oculomotor nerve. It supplies the rectus lateralis muscle, between the two heads of which it passes. Within the wall of the cavernous sinus it is joined by filaments from the carotid plexus of the cervical sympathetic and as it enters the orbit it communicates with a small filament from the ophthalmic nerve.

The **facial,** or seventh, **nerve** leaves the cranial cavity by way of the internal auditory meatus through which it passes above, and anterior to the auditory (*acoustic*) nerve. Within the meatus it lies first to the medial side of, and then directly over the auditory (*acoustic*) nerve. The facial nerve consists of a large *motor part*, or the facial nerve proper, and a small *sensory part*, commonly known as the *pars intermedia of Wrisberg.* Accompanied by the auditory (*acoustic*) nerve and the auditory (*internal auditory*) artery, the two parts pass, at the bottom of the meatus, to the facial, or Fallopian, canal, where the facial leaves the auditory (*acoustic*) nerve and follows the course of the canal, and, at a point where the latter bends backward, the *geniculum*, the two roots unite in a gangliform swelling, the geniculate ganglion. The facial nerve supplies the muscles of expression of the face, the stapedius muscle, the posterior belly of the digastric, and the stylo-hyoid muscle. It carries fibers of deep pressure sense in the face. Injuries to the nerve from mastoid operations are not infrequent, and inflamma-

tory reactions in the Fallopian (*facial*) canal give rise to *Bell's palsy*, a sponta-
neous type of facial paralysis resulting from exposure to cold or infection.   (For a
description of the course of the facial canal, see p. 500 Dissection of the middle
ear.)

The **auditory** (**acoustic**), or eighth, **nerve** leaves the cranial cavity through
the internal auditory meatus in company with the auditory (*internal auditory*)
artery, the facial nerve, and the pars intermedia.   Reaching the bottom of the
meatus, it divides into two branches, the cochlear and the vestibular, for the
supply of the cochlea, the vestibule, and the semicircular canals.

The **glossopharyngeal,** or ninth, **nerve,** the **vagus,** or tenth, **nerve,** and the
spinal accessory, or eleventh, **nerve,** all leave the cranial cavity by way of
the jugular foramen.   The glosso-pharyngeal has a separate sheath of dura mater
and arachnoid, and lies in front of the vagus and the spinal accessory nerves.
The sheath of dura mater of the vagus is common to it and the spinal accessory
nerve, but the two nerves have separate arachnoid sheaths.   (The nerve is
described in detail at p. 101.)   The spinal accessory nerve is made up of two parts:
a small portion *accessory* to, and running with the vagus, and a larger spinal portion, which rises from the spinal cord and enters the cranial cavity through the
foramen magnum, joining the accessory portion shortly after the latter emerges
from the medulla, and occupying the same sheath as the vagus.

The **hypoglossal,** or twelfth, **nerve** leaves the cranial cavity through the anterior condyloid foramen (*hypoglossal canal*).

The internal carotid artery.—With the cavernous sinus laid open and the
nerves within its wall exposed, before further disturbing the dura mater carefully
examine the internal carotid artery running in the medial wall of the sinus.
After its exit from the carotid canal, the curves which the artery makes in reaching the brain can now be seen to the best advantage.   Having emerged from the
carotid canal the artery turns upward, passing toward the posterior clinoid
process.   It next runs forward through the medial wall of the cavernous sinus to
reach the medial side of the anterior clinoid process, where it again turns upward
and pierces the dura mater on the medial aspect of the anterior clinoid process;
just before piercing the dura mater it gives off the ophthalmic branch.   The
cranial, or *terminal, portion* thus makes two bends, which give it the shape of the
letter S.   Running along with the artery and lateral to it is the abducent nerve.
The lining membrane of the sinus alone separates both the artery and the nerve
from the interior of the sinus.   Within the walls of the sinus the artery gives off
branches known as the *arteriæ receptaculi,* which supply the walls of the sinus,
the pituitary body (*hypophysis*), the Gasserian (*semilunar*) ganglion, and the dura
mater (through the anterior meningeal).   It is surrounded by filaments of the

cervical sympathetic which form two plexuses, the carotid lateral to, and the cavernous medial to the artery. The carotid plexus communicates with the abducent nerve and the Gasserian (*semilunar*) and Meckel's (*spheno-palatine*) ganglia; the cavernous plexus communicates wth the oculomotor, trochlear, and ophthalmic nerves, and furnishes the sympathetic root to the ophthalmic or lenticular (*ciliary*) ganglion.

DISSECTION.—The dura mater should now be dissected from the sides and base of the skull; it will be found closely adherent to the latter, requiring care in its removal in order to avoid injuring the following structures: the Gasserian (*semilunar*) ganglion, the superior maxillary (*maxillary*), and inferior maxillary (*mandibular*) nerves, which are branches from the ganglion, the greater superficial petrosal, the external superficial petrosal, when present, and the motor root of the trigeminal nerve. The last named and the greater superficial petrosal nerve run beneath the ganglion.

The **Gasserian** (**semilunar**) **ganglion** occupies a depression on the superior surface of the petrous portion of the temporal bone near the apex, and rests to a slight extent on the cartilage filling the middle lacerated foramen (*foramen lacerum*). It thus is in intimate relation with the internal carotid artery and the cavernous sinus. It is crescentic in outline, its concavity being directed backward and its convexity forward and laterally. It measures about one and a half to two centimeters in width, and about one centimeter in length. Its superior and inferior surfaces are slightly convex. It occupies an interval between the endosteal and meningeal layers of the dura mater (Meckel's space); the endosteal layer of the dura mater must therefore be divided in attempting its removal through the side or base of the skull. From the convexity of the ganglion arise the ophthalmic, the superior maxillary (*maxillary*), and inferior maxillary (*mandibular*) nerves; the first two are sensory nerves throughout, while the inferior maxillary (*mandibular*) nerve is sensory until it reaches the outside of the skull where it is joined by the motor root of the trigeminal nerve, which leaves the cranial cavity with it by way of the foramen ovale; the inferior maxillary (*mandibular*) then becomes a mixed nerve.

The **superior maxillary** (**maxillary**) **nerve,** intermediate in size between the ophthalmic and the inferior maxillary (*mandibular*), leaves the cranium by way of the foramen rotundum.

The **inferior maxillary** (**mandibular**) **nerve,** the largest branch of the trigeminal, leaves the cranial cavity by way of the foramen ovale which also transmits the lesser superficial petrosal nerve and the small meningeal (*accessory meningeal*) artery.

OPERATION ON THE GASSERIAN (SEMILUNAR) GANGLION

In Major Trigeminal Neuralgia permanent relief is offered by the Spiller-Frazier operation.   In this operation the sensory root is divided just behind the ganglion.   Regeneration never occurs after this solution of continuity.   However, if any of the three branches are divided peripheral to the ganglion there will be a regeneration of the nerves within a year, with return of symptoms.   This fact has led to the abandoning of neurectomies for trigeminal neuralgia, as the results are little better than those obtained from a successful alcoholic injection,   Unnecessary trauma to the ganglion at the operation should be carefully avoided.   It is often found possible to section the sensory root without disturbing the motor branch.   In order to avoid atrophic keratitis, it is extremely important to leave intact the necessary supply to the eye through the ophthalmic division.   Since less than nine per cent of cases of trigeminal neuralgia occur in the ophthalmic division, it is often possible to preserve the fibers in this posterior root which supply the eye by means of the first division.

The operation consists in avulsion of the lateral and lower two-thirds of the posterior root, which produces anesthesia in the second and third divisions of the trigeminal nerve without disturbing the function of the first, or ophthalmic, branch.   The procedure is undertaken through a small sickle-shaped incision within the hair line in the temporal region.   The base of the skin incision is carried down to the zygomatic process but no further, as there is considerable danger of injury to the upper branch of the facial nerve supplying the frontalis (*frontal belly of epicranius*) below this level.   The ascending limb is carried up about four centimeters just in front of the ear, before making the anterior curve which should not be carried beyond the hairline of the temporal side of the forehead.

The skin is completely dissected free from the underlying fascia, and a small nick parallel with the zygomatic process is made at the base in order that this flap may be folded back in the direction of the cheek.

The temporal fascia and muscle are then divided in the anterior aspect of the wound by a straight incision carried down in the direction of the fibers as deep as the underlying temporal bone.   A transverse cut of all the muscle structures is then made at the base of the opening along the zygomatic process, this time from before backward.

This should give a field of exposure of the temporal bone about the size of a silver dollar.   The bone is then opened by means of a Hudson drill, and the opening enlarged with rongeurs to the base of the middle fossa.   Careful freeing of the dura is necessary to avoid laceration.   A small opening is then made in the dura and the arachnoid to allow the escape of cerebro-spinal fluid, which produces enough reduction of brain volume to permit the elevation of the temporal lobe. The dura of the middle fossa is carefully elevated and the approach made to the ganglion along the floor.

The middle meningeal artery must be carefully sought and plugged with cotton at its point of emergence through the foramen spinosum. The artery is then severed, and further elevation of the dura will disclose the third division of the trigeminal nerve as it leaves through the foramen ovale. The dural sheath of the nerve must be divided and the overlying dural envelope pushed up to expose the ganglion. Care should be taken not to include the sheath of the ganglion in this exposure. Following the posterior border of the ganglion, the sensory root will be exposed as it passes into Meckel's cave; cerebro-spinal fluid is usually here encountered as the root comes into view. By means of a nerve hook the lower and lateral two-thirds of the root are then divided or avulsed. The motor root should be seen lying behind and assuming a more perpendicular course. It may be demonstrated by Faradic stimulation with the electrode. This filament should be carefully preserved, as well as the upper and medial third of the root, in cases where the ophthalmic division is not involved.

The eye requires constant attention during the first week following the operation, and the lid should be closed with adhesive to prevent the occurrence of keratitis. Should a corneal ulcer arise, immediate suture of the lid must be undertaken and the eyelid kept closed for from three to six months.

DISSECTION.—Divide the larger, or sensory, root of the trigeminal nerve, lift the Gasserian (*semilunar*) ganglion, and displace it forward and downward so as better to expose the smaller motor root and the greater superficial petrosal nerve, both of which lie beneath the ganglion. The motor root of the trigeminal nerve can be traced to the foramen ovale, where, with the inferior maxillary (*mandibular*) nerve, it makes its exit from the skull.

The **greater superficial petrosal nerve** arises partly from the geniculate ganglion of the facial nerve, and will be seen emerging from the hiatus of Fallopius (*hiatus of facial canal*). Since the nerve contains both motor and sensory fibers, it will be seen that the entire nerve could not originate from the geniculate ganglion, but that the motor fibers merely pass through it. Thence it runs in a small groove on the side of the superior surface of the petrous portion of the temporal bone beneath the Gasserian (*semilunar*) ganglion to reach the cartilage which fills the middle lacerated foramen (*foramen lacerum*). It then crosses the lateral side of the internal carotid artery to reach the posterior opening of the Vidian (*pterygoid*) canal where it meets the great deep petrosal from the carotid sympathetic plexus to form the Vidian nerve (*nerve of the pterygoid canal*).

PLATE XIV.

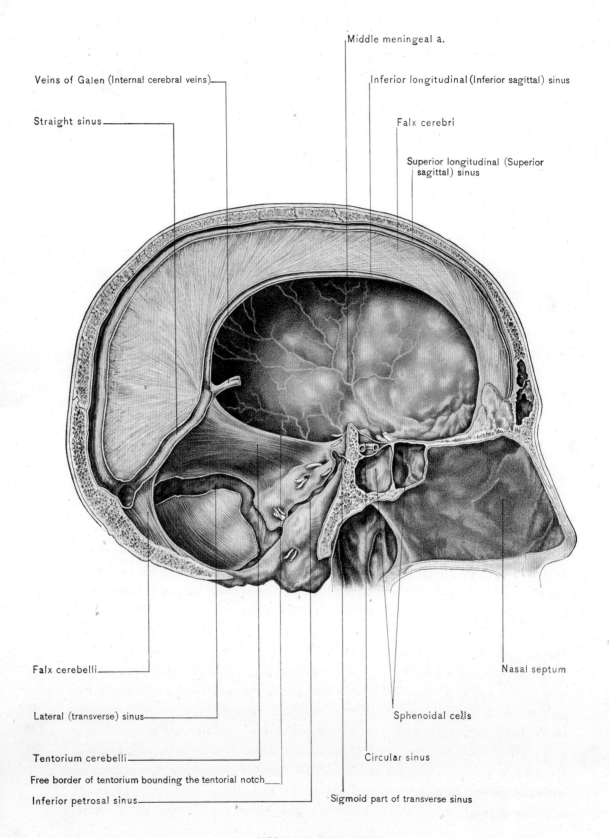

Middle meningeal a.

Veins of Galen (Internal cerebral veins)

Inferior longitudinal (Inferior sagittal) sinus

Straight sinus

Falx cerebri

Superior longitudinal (Superior sagittal) sinus

Falx cerebelli

Nasal septum

Lateral (transverse) sinus

Sphenoidal cells

Tentorium cerebelli

Circular sinus

Free border of tentorium bounding the tentorial notch

Inferior petrosal sinus

Sigmoid part of transverse sinus

MIDDLE MENINGEAL ARTERY.

The **lesser superficial petrosal nerve** is made up of fibers from the facial and the glosso-pharyngeal nerves.   It is really a continuation of the tympanic nerve, which is formed by a re-assembling of the fibers of that plexus, supplemented by a filament from the geniculate ganglion of the facial.   It emerges from the facial canal by way of a small foramen situated lateral to the hiatus of Fallopius (*hiatus of facial canal*), and passes through a small foramen situated between the foramina ovale and spinosum or through a fissure between the greater wing of the sphenoidal and the petrous portion of the temporal bone or through the foramen ovale.

The **external superficial petrosal nerve** leaves the facial nerve and canal by way of a small foramen placed lateral to the foramen for the lesser superficial petrosal nerve, on its way to join the plexus of the cervical sympathetic upon the middle meningeal artery.   This nerve is seldom found in the dissection of the interior of the base of the cranium, for in lifting up the endosteal layer of the dura mater the petrosal nerves are very apt to be severed unless the utmost care is observed.

The **Meningeal Arteries,** the anterior, the middle, the small (*accessory*), and the posterior meningeal, run between the skull and the dura mater, and are apt to be destroyed, or at least cut, when removing the dura mater; notwithstanding this, they can be traced by the grooves in the bones which they occupy. The greater part of the anterior branch of the middle, and the terminal part of the posterior meningeal arteries were described when removing the calvaria.

The **middle meningeal artery** (Plate XIV) is the largest and most important of the meningeal arteries.   As seen when dissecting the pterygo-maxillary region, both the middle and the small (*accessory*) meningeal are branches of the internal maxillary artery.   The middle meningeal artery runs between the two roots of the auriculo-temporal nerve and enters the cranial cavity by way of the foramen spinosum.   It occupies a groove in the greater wing of the sphenoidal bone, and almost immediately divides into an anterior and a posterior branch. Small branches of the middle meningeal artery pierce the cranial bones and anastomose with the vessels of the scalp.

The *anterior branch* runs through a groove across the greater wing of the sphenoidal, and continues into another groove in the antero-inferior angle of the parietal bone.   The commencement of this latter groove for a distance of seven to fourteen millimeters (one-fourth to one-half inch) is often bridged over by a thin plate of bone, and is thus converted into a canal.   The vessel continues along the groove near the anterior border of the parietal bone, runs almost parallel with the coronal suture to within a short distance of the superior longitudinal (*superior sagittal*) sinus, and gives off branches which run upward to the vertex and backward toward the occipital bone. The spheno-parietal sinus sometimes accompanies the artery for a part of its course, and may consequently be injured in fracture or during surgical manipulations.

The *posterior branch*, the smaller of the two, crosses the squamous portion of the temporal bone along the line of junction of the squamous with the petrous portion, and then passes upon the postero-inferior angle of the parietal bone, where it divides into its branches.

Extradural hemorrhage.—Owing to the relation of the anterior branch of the middle meningeal artery to the antero-inferior angle of the parietal bone, fracture of this part of the skull is apt to result in hemorrhage between the bone and the dura mater. It has already been noted that the dura mater is loosely attached to the vault of the cranium; this accounts for the size of the large extradural blood-clots occasionally seen. From the relation of the posterior branch of the middle meningeal artery to the motor area of the brain, it can readily be understood why symptoms due to pressure of an extradural clot are largely, if not altogether, motor. These cases constitute an especially favorable class for decompression, which should be done as soon as the diagnosis is made. If upon the removal of the clot the bleeding has not ceased, the vessel should be tied or clamped with a silver clip. It is sometimes necessary to tie both the anterior and the posterior branches.

Point for trephining.—The point of election for applying the trephine in a suspected case of extradural hemorrhage, meningeal in origin, is at a point about four centimeters (one and a half inches) behind, and two and a half centimeters (one inch) above the external angular (*zygomatic*) process of the frontal bone. When a simple or a compound depressed fracture is associated with the hemorrhage, the trephine should be applied near the fracture. To reach the posterior branch, the trephine should be applied immediately below the parietal eminence, and on the same horizontal level as in the preceding operation. The opening can subsequently be enlarged downward or backward and the vessel thus brought into view.

Branches of the middle meningeal artery.—The middle meningeal artery gives off branches within the cranial cavity to the Gasserian (*semilunar*) ganglion; a *petrosal branch*, which enters the hiatus of Fallopius (*hiatus of facial canal*) to supply the facial nerve and anastomoses with the stylo-mastoid branch of the posterior auricular artery; a *lacrimal*, or *orbital*, *branch* which enters the orbit by way of the sphenoidal fissure, or by a separate canal in the greater wing of the sphenoidal bone, and anastomoses with the ophthalmic artery; a *tympanic branch* to the tensor tympani muscle, and *branches* which leave the cranial cavity through foramina in the greater wing of the sphenoidal bone to anastomose in the

PLATE XV.

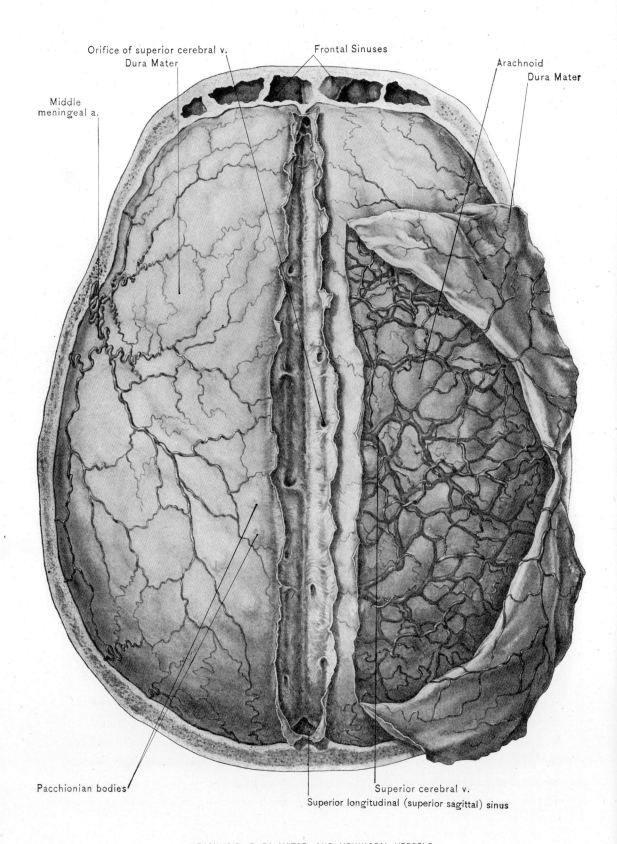

Orifice of superior cerebral v.
Dura Mater

Frontal Sinuses

Arachnoid
Dura Mater

Middle
meningeal a.

Pacchionian bodies

Superior cerebral v.

Superior longitudinal (superior sagittal) sinus

ARACHNOID, DURA MATER, AND MENINGEAL VESSELS.

temporal fossa with the deep temporal arteries. It is accompanied by two veins which empty into the internal maxillary vein.

The **anterior meningeal arteries** are branches of the ethmoidal arteries; they supply the dura mater of the anterior cranial fossa in the region of the median line. The arteria receptaculi, anterior meningeal branches, derived from the cavernous portion of the internal carotid artery, supply the dura mater of the middle cranial fossa, and sanatomose with the anterior ramus of the middle meningeal artery. The dura mater of the middle cranial fossa is supplied chiefly by the *small (accessory) meningeal artery*, a branch of the internal maxillary, which enters the cranial cavity by way of the foramen ovale, and one or two branches from the ascending pharyngeal artery, which enter the cranial cavity through the middle lacerated foramen (*foramen lacerum*).

The **posterior meningeal arteries** are the cranial branches of the ascending pharyngeal, the occipital, and the vertebral arteries. Those arising from the ascending pharyngeal and the occipital arteries enter the cranial cavity by way of the posterior lacerated, or jugular, foramen, and those from the vertebral artery by way of the occipital foramen, or foramen magnum; they supply the dura mater of the occipital, or posterior cranial, fossa. The ascending pharyngeal artery also sends a meningeal branch through the middle lacerated foramen (*foramen lacerum*), and an occasional one through the anterior condyloid foramen.

The **meningeal veins,** with the exception of those accompanying the middle meningeal artery, empty into the sinuses.

The brain having been hardened by one of the processes already mentioned at page 47 can now be studied in detail.

THE ARACHNOID (Plate XV)

The **arachnoid** (**arachnoidea**), the intermediate of the three enveloping membranes of the brain, is a delicate connective tissue membrane, lying between the dura mater and the pia mater. Like the dura mater, it sends processes into the longitudinal and transverse fissures, between the hemispheres of the cerebellum, and, to a slight extent, into the fissure of Sylvius (*lateral fissure*). It also surrounds the nerves, for which it forms tubular sheaths as far as their points of exit from the skull. Unlike the pia mater, it does not dip into the sulci, or fissures, between the convolutions, but passes directly from one convolution to the other, bridging over the sulci, leaving a triangular interval between it and the fold of the pia mater which dips into the sulcus. It forms a loose investment for the brain, and is continued downward over the spinal cord. Being a serous membrane, it presents to the naked eye a smooth, polished surface. It is connected by delicate connective tissue with both the dura mater and the pia mater, but much more intimately with the latter, especially over the summits of the convolutions where they form practically a single membrane.

The intimate connection between the arachnoid and the pia mater makes the independent removal of the former very difficult.   In some places the numerous trabeculæ uniting the two consist of a delicate reticulum, forming the loose subarachnoidal tissue, while at the base of the brain the space is wide and only a few trabeculæ are found.   The arachnoid and pia mater can be separated, however, by inflating the subarachnoid space with air by means of a blowpipe.

The Subdural Space.—The space between the dura mater and the arachnoid is known as the subdural space; it contains a small amount of fluid, and does not communicate with the subarachnoid space or with the ventricles, through any demonstrable openings.   It is, however, probable that subarachnoidal fluid finds its way between the cell spaces in the arachnoid into the subdural space.

The Subarachnoid Space.—The space between the arachnoid and the pia mater is known as the subarachnoid space.   In places this space consists merely of trabeculæ and resembles a sponge more than a free reservoir.   The space is most pronounced at the base of the brain.   Here the arachnoid membrane is thicker than elsewhere, and bridges over the interval between the temporal lobes and the space between the hemispheres of the cerebellum, partially occupied by the medulla oblongata.   By the intervention of the pons this general subarachnoid space is subdivided into the *anterior* and the *posterior space.*   The posterior space communicates with the subarachnoid space of the spinal cord and with the fourth ventricle of the brain through a small opening in the roof of the latter, *the foramen of Magendie (median aperture of fourth ventricle),* and through the *foramina of Luschka (lateral apertures of fourth ventricle),* located at each lateral recess of the fourth ventricle in the neighborhood of the vago-glosso-pharyngeal nerves.   This space contains the cerebro-spinal fluid, so that the brain may be said to lie on a water-bed.   Projecting into this space are seen the larger blood-vessels on their way toward the brain; the lymphatics of the brain and spinal cord empty into this space, which is in communication with the perilymph of the internal ear and with the lymphatics of the nose.

Subarachnoid cisterns is the name given to the more spacious portions of the subarachnoid space.   Several spaces are recognized according to locality, the largest being the *cisterna magna (cisterna cerebello-medullaris),* situated between the adjacent surfaces of the medulla oblongata and cerebellum. It is the upward continuation of the posterior portion of the spinal subarachnoid space, being continuous with it through the foramen magnum.   The *cisterna pontis* is the continuation of the anterior portion of the spinal subarachnoid space upon the anterior surface of the medulla oblongata and the pons; it communicates freely around the medullo-pontine furrow, or sulcus, with the cisterna magna (*cisterna cerebello-medullaris*) which is situated above and behind the medulla oblongata. The *cisterna basalis* (*cisterna interpeduncularis*) is that part of the subarachnoid space situated between the tips of the temporal lobes and the crura cerebri (*cerebral peduncles*) and in front of the pons; into it project the circle of Willis (*circulus arteriosus*) and the vessels connected with this circle. Laterally, the cisterna basalis (*cisterna interpeduncularis*) extends into the Sylvian fissures (*lateral fissures*), forming the *cistern of the lateral fissure*; while anteriorly it extends into a minor space in front of the optic chiasm forming the *cistern of the terminal lamina*, and thence further forward into the great longitudinal fissure, over the convex dorsal surface of the corpus callosum, to form the cistern of the corpus callosum. The space just back of the chiasm is known as the *cisterna chiasmatis*. Another large space is found above the corpus callosum; in the pia mater at the bottom of this space are the anterior cerebral arteries. Another space is seen between the superior vermis of the cerebellum and the corpora quadrigemina containing the veins of Galen (*internal cerebral veins*).

The **cerebro-spinal fluid** assists in protecting the brain and spinal cord from violent shocks and vibrations. It is a serous fluid, but, unlike ordinary serum, it does not coagulate spontaneously upon standing, and is not readily absorbed when injected into the tissues. It is secreted by the cells of the ependyma over the fringe-like, vascular processes of the choroid plexuses of the lateral, third, and fourth ventricles, and probably also by the cells of the arachnoid. The fluid passes from the lateral ventricles to the third ventricle through the foramina of Monro (*interventricular foramina*), from the third to the fourth ventricle through the aqueduct of Sylvius (*aqueduct of cerebrum*), and from the fourth ventricle through the foramen of Magendie (*median aperture of fourth ventricle*) and the foramina of Luschka (*lateral apertures of fourth ventricle*) to the subarachnoid space of the brain and spinal cord; some of the cerebro-spinal fluid passes directly from the fourth ventricle to the central canal of the spinal cord. Through these three openings then, the ventricles and their cerebro-spinal fluid, which originates in the choroid plexus, communicate with the subarachnoid space. A path is thus provided for the release of intraventricular tension by allowing this fluid to escape into the basal cisterns and the subarachnoid space of the cord. By exudation of plastic lymph or congenital anomalies or as a result of pressure by tumors, one or another of the openings may become closed and an internal hydrocephalus result. Dandy has recently made use of alterations in the size and position of the ventricles as an aid in diagnosing brain tumors. The normal quantity of cerebro-spinal fluid in the adult is from sixty to one hundred and fifty cubic centimeters. About half of the fluid is said to be in the spinal portion of the subarachnoid space; the lateral ventricles contain about twenty to thirty cubic centimeters each.

The cerebro-spinal fluid which is constantly being secreted must have an adequate means for escape in order to maintain intracranial and intraspinal pressure within normal limits. This occurs through the prolongations of the arachnoid along the cranial and spinal nerves; these extensions of the subarachnoid space are in communication with the lymph vessels in the sheaths of those nerves, and in this manner the fluid reaches the general lymphatic system of the body; and by way of the Pacchionian bodies it escapes directly into the sinuses of the dura mater, as well as into the large cortical veins by means of small openings in their walls.

Choked Disc, also known as optic neuritis and papillitis, occurs in conditions which are associated with increased intracranial pressure. It is found in a large percentage of brain tumors, in basal meningitis, especially tuberculous, and may be present in brain abscess. It is frequently bilateral, but often more advanced on one side than on the other. It occurs also in chronic nephritis, diabetes, hydrocephalus, and meningeal hemorrhage. The sheath of the optic nerve becomes distended, causing a congestion of the veins of the optic disc (choked disc), an important diagnostic sign. Inflammation may produce a neuroretinitis or neuritis closely simulating a papilledema in the early stages of the latter. The disc is more injected and a deeper red, and the margins are not inclined to show the translucent, fluffy appearance seen in choked disc.

Hydrocephalus.—This condition has been divided into two types: **Internal** and **External.**

Internal Hydrocephalus.—Having traced the course of the spinal fluid, it is evident that any obstruction in the region of the fourth ventricle, the aqueduct of Sylvius (*aqueduct of the cerebrum*), the third ventricle, or the foramina of Monro (*interventricular foramina*), will obstruct the fluid secreted in the lateral ventricles, so that pressure will become increased and gradually produce an enlargement of the head and thinning of the brain structures, especially over the cortex. In some cases where the hydrocephalic process has been of long duration, the cortex may become so thin that it resembles a transparent membrane. Usually the temporal lobes and the basal ganglia do not suffer to the same extent as the frontal and parietal regions. The choroid plexus, which secretes cerebro-spinal fluid, has been likened to the kidney in its ability to continue secreting in the face of tremendous pressure, so that the brain in hydrocephalus may resemble the picture of hydronephrosis where complete destruction of the kidney has occurred.

External Hydrocephalus arises when the absorptive mechanism for the outlet of the cerebro-spinal fluid is occluded, or the pathways which normally conduct the fluid over the cortex become obstructed. Meningitis, exudates, hemorrhages, and traumatic lesions produce this type of hydrocephalus, whereas tumors, occlusion of the aqueduct of Sylvius (*aqueduct of the cerebrum*), and arachnoiditis of the basal cistern produce internal hydrocephalus.

In internal hydrocephalus some encouraging results have been obtained from callosal puncture, produced by a curved cannula passed down along the falx at a point two and a half centimeters (one inch) in front of the midpoint, measured between the glabella and the inion. A small incision in the scalp across the midline and at right angles to the longitudinal (*sagittal*) sinus, is first made. A point about three centimeters from the midline on either side, preferably the right, is then chosen for trephining. This is necessary to avoid injury to the longitudinal (*sagittal*) sinus by the drill. The bone is then carefully rongeured away to the midline over the sinus. A small dural opening is made, just large enough to permit the introduction of the cannula, to the lateral side of the sinus. The large cortical veins must be looked for and avoided in making the dural incision and in passing the cannula. The cannula is then introduced and directed towards the falx until this structure is determined by resistance; the beak is then turned downward with the same motion as is used in passing an urethral sound. The cannula is advanced until it reaches the corpus callosum between the hemispheres, and after piercing this structure cerebro-spinal fluid will be encountered. By moving the beak of the cannula backward and forward an opening of about two centimeters is torn, so as to permit the escape of the cerebro-spinal fluid over the cortex. The dural opening is then carefully closed, the bone fragments replaced, the pericranium sutured over the fragments, and the skin closely approximated to prevent the possibility of cerebro-spinal fluid leakage.

In advanced cases of hydrocephalus where the cortex is quite thin, a number twelve cystoscope may be passed through the trephine opening and the dural incision in the region of the right parietal lobe, well behind the Rolandic (*central*) fissure. It is then possible to see the interior of the ventricle. The instrument may be passed forward through the foramen of Monro (*interventricular foramen*), and by means of the beak an opening carefully punched through the floor of the third ventricle. This procedure has met with some success.

A further method which recently has been advocated is that of approaching the lateral ventricle from the occipital region just above the tentorium and below the occipital pole on its medial aspect, near the region of the brain stem, and by gentle and careful pressure the velum interpositum is broken through, so as to make a new outlet from the ventricle to the cortex.

Catheterization of the aqueduct of Sylvius (*aqueduct of the cerebrum*) has been found to be extremely dangerous and is not at present an accepted method of relief.

At best these procedures offer little when the cases have developed a marked hydrocephalus, as the destruction of the brain tissue is so great that the individuals frequently never reach normal adult mentality.

In external hydrocephalus removal of the fluid must be accomplished in other ways, since the channels of absorption have been obstructed or closed. Dehydration by the use of magnesium sulphate and the strict control of fluid intake has been found of some value, especially in cases where, following acute traumatic injuries, temporary disturbance of the absorptive factors has given rise to acute pressure of the external hydrocephalic type. Those cases of active meningitis or exudates are usually self-limiting, and if re-establishment of cerebro-spinal fluid circulation occurs after the subsidence of the inflammation, the patient will survive without further operative measures.

Spinal drainage may be undertaken to combat the acute phase of the pressure, provided due regard is taken to avoid the removal of large amounts of fluid when the pressure is high, which would have a distinct tendency to produce respiratory failure by herniation of the occipital lobes through the foramen magnum, thus causing direct pressure upon the medulla and the respiratory centers.

The **lymphatics** of the brain open into the subarachnoid space and the ventricles.

The **Pacchionian bodies,** enlargements of the normal villi of the arachnoid (described at p. 39), project from the surface of that membrane, and may perforate the overlying dura mater and cause absorption of the bone in their vicinity.

DISSECTION.—The next step in the dissection consists in removing the arachnoid from the base of the brain, in order to study the arteries entering the cranial cavity to supply the brain, and the formation of the arterial circle of Willis (*circulus arteriosus*).

THE ARTERIES OF THE BRAIN

The **circle of Willis (circulus arteriosus),** also known as the polygon of Willis (Plate XVI), lies in the pia mater and projects into the subarachnoid space. It is the anastomosis at the base of the brain formed by branches of the internal carotid and basilar arteries. It forms a heptagonal figure, although it is usually not exactly symmetrical. This arrangement serves to equalize the

PLATE XVI.

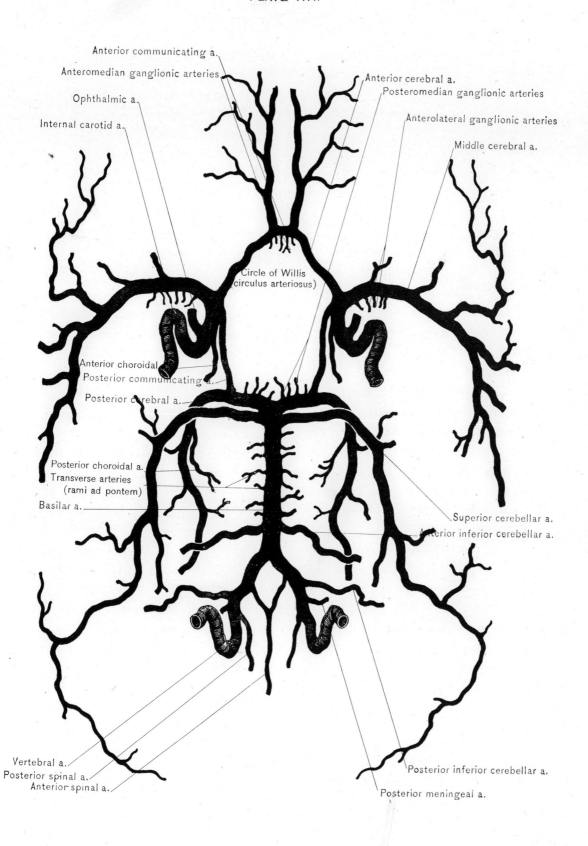

Anterior communicating a.

Anteromedian ganglionic arteries

Ophthalmic a.

Internal carotid a.

Anterior cerebral a.

Posteromedian ganglionic arteries

Anterolateral ganglionic arteries

Middle cerebral a.

Circle of Willis
(circulus arteriosus)

Anterior choroidal

Posterior communicating a.

Posterior cerebral a.

Posterior choroidal a.

Transverse arteries
(rami ad pontem)

Basilar a.

Superior cerebellar a.

Anterior inferior cerebellar a.

Vertebral a.

Posterior spinal a.

Anterior spinal a.

Posterior inferior cerebellar a.

Posterior meningeal a.

CIRCLE OF WILLIS (CIRCULUS ARTERIOSUS) AND ARTERIES OF BRAIN.

flow of blood derived from the two internal carotid arteries and the basilar artery. Without this or some similar arrangement ligation of the common carotid, internal carotid, or vertebral artery would probably always result in softening of the brain.   A further anastomosis exists between the branches of the posterior, the middle, and the anterior cerebrals which communicate on the lateral surface of the hemisphere.   The circle of Willis (*circulus arteriosus*) is formed by the *two posterior cerebral arteries*, which are the terminal divisions of the basilar, the *two internal carotid arteries*, the *two posterior communicating branches* of the internal carotid arteries, which connect the latter with the posterior cerebral arteries, the *two anterior cerebral arteries*, branches of the internal carotid arteries, and the *anterior communicating artery*, a transverse branch which connects the anterior cerebral arteries.   It is in relation with the several structures which are situated in the interpeduncular space and form the floor of the third ventricle.   It surrounds the posterior perforated space and the floor of the thalamencephalon.

The arteries which enter the cranial cavity for the supply of the brain are the two internal carotid and the two vertebral.

The **internal carotid artery,** one of the two terminal branches of the common carotid, enters the cranial cavity by way of the carotid canal (to whose direction it conforms), passing at first vertically upward and then bending and running forward and medialward to pierce the cartilage which fills the middle lacerated foramen (*foramen lacerum*), and ascends on the side of the body of the sphenoidal bone along the medial wall of the cavernous sinus (see p. 56).   Upon the inner aspect of the anterior clinoid process it pierces the dura mater, gives off the ophthalmic artery, and passes between the optic and the oculomotor nerves. Having reached the anterior perforated space at the medial extremity of the fissure of Sylvius (*lateral fissure*), it gives off the posterior communicating and the anterior choroid arteries, and divides into the anterior and middle cerebral arteries.   The artery is not often wounded because of its deep position, although an aneurysm of its upper portion is not uncommon.

The **anterior cerebral artery,** the smaller of the terminal branches, runs forward and medialward across the anterior perforated space and the lamina cinerea (*lamina terminalis*), and between the optic and the olfactory nerves, to reach the longitudinal fissure.   Here it is joined to the anterior cerebral artery of the opposite side by a transverse branch, the anterior communicating artery. This is an important connection because through it the internal carotids of the two hemispheres anastomose.   It now curves around the genu of the corpus callosum, and runs backward along the upper surface of the corpus callosum and at the bottom of the longitudinal fissure of the cerebrum as far as the splenium of the corpus callosum, where it anastomoses with the posterior cerebral artery.

At its commencement the anterior cerebral artery gives off a few anteromedian branches to the anterior extremity of the caudate nucleus. At the
bottom of the longitudinal fissure it gives off branches to the corpus callosum,
the frontal lobe, the marginal (*medial part of superior frontal*) gyrus, the quadrate
lobule (*precuneus*), and the gyrus fornicatus, or limbic lobe.

The **anterior communicating artery,** the shortest artery in the body, lies on
the lamina cinerea (*lamina terminalis*) in front of the optic commissure, and
connects the two anterior cerebral arteries across the longitudinal fissure. It also
gives off *anteromedian ganglionic branches* which pierce the lamina cinerea
(*lamina terminalis*), and a small branch to the anterior extremity of the corpus
callosum. Sometimes this vessel is absent, and then the two anterior cerebral
arteries either have no connection or they form a common trunk, and then divide.

The **middle cerebral artery** (Plate XVII), the largest of the terminal
branches of the internal carotid, runs lateralward and deep within the fissure of
Sylvius (*lateral fissure*). It supplies the motor area of the brain. It gives
off branches which supply the caudate and lenticular (*lentiform*) nuclei, the internal
capsule, the optic thalamus, and the surface of the brain, as follows: small
branches which pass through the bottom of the fissure of Sylvius (*lateral fissure*)
to the head of the caudate nucleus; anterolateral branches which pass through
the anterior perforated space (*substantia perforata anterior*) and supply the body
and tail of the caudate nucleus, the internal capsule, and the optic thalamus; a
branch, the lenticulo-striate, which passes through an aperture in the anterior
perforated space and supplies the lenticular (*lentiform*) and caudate nuclei.
The lenticulo-striate artery is often called the *artery of cerebral hemorrhage* (Char-
cot) since it is so frequently found ruptured in apoplexy. Finally, opposite the
island of Reil (*insula*), the middle cerebral artery gives off *cortical branches* which
supply the operculum and the temporal and parietal lobes, especially the supramarginal and the angular gyri, and the first temporal convolution.

The **posterior communicating artery** arises from the posterior surface of the
internal carotid opposite the sella turcica, and runs directly backward, parallel
to, and on the medial side of the oculomotor nerve beneath the optic tract to
join the posterior cerebral artery. It varies in size; sometimes it is so large as
to give the impression of being a continuation of the posterior cerebral artery.
The vessels of the two sides often differ greatly in size. The artery gives off
branches to the uncinate convolution (*hippocampal gyrus*), with which it is in relation, and a branch, the middle thalamic, which passes vertically through the
hippocampal fissure to the optic thalamus.

The **anterior choroidal artery** is a branch given off by the internal carotid
just distal to the posterior communicating artery. It passes backward and

PLATE XVII.

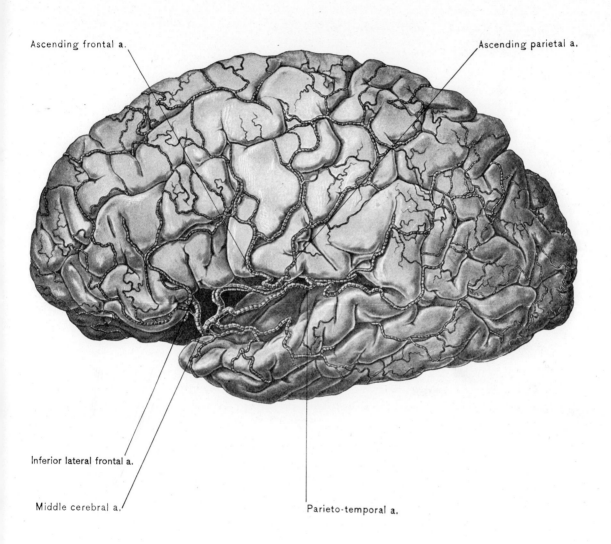

Ascending frontal a.

Ascending parietal a.

Inferior lateral frontal a.

Middle cerebral a.

Parieto-temporal a.

MIDDLE CEREBRAL ARTERY.

lateralward under the tip of the temporal lobe of the cerebrum, to enter the descending cornu of the lateral ventricle on its way to supply the hippocampus major and the corpus fimbriatum. It is then continued upward and forward as the artery of the choroid plexus of the lateral ventricle, and anastomoses at the foramen of Monro (*interventricular foramen*) with the artery of the choroid plexus of the third ventricle.

The **vertebral artery,** a branch of the first portion of the subclavian, enters the cranial cavity by way of the foramen magnum, and runs upward around the medulla oblongata, between the hypoglossal nerve and the anterior root of the first cervical, or suboccipital, nerve. Thence it runs forward along the medulla oblongata to the medial side of the hypoglossal nerve, and joins the vertebral artery of the opposite side at the lower border of the pons, to form a single trunk, the basilar artery. The branches given off from the vertebral artery within the cranial cavity are the posterior meningeal, the anterior and posterior spinal, and the posterior inferior cerebellar artery.

The **posterior meningeal artery** arises from the vertebral artery opposite the foramen magnum, just after the artery has pierced the dura mater, and supplies the bone and dura mater of the occipital fossa.

The **anterior spinal artery** arises from the vertebral artery near its termination in the basilar, and joins the anterior spinal artery of the opposite side at about the level of the foramen magnum to form a common median trunk, which passes through the foramen magnum and runs downward along the anterior median fissure of the spinal cord, in the pia mater. In its course it is reinforced by successive branches at the level of each vertebra. These branches are derived from the vertebral, the ascending cervical, the intercostal, the lumbar, the ilio-lumbar, and the lateral sacral arteries, all of which enter the spinal canal by way of the intervertebral foramina, and by their medial union form a continuous anterior spinal artery which extends along the entire length of the anterior median fissure of the spinal cord.

The **posterior spinal artery,** smaller than the anterior, arises from the vertebral artery at the side of the medulla oblongata, and passes backward to the side of the posterior surface of the spinal cord, where it divides into two branches, one of which descends behind, and the other in front of the posterior roots of the spinal nerves. Like the anterior spinal, it is reinforced at the successive vertebral levels by branches derived from the vertebral, the intercostal, the lumbar, the lateral sacral, and the common trunk of the anterior spinal artery by branches which run around the sides of the spinal cord.

The **posterior inferior cerebellar artery** arises from the vertebral near its termination (sometimes this branch may arise from the basilar artery); it winds backward and upward around the medulla oblongata, between the vagus and spinal accessory (*accessory*) nerves; it then runs over the inferior cerebellar peduncle (*restiform body*) to the under surface of the cerebellum, there to divide into a lateral and a medial branch. *The lateral branch* traverses the under surface of the hemisphere of the cerebellum, which it supplies, and running along the lateral margin of the cerebellum, anastomoses with the superior cerebellar artery. *The medial branch*, practically the continuation of the main vessel, runs in the groove between the hemisphere of the cerebellum and the vermiform process (*vermis cerebelli*), both of which it supplies. The posterior inferior cerebellar artery also sends branches to the choroid plexus of the fourth ventricle, and anastomoses with the superior cerebellar artery.

The **basilar artery** (Plate XVIII), formed by the union of the two vertebral arteries at the posterior border of the pons, runs along the median line of the anterior, or lower, surface of the pons as far as its anterior, or upper, border, where it divides into two terminal branches, the *posterior cerebral arteries.* Running on each side of, and almost parallel with the basilar artery, are the abducent, or sixth, nerves. With the brain *in situ*, the basilar artery lies on the dorsal surface of the body of the sphenoidal bone. Its branches, named from behind forward, are: the transverse (*rami ad pontem*), the internal auditory, the anterior inferior cerebellar, the superior cerebellar, and the two terminal.

The **transverse arteries** consist of numerous small branches which arise from the basilar, pass lateralward over the pons, and supply the pons and the adjacent portion of the cerebrum.

The **internal auditory artery,** one on each side, arises from the basilar artery and may also arise from the transverse arteries. It accompanies the auditory nerve into the internal auditory (*acoustic*) meatus, where it runs between the facial and auditory (*acoustic*) nerves, and reaching the bottom of the meatus passes into the internal ear which it supplies.

The **anterior inferior cerebellar artery** arises from the basilar artery near its middle. Each artery passes lateralward and backward over the pons and the middle crus to the anterior inferior surface of the cerebellum to which it is distributed. It anastomoses with the superior cerebellar arteries.

The **superior cerebellar artery,** one on each side, arises from the basilar so near its bifurcation as sometimes to be mistaken for the posterior cerebral artery. It is separated from the posterior cerebral artery by the oculomotor nerve. It passes lateralward around the crura cerebri (*cerebral peduncles*), lying almost parallel to the trochlear nerves and behind the roots of the oculomotor nerve, and reaches the superior surface of the cerebellum. Here it divides into branches

PLATE XVIII.

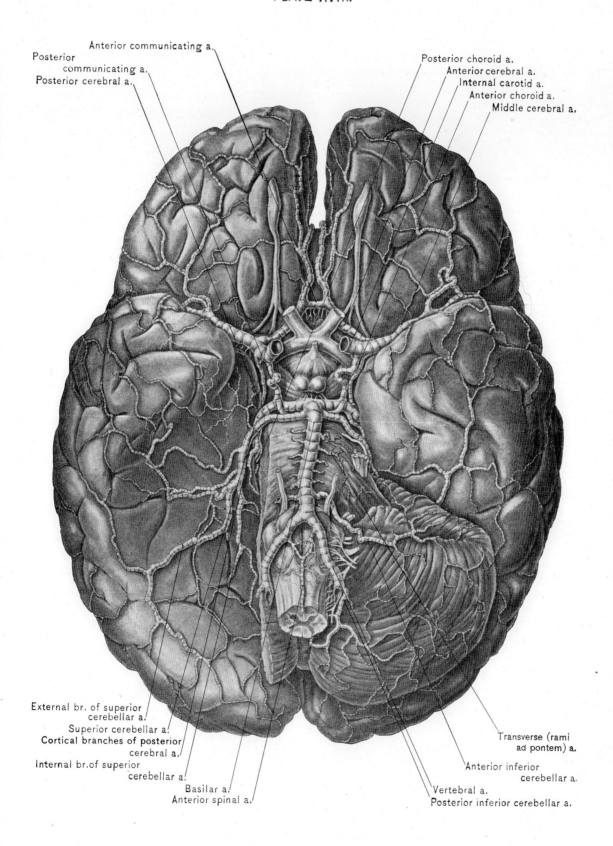

Anterior communicating a.

Posterior
communicating a.
Posterior cerebral a.

Posterior choroid a.
Anterior cerebral a.
Internal carotid a.
Anterior choroid a.
Middle cerebral a.

External br. of superior
cerebellar a.
Superior cerebellar a.
Cortical branches of posterior
cerebral a.
Internal br. of superior
cerebellar a.

Transverse (rami
ad pontem) a.

Anterior inferior
cerebellar a.

Basilar a.
Anterior spinal a.

Vertebral a.
Posterior inferior cerebellar a.

ARTERIES AT BASE OF BRAIN.

which anastomose with the corresponding artery of the opposite side and with the inferior cerebellar artery.

The **posterior cerebral artery,** the paired terminal branch of the basilar, winds around the crura cerebri (*cerebral peduncles*) and, running parallel with the superior cerebellar, from which it is separated by the oculomotor nerve, reaches the medial surface of the posterior part of the cerebrum. As already noted, it is joined to the internal carotid artery by the posterior communicating branch of the latter vessel. It supplies the occipital and temporal lobes, and anastomoses with the anterior and middle cerebral arteries.

Like the anterior and middle cerebral arteries, the posterior cerebral gives off central, or ganglionic, and cortical branches. The *central branches (posteromedial and posterolateral)* are small branches which pass through the posterior perforated space (*substantia perforata*) to supply the optic thalamus and the walls of the third ventricle, laterally giving off a *posterior choroidal branch* which passes through the transverse fissure to reach the velum interpositum (*tela choroidea of the third ventricle*) and the choroidal plexus; while others run to the optic thalamus, the crura cerebri (*cerebral peduncles*), and the corpora quadrigemina The *cortical branches,* which are terminal, are distributed to the adjacent parts of the temporal and occipital lobes.

Anastomoses of Cerebral Arteries.—There is no anastomosis between the cortical and the central branches of the arteries which supply the brain, therefore, these two sets of branches form two independent systems. The cortical branches, however, do anastomose with each other, but seldom sufficiently to nourish a portion of the brain from which the blood current through the main artery supplying it has been cut off. In other words, the central vessels differ from the vessels of the upper or lower extremity in not being able to establish a collateral circulation which will perform the office of the principal vessel in the event of its being seriously disabled. In this respect they resemble the vessels of the lungs, the kidneys, and the retina. The central branches do not anastomose with each other; therefore, obstruction of one of the chief vessels of the brain will result in softening of the region supplied by its central branches, although softening of the region supplied by its cortical branches does not necessarily follow. However, the communication of the larger vessels is usually sufficient to allow of the establishment of a collateral circulation after ligation of the carotid on one side.

Peculiarities of the Arteries to the Brain.—In studying the course of the four large arteries—the two internal carotids and the two vertebrals—which enter the cranial cavity to supply the brain, the dissector will notice the following peculiarities: first, their length and tortuosity; secondly, the free anastomosis of the four arteries by means of the circle of Willis (*circulus arteriosus*), and thirdly, the course of their numerous small branches through the third and innermost membrane of the brain, the pia mater, by duplications of which they reach the interior of the brain. The tortuosity of these arteries diminishes the force of the current of blood, thus lessening the danger of apoplexy, while through the circle of Willis (*circulus arteriosus*) the pressure in the four arteries is equalized.

THE VEINS OF THE BRAIN

The **veins of the brain** empty into the sinuses of the dura mater (see p. 36); they do not accompany the corresponding arteries.

The **veins of the cerebrum** consist of a superficial, or cortical, set which ramify in the pia mater and empty directly into the sinuses, and a central set which empty into the sinuses indirectly through the medium of the veins of Galen(*internal cerebral veins*).

The **cerebellar veins** which run over the superior surface of the cerebellum, empty into the veins of Galen (*internal cerebral veins*) and the straight sinus, while all of those which traverse the inferior surface of the cerebellum empty into the inferior petrosal, the lateral (*transverse*), and the occipital sinuses.

Absence of Valves.—The veins and sinuses of the brain are destitute of valves. Their absence may be compensated for in the superior longitudinal (*superior sagittal*) sinus by the presence of the chordæ Willisii, and by the fact that the veins which empty into this sinus pass from behind forward in a direction opposite to that of the blood current, and that in entering the sinus they pass obliquely through its wall.

THE PIA MATER

The **Pia Mater,** the innermost and most intimate investment of the brain, sends processes into all the fissures of the cerebrum and between most of the laminæ of the cerebellum. It is the vascular membrane of the brain, and carries the minute branches of the two internal carotids and the two vertebral arteries, and the veins which return the blood conveyed to the brain by these vessels, all of which are associated by delicate connective-tissue fibers. The connective-tissue element of the pia mater may be likened to a grape arbor, and the vessels running over and through the interstices, to the grape vine. Added to the above are numerous minute vessels, given off from the inner surface of the pia mater, which pass perpendicularly into the substance of the brain.

Only two of the processes of the pia mater receive special names—the **velum interpositum (tela choroidea of third ventricle)**, which reaches the interior of the brain by way of the transverse fissure, and the **choroid plexuses** of the third and fourth ventricles.   (The velum interpositum (*tela choroidea of third ventricle*) and the choroid plexus are descriedb with the ventricles of the brain.)   The portions of the pia mater which cover the crura cerebri (*cerebral peduncles*) and the pons differ from the rest of the membrane, inasmuch as they present a dense fibrous structure which contains but few vessels.

NERVE SUPPLY.—The pia mater is supplied with nerves by branches from the sympathetic, the trigeminal, and the glossopharyngeal nerves.

THE BRAIN

DISSECTION.—If the arachnoid and the pia mater have been allowed to remain in place thus far, they should now be removed, with the exception of that portion of the pia mater which is prolonged medialward between the splenium of the corpus collosum above, and the pineal body and the corpora quadrigemina below, to form the velum interpositum (*tela choroidea of third ventricle*) which is placed between the corpus callosum and the fornix above and the optic thalami, the pineal body, and the corpora quadrigemina below.   The removal of these membranes exposes the surface of the brain.   In dissecting them from the base of the brain care should be taken not to detach any of the cranial nerves.

Definition and Weight.—The brain, or encephalon, is the intracranial mass of nervous matter, or that portion of the cerebro-spinal axis which is contained within the cavity of the cranium.   Its average weight in the adult male is one thousand three hundred and seventy-five grams (forty-five ounces), and in the female one thousand two hundred and forty-five grams (forty-one ounces).

Divisions.—The brain is composed of four main portions: the cerebrum (large brain); the cerebellum (small brain), which is second in size; the pons Varolii (*pons*), which is third in size, and the medulla oblongata, the smallest, although physiologically the most important.

Position of the Pons.—Of these four portions the pons is the center around which the three remaining portions are not only grouped, but to which they are connected in the following manner: to the cerebrum by the crura cerebri (*cerebral peduncles*), to the cerebellum by the crura cerebelli, or middle peduncles of the cerebellum (*brachium pontis*), and to the medulla oblongata by the anterior pyramids (*pyramids*) and part of the lateral tracts.   The pons rests upon the posterior surface of the body of the sphenoidal bone and the superior part of the basilar process of the occipital bone.

Position of the Cerebrum.—The cerebrum occupies all the superior part of the cranial cavity, concealing from view the other portions of the brain, when viewed from above, and rests upon the floor of the anterior and middle fossæ of the skull and the tentorium cerebelli. The tentorium cerebelli, in addition to supporting the cerebrum, separates it from the cerebellum and protects the latter from pressure by the cerebrum.

Position of the Cerebellum.—The cerebellum occupies the space between the tentorium cerebelli and the floor of the posterior cranial fossa.

Position of the Medulla Oblongata.—The medulla oblongata is continuous below with the spinal cord, and, resting upon the posterior part of the basilar process of the occipital bone, it lies almost wholly within the cranial cavity.

Contour.—The brain is convex upon its superior and lateral surfaces, and irregular upon its inferior, or basilar, surface, where it conforms to the base of the skull.

Structures at the base of the brain (Plate XIX).—In dissecting the brain the most suitable article upon which to place it is an ordinary dinner plate covered with a thick layer of absorbent cotton or cheese-cloth wet with alcohol. This soft bed will prevent the convolutions from being flattened when the brain is laid on its superior surface to study the structures forming its base. These are the inferior surfaces of the frontal and temporal lobes of the cerebrum, which are irregular and conform to the inequalities of the base of the skull. With the brain arranged for dissecting the following structures should be carefully noted: the fissure of Sylvius (*lateral fissure*), which separates the frontal from the temporal lobe; the olfactory tracts and bulbs; the longitudinal fissure; the corpus callosum and its peduncles; the anterior perforated substances (*substantiæ perforatæ*); the optic commissure and the terminal parts of the optic tracts; the lamina cinerea (*lamina terminalis*), the tuber cinereum and a part of the infundibulum (*infundibulum hypothalami*) (the remaining part, with the pituitary body, is described at p. 94); the corpora albicantia, or corpora mamillaria; the posterior perforated substance (*substantia perforata*); the crura cerebri (*cerebral peduncles*); the pons; the middle crura (*brachium pontis*) of the cerebellum; the lateral hemispheres of the cerebellum; the medulla oblongata; the posterior extremity of the inferior vermiform process (*vermis cerebelli*) of the cerebellum, and, finally, the roots of the cranial nerves.

The **olfactory tract and bulb** are seen occupying the olfactory sulcus.

Frontal Lobe.—The inferior, or orbital, surfaces of the frontal lobes are triangular in shape, and separated in front by the longitudinal fissure. Their bases are directed backward, and are formed by the fissure sof Sylvius (*lateral fissures*). They present two well-pronounced sulci, the orbital and the olfactory. These, as will be seen later, divide them into their convolutions.

Temporal Lobe.—The inferior surface of the temporal, or temporo-sphenoidal, lobe is slightly convex anteriorly and concave posteriorly, and thus accommo-

PLATE XIX.

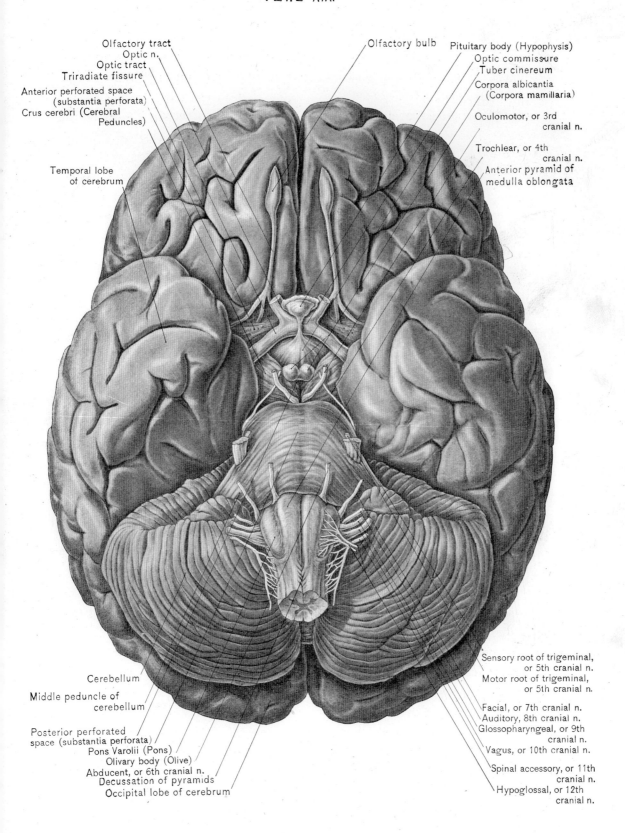

Olfactory tract
Optic n.
Optic tract
Triradiate fissure
Anterior perforated space
(substantia perforata)
Crus cerebri (Cerebral
Peduncles)

Temporal lobe
of cerebrum

Olfactory bulb
Pituitary body (Hypophysis)
Optic commissure
Tuber cinereum
Corpora albicantia
(Corpora mamillaria)

Oculomotor, or 3rd
cranial n.

Trochlear, or 4th
cranial n.
Anterior pyramid of
medulla oblongata

Cerebellum

Middle peduncle of
cerebellum

Posterior perforated
space (substantia perforata)
Pons Varolii (Pons)
Olivary body (Olive)
Abducent, or 6th cranial n.
Decussation of pyramids
Occipital lobe of cerebrum

Sensory root of trigeminal,
or 5th cranial n.
Motor root of trigeminal,
or 5th cranial n.

Facial, or 7th cranial n.
Auditory, 8th cranial n.
Glossopharyngeal, or 9th
cranial n.
Vagus, or 10th cranial n.

Spinal accessory, or 11th
cranial n.
Hypoglossal, or 12th
cranial n.

BASE OF BRAIN AND SUPERFICIAL ORIGIN OF CRANIAL NERVES.

dates itself anteriorly to the portions of the middle cranial fossa formed by the greater wing of the sphenoidal and the anterior surface of the petrous portion of the temporal bone, and posteriorly to the convex tentorium. It presents the termination of two well-pronounced sulci, the middle temporal and the inferior occipito-temporal (*inferior temporal*).

Fissure of Sylvius (**Lateral Cerebral Fissure**).—This fissure lies between the inferior surfaces of the adjacent frontal and temporal lobes. It is the largest of the primary fissures of the cerebrum, and through it runs the middle cerebral artery; into this fissure extends the lesser wing of the sphenoidal bone, and from the floor of its anterior portion projects the island of Reil (*insula*), or central lobe of the cerebrum.

The **longitudinal fissure** separates the two frontal lobes, and, on lifting the cerebellum, will be seen completely separating the two occipital lobes.

Corpus Callosum.—Careful separation of the frontal lobes will reveal the beak, or rostrum, of the corpus callosum; also the peduncles of the corpus callosum, two white bands which are continued backward and lateralward on each side of the rostrum across the anterior perforated substance (*substantia perforata*) to the commencement of the fissure of Sylvius (*lateral fissure*).

The **anterior perforated space** (**substantia perforata anterior**), one on each side, is situated at the inner extremity of the fissure of Sylvius (*lateral fissure*). It is triangular in shape, bounded in front by the frontal lobe and the root of the olfactory tract, laterally by the apex of the temporal lobe and the fissure of Sylvius (*lateral fissure*), and posteriorly by the optic tract, and is crossed by the peduncle of the corpus callosum and the lateral olfactory root or stria. It transmits small vessels, chiefly perforating branches of the middle cerebral artery, to the corpus striatum, which lies immediately above the space.

The **optic commissure,** or **chiasma,** from which arise the optic nerves, lies between the two anterior perforated spaces (*substantiæ perforatæ*) and behind the anterior inferior portion of the longitudinal fissure. It is formed by the union of the converging optic nerves anteriorly, and by the diverging optic tracts posteriorly. The latter are two cords composed of white matter running on the lateral side of the crura cerebri (*cerebral peduncles*).

The **interpeduncular fossa** is a lozenge-shaped or quadrilateral area, bounded anteriorly by the optic commissure, posteriorly by the pons and the optic tracts, and laterally by the crura cerebri (*cerebral peduncles*). It contains the tuber cinereum, the intradural portion of the infundibulum (*infundibulum hypothalami*), the corpora albicantia (*corpora mamillaria*), the posterior perforated space (*substantia perforata*), and the oculomotor nerves. These structures, except the last mentioned, form the floor of the third ventricle with the exception of its anterior part, which is formed by the structure next to be described—the lamina cinerea (*lamina terminalis*).

The **lamina cinerea** (**lamina terminalis**) lies above the optic commissure, and is a delicate membrane continuous with the anterior perforated spaces (*substantiæ perforatæ*). It can best be exposed by displacing the commissure backward, when it will be seen extending from the beak, or rostrum, of the corpus callosum, to which it is attached anteriorly, to the tuber cinereum, to which it is attached posteriorly.

The **tuber cinereum** is a gray eminence, situated behind the optic commissure and in front of the *corpora albicantia*, or corpora mamillaria. It is a hollow conical process continuous with the infundibulum, which connects the third ventricle with the pituitary body. The *infundibulum* (*infundibulum hypothalami*) pierces the diaphragma sellæ, a process of the dura mater which bridges the pituitary fossa. The cavity of the tuber cinereum may sometimes extend through the greater part of the infundibulum but near the pituitary body it is always occluded.

The **pituitary body,** or **hypophysis cerebri,** is the small body which occupies the pituitary (*hypophyseal*) fossa, or sella turcica, and is covered superiorly by the diaphragma sellæ. It is composed of an anterior and a posterior lobe, which differ in size, structure, and origin. The *anterior lobe*, much the larger, is of a reddish-gray color, and is an isolated process of the wall of the buccal cavity of the embryo. The *posterior lobe*, yellowish-gray in color, is lodged in a depression in the anterior lobe, and is a process of the brain. It is the only part of the pituitary body structurally continuous with the infundibulum, which, as we have seen, in passing from the floor of the third ventricle to the pituitary body, pierces the diaphragma sellæ. (For operative procedure see under frontal lobe tumors, p. 117.)

The **corpora albicantia** (**corpora mamillaria**), two knobs situated behind the tuber cinereum, consist each of two nuclei, a medial, forming the greater part, and a lateral, giving rise to several tracts: the bundles of Vicq d'Azyr (*fasciculus mamillo-thalamicus*) from the optic thalamus, which reach the base of the brain, the fasciculus tegmento-mamillaris, and the peduncles of the corpora mamillaria The majority of the fornix fibers terminate in these bodies.

The **posterior perforated space** (**substantia perforata posterior**) is triangular in shape, its base corresponding to the corpora albicantia (*corpora mamillaria*); its apex, to the pons, and its sides, to the crura cerebri (*cerebral peduncles*). It gives passage to posteromedian ganglionic branches of the posterior cerebral and posterior communicating arteries, which run to the optic thalami.

The **crura cerebri** (**cerebral peduncles**) are two large cylindrical masses of white and gray matter. They are about eighteen millimeters (three-fourths

of an inch) long.   They are broader anteriorly than posteriorly and are composed
of the longitudinal fibers of the pons, together with some fibers from the cerebellum.   They commence at the anterior border of the pons, from which they
emerge, and then pass forward and laterally, traversing the superior occipital
foramen in the tentorium cerebelli in company with the superios peduncles of
the cerebellum (*brachia conjunctiva*), the oculomotor and trochlear nerves, and
the basilar artery.   Each peduncle enters the anteromedial aspect of the corresponding temporal lobe.   The optic tract and the trochlear nerve pass around the
lateral border of the corresponding crus cerebri (*cerebral peduncle*), while the oculomotor nerve winds around the medial border.   Later on, when making sections
of the brain to study the arrangement of its interior, the crura cerebri (*cerebral
peduncles*) will be cut across, when the *substantia niger*, a pigmented gray nucleus
in the interior of each peduncle, will be exposed.   The nucleus separates
the fibers of the crura cerebri (*cerebral peduncles*) into two sets: the lower and
smaller one being the *crusta* and the upper and larger, the *tegmentum*.

The **pons varolii** (**pons**) is the bridge across the interval between the two
eerebellar hemispheres.   It is composed chiefly of white matter, and is situated
behind the crura cerebri (*cerebral peduncles*), in front of the medulla oblongata,
and between the hemispheres of the cerebellum.   It is about twenty-five millimeters (one inch) long, and rather more than this in width; from its dorsal to
its ventral surface it measures about eighteen millimeters (three-fourths of an
inch).   Its ventral surface is markedly convex transversely, and presents an
anteroposterior median groove, *sulcus basilaris*, which accommodates the basilar
artery.   It consists principally of two sets of fibers, a transverse, or superficial,
and a longitudinal, or deep, set.   The former set extends laterally into each
hemisphere of the cerebellum, forming the *middle cerebellar peduncles* (*brachia
pontis*), or great transverse commissure, of the cerebellum; the latter set, the
superior cerebellar peduncles (*brachia conjunctiva*), extends forward and lateralward and helps to form the crura (*peduncles*) of the cerebrum.   Making their
exit through the sides of the pons, are the trigeminal nerves.   The upper surface
of the pons forms a part of the floor of the fourth ventricle.

The **medulla oblongata,** the smallest of the four divisions of the brain, is
the enlarged upper end of the spinal cord.   It extends from the lower border of the
pons, from which it is separated by a transverse groove, to the attachment of
the upper root bundles of the first cervical nerves.   Its superior surface lies in the
depression between the hemispheres of the cerebellum.   It is pyramidal
in shape; it is about thirty-two millimeters (one and a quarter inches) long, eighteen
millimeters (three-quarters of an inch) wide at its broadest part, which is its upper
portion, and twelve millimeters (one-half inch) in thickness.   It forms part of

the sides, and the largest and most important part of the floor of the fourth ventricle. Its further description will be deferred until the dissection of the cerebrum is completed.

The **hemispheres of the cerebellum** are situated chiefly upon each side of the medulla oblongata. The arrangement of the gray matter which forms the surface of the cerebellum differs from that of the cerebrum in that it is disposed in convolutions, or gyri, separated by fissures, while in the cerebellum it is arranged in closely applied laminæ, and in that the upper and lower surfaces of the hemispheres are divided into lobes. (These will be described with the dissection of the cerebellum.) By lifting up the medulla oblongata, the depression, or valley, between the two hemispheres of the cerebellum will be partly exposed. There will also be seen the inferior surface of the middle lobe, or inferior vermiform process (*vermis cerebelli*), that portion of the cerebellum which forms the roof of the fourth ventricle; projecting beyond the medulla oblongata is the posterior extremity of the inferior vermiform process (*vermis cerebelli*) of the cerebellum, called the tuber vermis, or tuber valvulæ.

Next examine the roots of the cranial nerves anteroposteriorly in the order in which they are named below.

THE ORIGINS OF THE CRANIAL NERVES (Plate XIX)

The **olfactory,** or **first cranial, nerve** is devoted to the special sense of smell. It is composed of about twenty filaments which pass upward from the plexuses in the nasal mucous membrane through the foramina in the lamina cribrosa to pierce the meninges and terminate in glomeruli in the olfactory bulb. The nerves are non-medullated. The olfactory bulbs and tracts are not a part of the olfactory nerves, but of the brain. The olfactory impulses are transmitted through the initial cells which lie in the bulb, and whose axones form the olfactory tracts to the olfactory trigone. Here the tract breaks up into three roots: the lateral olfactory stria, which extends through the fornix to the end of the gyrus hippocampi; the medial olfactory stria, which passes toward the subcallosal gyrus, over the corpus callosum and thence to the hippocampus; the olfactory bundle of the hippocampus, which extends to the septum lucidum where it is augmented by additional fibers from the septum and then passes posteriorly through the fornix to the hippocampus.

The **optic,** or **second cranial, nerve,** which also represents a portion of the brain, is the nerve of vision, and consists of nerve fibers which arise from the ganglion cells of the retina and which converge to the optic papilla where they form the optic nerve. At the optic chiasma the nasal portions of the fibers pass to the optic tract of the opposite side, and the temporal portions pass backward

PLATE XX.

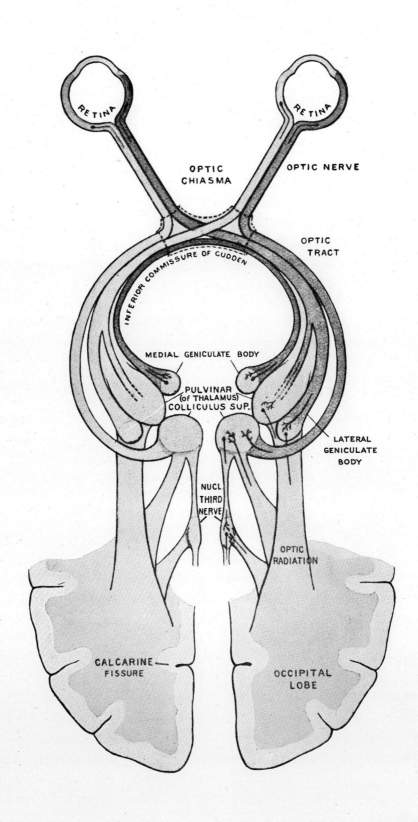

DIAGRAM OF THE CENTRAL CONNECTIONS OF THE OPTIC NERVE AND OPTIC TRACTS.   (AFTER CUNNINGHAM)

through the optic tract of the same side. The *optic tract* ends within the lateral geniculate body, the pulvinar, the superior colliculus of the corpora quadrigemina, and the optic thalami. On account of the course of the nerve-fibers from the optic nerves to the tracts, a lesion of one optic tract causes **hemianopsia,** or obliteration of vision in the corresponding halves of both eyes; for example, a lesion of the left optic tract will cause loss of vision in the left half of both retinae or the right half of the fields of vision. Likewise, a lesion at the chiasma due to a pituitary tumor produces a bitemporal hemianopsia, that is, the fibers supplying the nasal half of each retina are destroyed, with consequent loss of vision in each temporal field. (Plate XX.)

The **oculomotor,** or **third cranial, nerve,** arises superficially from a groove on the medial side of the crus cerebri (*cerebral peduncle*), just anterior to the pons, and has its deep origin from a nucleus ventral to the aqueduct of Sylvius (*cerebral aqueduct*) within the floor of the central gray substance. It is a motor nerve, and supplies all the muscles of the eyeball, including the levator palpebræ superioris, except the superior oblique, the lateral rectus, and the radiating fibers of the iris.

The **trochlear,** or **fourth cranial, nerve,** is the smallest of the cranial nerves, and arises at the side of the frenulum veli from the anterior end of the anterior medullary velum, immediately behind the corpora quadrigemina. In the substance of the anterior medullary velum, it decussates with its fellow of the opposite side. The deep origin is from the *trochlear nucleus* in the floor of the aqueduct of Sylvius (*cerebral aqueduct*), and in close relation with the nucleus of the oculomotor nerve.

The **trigeminal,** or **fifth cranial, nerve,** the largest of the cranial nerves, possesses two roots—a larger, posterior, or sensory, root which enters the brain stem through the side of the anterior third of the pons, and a smaller, anterior, or motor, root which emerges from the pons just in front of, and ventral to the sensory root. These roots can be traced to the floor of the fourth ventricle and to the gray matter in the lower part of the medulla oblongata and in the upper part of the spinal cord. It is the only cranial nerve which resembles a spinal nerve in arising by two roots, a posterior, or sensory, and an anterior, or motor, and in having a ganglion, the Gasserian (*semilunar*) ganglion, on the posterior root. It distributes sensory filaments to the dura mater, pia mater, orbit, eyelids, nose, gums, teeth, tonsils, palate, sphenoidal and ethmoidal cells, frontal and maxillary sinuses, nasal fossæ, pharynx, articulation of the mandible, the ear, the parotid gland, the anterior two-thirds of the scalp, the forehead, and face; gustatory filaments by way of the chorda tympani to the anterior two-thirds of the tongue, and motor filaments along its third division to the four muscles of mastication, the temporal, masseter, and external and internal pterygoids.

The **abducent,** or **sixth cranial, nerve** emerges from the anterior pyramid of the medulla oblongata and the interval between the anterior pyramid and the olive, close to the lower margin of the pons. Its deep origin is from the floor of the fourth ventricle. It is a motor nerve, and supplies the lateral rectus muscle of the eyeball.

The **facial,** or **seventh cranial, nerve** consists of two portions, a large motor, and a small sensory part. The *sensory part,* or *pars intermedia of Wrisberg,* terminates in the forepart of the nucleus of the glossopharyngeal nerve, in the floor of the fourth ventricle. It enters the brain stem at the lower border of the pons, lateral to the facial nerve proper and between the olivary and restiform bodies. The *pars intermedia of Wrisberg* is considered a portion of the glosso-pharyngeal, or ninth cranial, nerve, its nucleus being continuous with the nucleus of that nerve. Its fibers leave the trunk of the facial as the chorda tympani nerve, which later joins the mandibular branch of the trigeminal and passes by way of the lingual to supply the anterior two-thirds of the tongue with the sensa-tion of taste. Thus, all of the special sensory fibers to the tongue are derived from the glossopharyngeal nerve. The motor portion, or *facial nerve proper,* has its deep origin in a nucleus situated laterally in the reticular formation at the level of the lower pons, dorsal to the superior olive and between the root of the abducent and spinal portion of the trigeminal. From the nucleus the fibers pass medially and dorsally to the floor of the fourth ventricle, thence winding around the nucleus of the abducent nerve. It emerges from the medulla oblongata in the groove between the olivary and restiform bodies. The range of distribution of the facial nerve is large, and its connections with other nerves are numerous. It supplies the stapedius muscle, gives off the chorda tympani nerve, the posterior auricular nerve, the nerve to the posterior belly of the digastric, and a branch to the stylo-hyoid muscle. In addition, it supplies the muscles of expression and the buccinator muscle. It also carries fibers of deep pressure sense from the face and must therefore, to some degree, be considered a mixed nerve.

The **auditory,** or **eighth cranial, nerve** is a purely sensory nerve. It really consists of two nerves, the vestibular and the cochlear, or auditory nerve proper. The vestibular nerve terminates in the floor of the fourth ventricle, the nuclei being grouped as the medial, the lateral (*Deiter's*), the superior, and the nucleus of the spinal root of the vestibular nerve. The cochlear nerve terminates in its ventral and dorsal nuclei. The auditory nerve passes through the internal auditory meatus with the facial nerve and the internal auditory artery, courses medially and downward, arches ventrally around the restiform body and enters the medulla at the inferior border of the pons, just to the lateral side of the facial nerve. The cochlear nerve supplies the cochlea, and is the nerve of the sense of hearing. The vestibular nerve supplies the vestibule and the semicircular canals; it is associated with maintenance of equilibrium of the body.

The **glossopharyngeal,** or **ninth cranial, nerve** is a mixed sensory and motor nerve. It is attached to the medulla by several roots in the posterolateral sulcus, dorsal to the anterior end of the olivary body. They are united in a single trunk just in front of the cerebellum. The motor fibers arise from the nucleus ambiguus in the lateral funiculus of the medulla. The sensory fibers have their termination in the glossopharyngeal nucleus, that is, in the nucleus alæ cinereæ and the nucleus of the tractus solitarii. This nerve is distributed to the tympanum, the stylo-pharyngeus muscle, the mucous membrane of the pharynx, the tonsil, and the back of the tongue. Its sensory fibers include the fibers of the special sense of taste, supplying the circumvallate papillæ at the back of the tongue.

The **vagus,** or **tenth cranial, nerve** is also both sensory and motor. It is the longest of the cranial nerves and has the most extensive distribution. The right and left vagus are asymmetrical in the chest and abdomen. This nerve is attached to the medulla by fifteen or twenty small roots in the posterolateral sulcus just below the attachment of the glossopharyngeal nerve. They do not unite to form a trunk until they have pierced the pia mater. The central connections for the sensory fibers are: the nucleus of termination of the vagus in the nucleus alæ cinereæ in the floor of the fourth ventricle and in the nucleus tractus solitarii; and for the motor fibers the dorsal motor nucleus of the vagus, which lies in the ventromedial side of the nucleus alæ cinereæ, and the nucleus ambiguus. It supplies the dura mater, the external ear, the pharynx, the larynx, the esophagus, the trachea, the lungs, the heart, and some of the abdominal viscera—the liver and the alimentary tract.

The **spinal accessory,** or **eleventh cranial, nerve** has purely motor fibers. It consists of two portions: an accessory, or upper, and a spinal, or lower. The **accessory portion,** the smaller of the two, arises from the floor of the fourth ventricle in common with the glossopharyngeal and the vagus. It emerges by fine filaments from the side of the medulla oblongata below the origin of the vagus nerve, but through the same groove. The **spinal portion** emerges by several filaments from the side of the spinal cord, between the ligamentum denticulatum and the posterior roots of the spinal nerves, as low down as the sixth cervical nerve. It gains entrance to the cranial cavity by way of the foramen magnum of the occipital bone, and passes out through the middle compartment of the jugular, or posterior lacerated, foramen. In the latter situation the accessory portion leaves it to join the ganglion of the trunk of the vagus and to be distributed to the areas supplied by the vagus. The spinal portion of the nerve supplies the trapezius and sterno-mastoid muscles.

The **hypoglossal,** or **twelfth cranial, nerve** a motor nerve, issues from the side of the medulla oblongata by several filaments which emerge through the groove between the anterior pyramid and the olivary body. Its origin is from an elongated nucleus lying in the floor of the central canal in the lower half of the medulla and in the floor of the fourth ventricle. The filaments of this nerve are collected into two bundles which perforate the dura mater separately before passing through the anterior condyloid foramen (*hypoglossal canal*), in which they unite to form the trunk of the nerve. It supplies the extrinsic muscles of the tongue, the genio-glossus, hyo-glossus, and the stylo-glossus. Through fibers derived probably from the vagus or the cervical sympathetic nerves it supplies a meningeal branch to the dura mater, and through fibers derived from the first three cervical nerves it supplies motor branches to the genio-hyoid, sterno-hyoid, sterno-thyroid, omo-hyoid, and thyro-hyoid muscles. It is frequently used in facio-hypoglossal anastomosis; being close to the facial nerve it has the preference in this procedure. The fact that it is entirely motor and when used for anastomosis the resultant hemiatrophy of the tongue is not apparent, leaving no speech defect where the other side remains intact, there is perhaps no better nerve available for such an anastomosis than the hypoglossal.

THE CEREBRUM (Plates XXI; XXII; XXIII)

With the brain laid on its base examine its upper surface. This surface is formed entirely by the cerebrum, and consists of two halves, or hemispheres, separated from each other in the median line by the longitudinal fissure. This and the transverse fissure are the two largest fissures of the brain.

The Longitudinal Fissure.—By gently separating the hemispheres the longitudinal fissure will be seen to reach the base of the brain both anteriorly and posteriorly, while the intervening portion is rendered more shallow by a transverse band of white matter, the *corpus callosum*, which may therefore be said to form its floor; it is the chief connection between the two cerebral hemispheres. Running through the bottom of the fissure anteroposteriorly, and over the superior surface of the corpus callosum, are the anterior cerebral arteries. The longitudinal fissure also lodges the falx cerebri and its contained sinuses, the superior longitudinal (*superior sagittal*), and the inferior longitudinal (*inferior sagittal*).

The transverse fissure separates the posterior ends of the hemispheres of the cerebrum from the cerebellum; it accommodates the tentorium cerebelli and its contained sinuses, the lateral (*transverse*), the superior petrosal, and,

PLATE XXI.

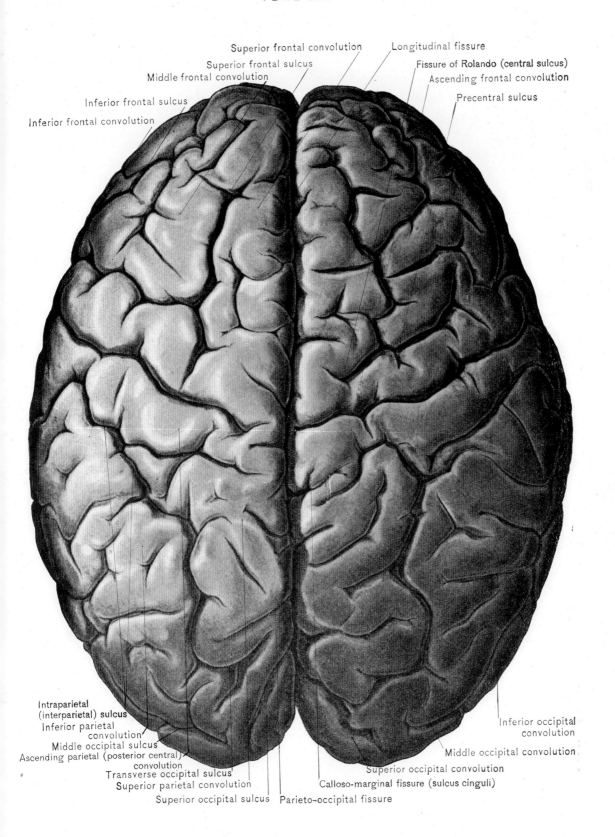

Superior frontal convolution

Longitudinal fissure

Superior frontal sulcus

Fissure of Rolando (central sulcus)

Middle frontal convolution

Ascending frontal convolution

Inferior frontal sulcus

Precentral sulcus

Inferior frontal convolution

Intraparietal (interparietal) sulcus

Inferior parietal convolution

Middle occipital sulcus

Ascending parietal (posterior central) convolution

Transverse occipital sulcus

Superior parietal convolution

Superior occipital sulcus

Parieto-occipital fissure

Calloso-marginal fissure (sulcus cinguli)

Superior occipital convolution

Middle occipital convolution

Inferior occipital convolution

SUPERIOR SURFACE OF CEREBRUM.

PLATE XXII.

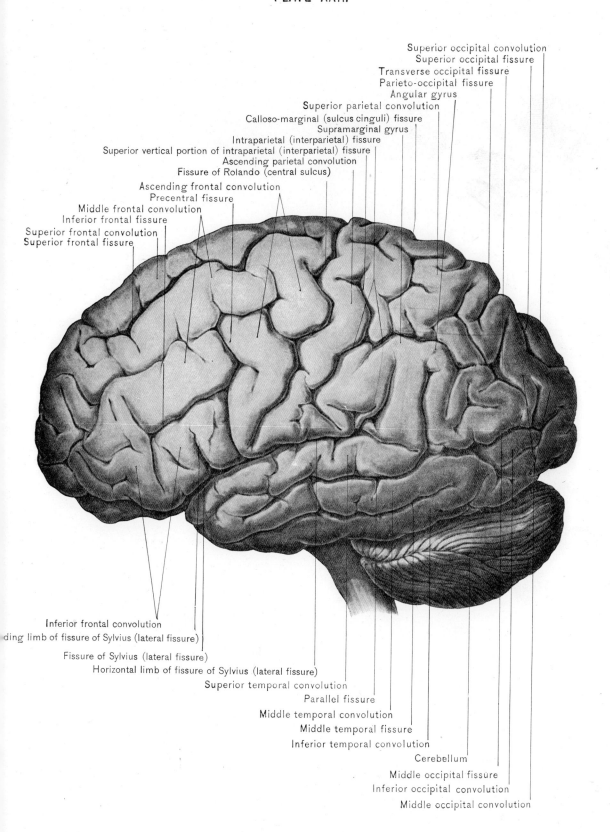

Superior occipital convolution
Superior occipital fissure
Transverse occipital fissure
Parieto-occipital fissure
Angular gyrus
Superior parietal convolution
Calloso-marginal (sulcus cinguli) fissure
Supramarginal gyrus
Intraparietal (interparietal) fissure
Superior vertical portion of intraparietal (interparietal) fissure
Ascending parietal convolution
Fissure of Rolando (central sulcus)
Ascending frontal convolution
Precentral fissure
Middle frontal convolution
Inferior frontal fissure
Superior frontal convolution
Superior frontal fissure

Inferior frontal convolution
ding limb of fissure of Sylvius (lateral fissure)
Fissure of Sylvius (lateral fissure)
Horizontal limb of fissure of Sylvius (lateral fissure)
Superior temporal convolution
Parallel fissure
Middle temporal convolution
Middle temporal fissure
Inferior temporal convolution
Cerebellum
Middle occipital fissure
Inferior occipital convolution
Middle occipital convolution

EXTERNAL SURFACE OF CEREBRUM.

PLATE XXIII.

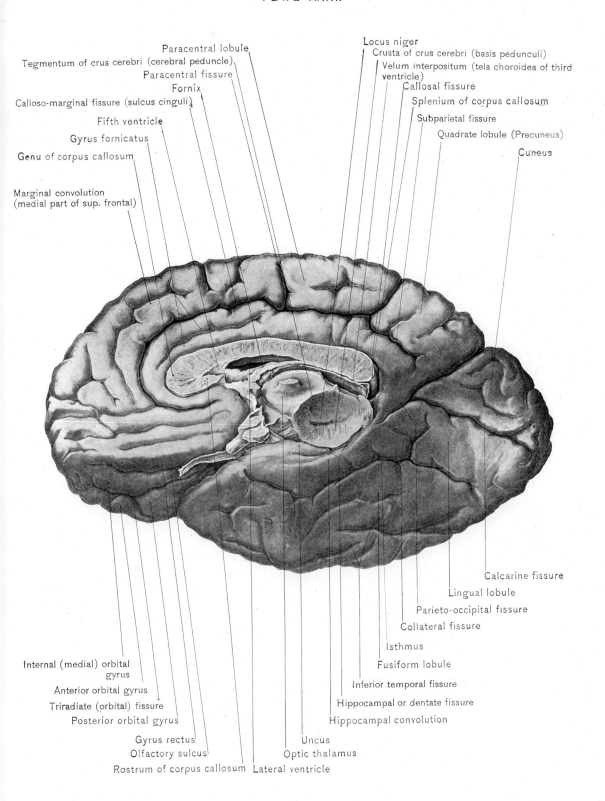

Locus niger
Crusta of crus cerebri (basis pedunculi)
Velum interpositum (tela choroidea of third ventricle)
Callosal fissure
Splenium of corpus callosum
Subparietal fissure
Quadrate lobule (Precuneus)
Cuneus

Paracentral lobule
Tegmentum of crus cerebri (cerebral peduncle)
Paracentral fissure
Fornix
Calloso-marginal fissure (sulcus cinguli)
Fifth ventricle
Gyrus fornicatus
Genu of corpus callosum
Marginal convolution (medial part of sup. frontal)

Calcarine fissure
Lingual lobule
Parieto-occipital fissure
Collateral fissure
Isthmus
Fusiform lobule
Inferior temporal fissure
Hippocampal or dentate fissure
Hippocampal convolution

Internal (medial) orbital gyrus
Anterior orbital gyrus
Triradiate (orbital) fissure
Posterior orbital gyrus
Gyrus rectus
Olfactory sulcus
Rostrum of corpus callosum   Lateral ventricle
Uncus
Optic thalamus

MEDIAN AND INFERIOR SURFACES OF CEREBRUM.

at its union with the falx cerebri, the straight sinus. Its deep portion transmits the pia mater into the interior of the cerebrum, where that membrane forms the ✓ velum interpositum (*tela choroidea of third ventricle*).

Convolutions and Fissures.—The surfaces of the hemispheres of the cerebrum are composed of convolutions or gyri, elevations of gray matter which are separated by fissures or sulci. The greater the development of the hemisphere, the more numerous are the fissures and convolutions, as the increased depth and number of the fissures afford additional surface. The gyri and sulci are the result of unequal growth, the surface increasing more rapidly than the central portion. In studying the fissures and convolutions from the fresh brain for the first time, that of a new-born child answers best, as the arrangement of these structures is somewhat simpler and agrees better with the description of the brain given in text-books.

Dissection.—Before studying the component parts of the brain by making sections, it is better carefully to study the surface anatomy of the hemispheres of the cerebrum. This entails separating the cerebrum from the remaining divisions of the brain and carrying an incision from the bottom of the longitudinal fissure through the median line of the corpus callosum and the structures in the median line of the cerebrum under the corpus callosum; in this way the three surfaces of each hemisphere of the cerebrum can be examined to the best advantage. To separate the cerebrum from the remainder of the brain, it is necessary to divide the crura cerebri (*cerebral peduncles*) and superior peduncles (*brachia conjunctiva*) of the cerebellum, the latter being exposed by lifting up the posterior lobes of the cerebrum. In order to do this, and also to obtain the best idea of the topographic relations of the different parts of the brain, the dissector should have at least two good brains at his disposal.

Surfaces.—Each hemisphere of the cerebrum presents three surfaces: a dorsolateral, a median, and a basilar. The basilar surface rests in the anterior and middle cranial fossæ and upon the tentorium cerebelli.

Arrangement of the Convolutions.—The surfaces of the hemispheres of the cerebrum are composed of gray matter arranged in folds, elevations, convolutions, or gyri; these, in turn, are separated by furrows, fissures, valleys, or sulci, varying in length, depth, as well as in importance. The deepest furrows, which are constant, separate the principal convolutions from each other, and are known as fissures; the remainder, as sulci. While the features of the principal convolutions are always arranged with considerable uniformity, numerous variations exist in the arrangement of the secondary and tertiary convolutions. The general arrangement of the fissures and convolutions of the two hemispheres is practically symmetrical, although slight differences always occur.

The **cerebral fissures,** besides being classified as primary and secondary, are subdivided into complete and incomplete fissures. *Complete fissures* extend through almost the entire thickness of the cerebrum, thus producing elevations in the lateral ventricles; examples of such fissures are the hippocampal and portions of the collateral and calcarine fissures. *Incomplete fissures* are furrows of variable depth, which do not cause protrusions in the ventricles.

It is by means of the convolutions and fissures of the brain that the amount of gray matter is greatly increased, without unduly augmenting the size of the brain; furthermore, the pia mater is thus enormously increased in extent, because it follows the windings of the gyri and fissures, and its vessels, which supply the cortex, are enabled to break up into fine branches before penetrating the brain tissue.

The **Cerebral Lobes.**—Each hemisphere of the cerebrum is incompletely divided by the deeper, and therefore the more important, of the fissures into the following lobes: the frontal, the parietal, the temporal, and the occipital. In addition to these four lobes there is a fifth lobe, the central lobe, or island of Reil (*the insula*); but as this projects into the bottom of the fissure of Sylvius (*lateral fissure*), and cannot be seen without drawing apart the sides of the latter, it will be described with the fissures. The individual lobes are distinct from each other on certain surfaces only, while on other surfaces they merge into each other without having definite boundaries. The fissures being the landmarks which serve as guides in mapping out the hemispheres into districts, or lobes, and also in locating the individual convolutions, the first task in the study of the surfaces of the hemispheres of the cerebrum will be to locate the principal fissures.

The **Principal Fissures of the Cerebrum** (Plate XXIV) are the fissure of Rolando (*the central sulcus*), the fissure of Sylvius (*lateral fissure*), and the parieto-occipital fissure. The fissure of Sylvius (*lateral fissure*) is found partly on the inferior, or basilar, and chiefly on the convex, or lateral, surface of the cerebrum; the fissure of Rolando (*the central sulcus*), only on the lateral surface of the cerebrum, and the parieto-occipital fissure, chiefly on the median surface, but also on the lateral surface.

The **fissure of Sylvius (lateral cerebral fissure)** is the most conspicuous fissure of the hemisphere. It corresponds in direction with the posterior border of the lesser wing of the sphenoidal bone, and contains the middle cerebral artery. The fissure commences on the inferior surface of the hemisphere at the anterior perforated space (*substantia perforata*) in a depression known as the vallecula Sylvii (*lateral cerebral fossa*). Its first part, or *stem,* then extends lateralward to the lateral surface of the hemisphere and forms a deep cleft which separates the

PLATE XXIV.

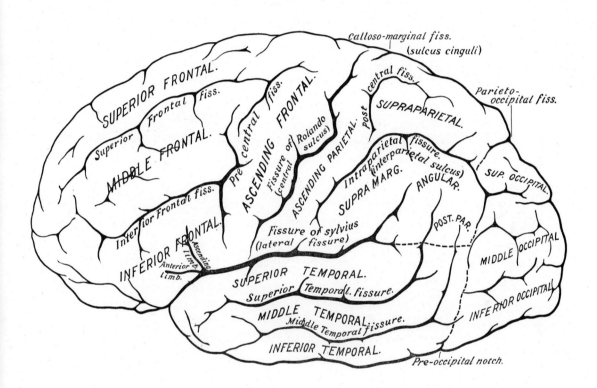

DIAGRAM OF LATERAL SURFACE OF CEREBRUM.

III

PLATE XXV.

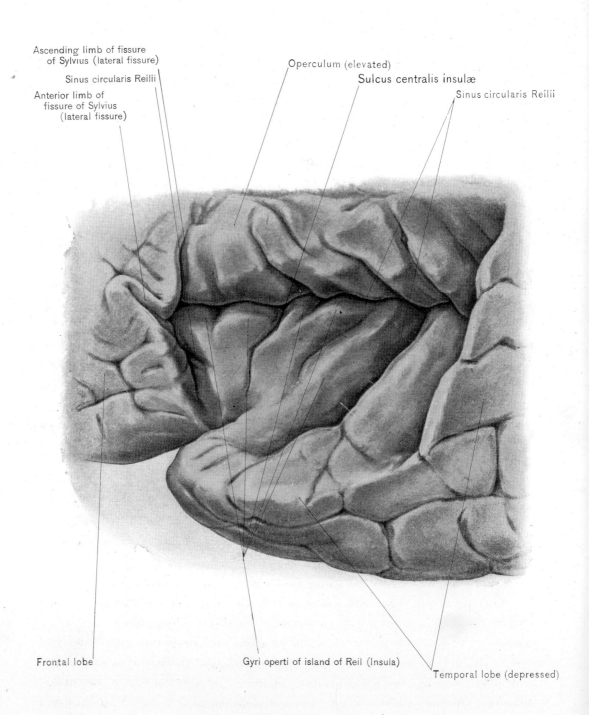

Ascending limb of fissure
of Sylvius (lateral fissure)

Sinus circularis Reilii

Anterior limb of
fissure of Sylvius
(lateral fissure)

Operculum (elevated)

Sulcus centralis insulæ

Sinus circularis Reilii

Frontal lobe

Gyri operti of island of Reil (Insula)

Temporal lobe (depressed)

ISLAND OF REIL (INSULA).

orbital area from the underlying temporal lobe. Reaching the surface at the Sylvian point, it divides into three limbs: an anterior ascending, a posterior, and an anterior horizontal limb. The anterior ascending limb passes upward and slightly forward for about ten millimeters (one-half inch) into the frontal lobe in front of the precentral fissure from which it is separated by the posterior part of the third frontal gyrus. The anterior horizontal limb extends forward and upward into the inferior frontal gyrus. The posterior limb runs backward and upward forming the boundary between the anterior portions of the temporal and parietal lobes, separating these two lobes by a deep cleft which usually ends behind the ascending limb. Sometimes the fissure divides into two short arms, one of which ends in the parietal lobe and the other curves downward into the temporal lobe.

The **island of Reil**, or **central lobe** (**insula**) (Plate XXV), is seen in the bottom of the fissure of Sylvius (*lateral fissure*) at the angle of separation of the ascending and the posterior limbs, by drawing the sides of the horizontal limb of the fissure of Sylvius (*lateral fissure*) widely apart and lifting the operculum. It comprises a series of from five to seven small convolutions, surrounded by a limiting sulcus (sulcus circularis Reilii). The convolutions of this lobe are arranged so that they radiate from the apex, which looks downward and forward. A fissure, the *sulcus centralis insulæ*, running in about the same direction as the fissure of Rolando (*central sulcus*), divides it into an anterior and a posterior portion. Additional smaller fissures are seen between the convolutions of the island of Reil (*insula*).

The **operculum** is that portion of the hemisphere of the cerebrum formed by the base of the inferior frontal convolution, the lower end of the ascending frontal, and the lower part of the ascending parietal convolution, it thus immediately overhangs the island of Reil (*insula*). The latter is lateral to the corpus striatum, and its fissures accommodate some of the branches of the middle cerebral artery.

The **Calloso-marginal Fissure** (**Sulcus Cinguli**) Plate XXIII.—Before attempting to trace the course of the fissure of Rolando (*central sulcus*), examine the inner surface of the hemisphere of the cerebrum and locate the callosomarginal fissure (*sulcus cinguli*), a secondary fissure running above the corpus callosum. It lies midway between the superior surface of the latter and the superior border of the hemisphere, and terminates upon the lateral surface of the hemisphere near this border and almost opposite the posterior end of the corpus callosum. As the calloso-marginal fissure (*sulcus cinguli*) is very rarely bridged over by a secondary convolution, there should be no difficulty in locating it.

The **fissure of Rolando,** or **central sulcus,** is one of the most important landmarks on the convex surface of the brain; running as it does through the motor

area of the cortex of the cerebrum, it becomes an indispensable guide for intracranial operations and localization. It commences at the upper border of the
hemisphere of the cerebrum just lateral to the longitudinal fissure and immediately in front of the terminal part of the calloso-marginal fissure (*sulcus
cinguli*). From here it runs obliquely downward and forward over the lateral
surface of the hemisphere, at an angle of about seventy-one and seven-tenths
degrees, to the anterior part of the longitudinal fissure, the Rolandic angle, terminating a slight distance above the horizontal limb and about twenty-five millimeters (one inch) behind the ascending limb of the fissure of Sylvius (*lateral fissure*).
The fissure of Rolando (*central sulcus*) presents two more or less distinct bends,
called its knees or genua; the superior genu, located at the junction of its middle
and upper thirds, has its convexity projecting backward; the inferior genu is
somewhat nearer the lower extremity of the fissure; its convexity points forward. As the frontal lobes increase in size and the brain in general attains
higher development, the fissure runs proportionately more obliquely backward.

The **parieto-occipital fissure,** the smallest of the principal fissures of the
cerebrum, is best seen as a deep cleft, the medial *parieto-occipital fissure,*
on the medial surface of the hemisphere of the cerebrum about thirty-
seven millimeters (one and a half inches) behind the corpus callosum. It begins
on the inferior occipito-temporal surface at the junction of the apex of the lingual
lobule with the isthmus of the gyrus fornicatus, or limbic lobe, and runs backward
and upward to reach the upper border of the hemisphere; thence it runs lateralward and forward on the lateral or convex surface for about twenty-five
millimeters (one inch), and midway between the central sulcus and the posterior
extremity of the cerebrum. It is joined by a secondary, nearly horizontal fissure, the *calcarine fissure,* the two together forming a T, whose posteriorly
directed diverging limbs enclose a wedge-shaped part of the occipital lobe, the
cuneus. On its *lateral,* convex portion, the fissure continues transversely
lateralward for about twelve millimeters (one-half inch), forming the *lateral
parieto-occipital fissure,* which sometimes appears merely as a slight indentation
upon the convex surface of the hemisphere.

The **frontal lobe,** the largest of the cerebral lobes, includes about one-third
of the cerebrum, or that portion of the hemisphere in front of, and above the main
part of the fissure of Sylvius (*lateral fissure*), and the portion in front of the
fissure of Rolando (*central sulcus*); upon the median surface it includes the corresponding portion of the hemisphere above the calloso-marginal fissure (*sulcus
cinguli*). There is generally no line of demarcation between the frontal and parietal lobes upon the mesial surface of the hemisphere, but extension of the
fissure of Rolando (*central sulcus*) into the longitudinal fissure (a condition

which sometimes occurs) designates the posterior limit of the frontal lobe on this surface.

Frontal Lobe Tumors.—Tumors in the frontal lobe, besides producing the usual signs of intracranial pressure, such as choked disc, headache, vomiting, and showing evidence of increase of spinal pressure, occasionally give symptoms which are characteristic of the frontal lobe. However, it is well to bear in mind that the involvement of the frontal lobe may be extensive without giving localizing symptoms. But when the tumor has extended, so that the connecting fibers between the two lobes in the corpus callosum are involved, mental deterioration and dementia become marked features. There may sometimes be a change in the patient's manner, such as jocosity, or tendency to be facetious with little regard for, or realization of the seriousness of his condition, or there may be a tendency toward irritability, with a sharp, scathing type of wit. Of value in establishing a frontal lobe localization is the loss of the sense of smell on the involved side. The choking may be greater on the side of involvement than on the opposite side, but this is not always the rule, and the reverse may be found ture in a definite percentage of cases. Abscess in the frontal lobe secondary to frontal sinus involvement is not uncommon, and is associated with a history of headache and loss of smell on one side, choked disc, and a possible Kernig's sign. Lumbar puncture in all cases of abscess is not without danger of rupturing the abscess, and must be undertaken with great care, being resorted to only when insufficient evidence is present to make a diagnosis. Bárány tests likewise should be avoided, because turning and douching may cause vomiting, favoring rupture of the abcess into the subarachnoid space, with fatal meningitis as the result.

The **operation** for exploration of the frontal lobes, as well as the approach to the pituitary region, consists of a skin flap carried from a point just below the lateral extent of the eyebrow on the supra-orbital ridge to the base of the nose. The incision is then carried back from the root of the nose exactly in the midline to a point just behind the measurement for the Rolandic fissure (*central sulcus*). The skin incision is then swung at right angles down over the parietal region, so that the base of the incision extends to a point just behind and above the tip of the ear. This allows for a large cranioplastic flap whose base may be broken across the thinned-out portion of the temporal bone. It is important that the trephine openings on the midline should be at least two centimeters from this line, in order to avoid injuring the longitudinal (*sagittal*) sinus with the drill. The anterior limb of the bony opening should be made high enough just to avoid the frontal sinus. When the flap has been sawed free, a heavy object, such as the handle of a large chisel, is placed across the base of the flap from the ear to the lateral angle of the orbit. The bone flap is pried up from the midline and broken across the base by a sharp effort. This will expose the dura, and the underlying middle meningeal artery will probably be seen bleeding freely from several points where its diploic attachments have been torn. Occasionally the artery is severed at the base when the flap is broken back. In the latter case it may be tied. The next step in the operation consists of opening the dura, which should not be undertaken until all points of bleeding have been definitely controlled, so that closure of the wound can be made at any time without delay, should the patient's condition become unsatisfactory. In the presence of a tight brain no attempt should be made to open the dura until the ventricle on the opposite side has been tapped and drained, so as to insure sufficient room for manipulation of the frontal lobe. A dural flap is then made by carefully opening a small point on the dura near the anterior and mesial aspect of the field. This is carried down about one centimeter from the bony opening, and conforms closely to the shape of the bone flap. The cortex is then exposed, and the frontal lobe is explored on the under surface and along the midline for the presence of the tumor. If palpation does not reveal a tumor in the lobe itself, it is wise to examine the surface along the falx.

The approach to the pituitary area for a suprasellar growth is similar to the above, except that the frontal lobe is elevated gently and the exploration proceeds along the base of the anterior fossa, directing the elevation towards the midline. The olfactory nerve will be seen and divided. The optic nerve on the side of the operation will be encountered just anterior to the clinoids. The chiasma may be seen in the pituitary region, exposed by careful progress and gentle elevation.

Tumors of the motor area do not always present convulsions as the initial symptom with the signs of intracranial pressure. Progressive weakness of the hand or foot extending into the adjoining area, and later to the face, should be considered extremely significant. Irritating lesions of the cortex do produce convulsions of the Jacksonian type, arising in a group of muscles and rapidly spreading to the entire body, rarely bilateral. The operative procedure for tumors in the motor area is similar to that described under frontal lobe tumors. The cranioplastic flap, however, is designed so as to include the Rolandic area, and the base of the flap is broken across the temporal region as low as possible.

The **parietal lobe** (see also p. 128) includes that portion of the lateral surface of the hemisphere of the cerebrum above the horizontal limb of the fissure of Sylvius (*lateral fissure*) and a line representing the extension of the same limb backward to meet the posterior boundary of the lobe; also the portion behind the fissure of Rolando (*central sulcus*) and in front of the lateral portion of the parieto-occipital fissure. Upon the median surface, it includes that part of the hemisphere in front of the mesial portion of the parieto-occipital fissure; it is unlimited in front on this surface for want of a line of demarcation between it and the frontal lobe, but, as previously stated, by extending the fissure of Rolando (*central sulcus*) into the longitudinal fissure, its anterior superior limit would be represented.   The parietal lobe is only partly separated posteriorly from the occipital lobe by the lateral portion of the parieto-occipital fissure and the transverse occipital fissure; the latter is a secondary fissure which is not always present. From the temporal lobe, below, there is no attempt at complete separation.   At the lower margin of the lateral surface of the hemisphere of the cerebrum, between the occipital and temporal lobes, is the *pre-occipital notch* produced by a fold of dura over the parieto-mastoid suture and above the highest part of the lateral (*transverse*) sinus.   The upper part of a line drawn from the extremity of the lateral portion of the parieto-occipital fissure to the pre-occipital notch, together with the lateral portion of the fissure, will about represent the junction of the parietal and occipital lobes.   The lower part of the line will represent the line of junction of the occipital and temporal lobes.   This notch must not be confounded with another impression, sometimes described as the pre-occipital notch, produced by the superior border of the petrous portion of the temporal bone.

Parietal and temporal lobe tumors.—It is difficult to localize lesions in the right temporal lobe as this is a silent area of the brain.   Tumors occurring in this area in the majority of cases give rise only to symptoms of intracranial pressure.   Involvement of the parietal lobe close to the midline and high on the cortex frequently gives rise to a loss of sense of position, astereognosis, disturbance of the vibratory sense, as well as adiadokokinesis.   There may be some slight disturbance of touch, pain, and temperature on the opposite side.   This is only present in extensive lesions, and then the cognizational values of these senses alone is lost; that is, the appreciation of difference in temperature, differences between two points of the compass, in tactile sensation, and differences in intensity of pain between the two sides.

On the left side of the brain, temporal and parietal lobe tumors produce not only the positive symptoms noted above, but also various forms of aphasia. When the tumor is confined to, and invades the temporal lobe, auditory and jargon aphasia may develop.   Amnesia is sometimes a prominent factor in lesions which involve the lower surfaces of the temporal lobe.   Jargon aphasia is present in lesions around the supramarginal gyrus.   In this condition the patient is unable to say the words he desires, although if the words are supplied he may recognize them and show his understanding.   Because of the lack of words he talks in a round-about way or as though he were speaking in a peculiar jargon.   It is highly important to differentiate a condition in which the patient is unable to say the word he desires, though he recognizes that word when seen or heard, from the patient who is unable to say a word and also unable to recognize it as well. When pure motor aphasia is present, there is a lesion in Broca's (*parolfactory*) area or at the island of Reil (*insula*) and its adjoining convolution in the inferior frontal convolution. The patient shows a paralysis of word expression. He may understand clearly, be able to recognize the word or even write his communications, but the power of speech is entirely lost.

Temporal lobe tumors as they progress, especially the gliomas which invade the deeper structures of the brain, are inclined to produce visual field defects of the quadrant type, from destruction of the visual pathways which pass from the thalamus below the posterior horn of the lateral ventricle to swing back to the region of the cuneate lobe on the mesial aspect of the occipital pole. Therefore, a homonymous hemianopsia or homonymous quadranopsia should be carefully sought for where temporal lobe involvement is suspected.

The **occipital lobe** (Plate XXVI) includes that portion of the convex surface of the hemisphere of the cerebrum behind the lateral portion of the parieto-occipital fissure and a line connecting the extremity of this fissure with the pre-occipital notch. Upon the median surface of the hemisphere it includes that part posterior to the mesial portion of the parieto-occipital fissure. Upon the basilar surface there is no line of demarcation between it and the temporal lobe. (The inferior surface of this lobe is described with the same surface of the temporal, since two of the most important secondary fissures in this area occupy both of these lobes, and extend without breach of continuity from one to the other.)

Occipital Lobe Tumors.—Tumors of the occipital pole frequently give rise only to symptoms of intracranial pressure. Those on the right side of the brain may produce a left homonymous hemianopsia or visual hallucinations, but without further symptoms. So-called mind-blindness may occur when the lesion is deep seated. This is characterized by attacks of sudden loss of consciousness without convulsions, a condition in which the patient's mind becomes suddenly blank for a short period of time. Lesions of the left occipital pole are inclined to produce not only a right homonymous hemianopsia, but as they advance forward they may give rise to some form of aphasia, confusion of mind, active delirium, and visual hallucinations.

Visual hallucinations due to organic disease of the brain are of two types: a crude type, consisting of flashes of light, or colors, and a formed type which is composed of figures or objects. Where the tumor is confined to the occipital pole, without extension to the thalamus, the hallucinations which may occur are of the crude variety. Lesions of the temporal lobe invading the thalamus

PLATE XXVI.

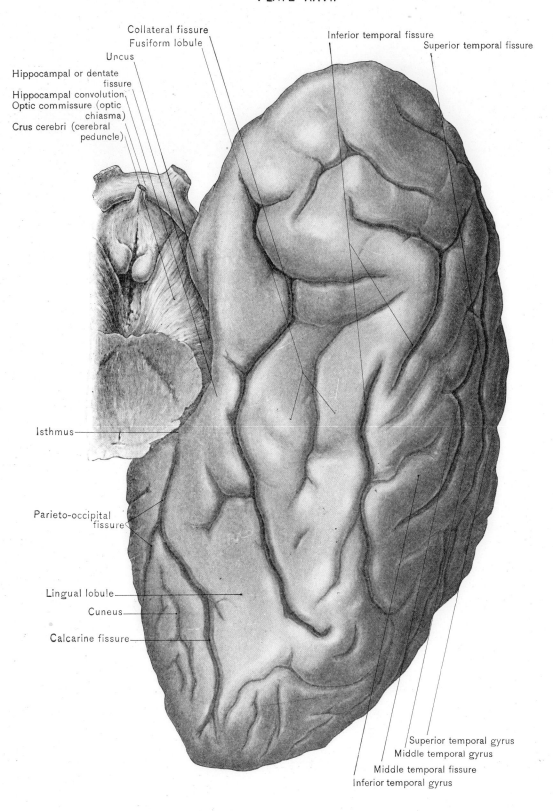

Collateral fissure

Fusiform lobule

Uncus

Hippocampal or dentate fissure

Hippocampal convolution

Optic commissure (optic chiasma)

Crus cerebri (cerebral peduncle)

Inferior temporal fissure

Superior temporal fissure

Isthmus

Parieto-occipital fissure

Lingual lobule

Cuneus

Calcarine fissure

Superior temporal gyrus

Middle temporal gyrus

Middle temporal fissure

Inferior temporal gyrus

INFERIOR SURFACE OF OCCIPITAL AND TEMPORAL LOBES.

or at the optic pathways produce form hallucinations, so that the patient will see objects, such as chairs, tables, men, dogs, horses, etc. The objects are never clear cut in their details. Sixty per cent are usually seen in the corresponding blind fields, about forty per cent may be referred to the homolateral side.

The operative procedure for exploration of the occipital lobe consists of a cranioplastic flap, so designed that the anterior limb extends along the line of the Rolandic fissure (*central sulcus*) and back along the midline to a point about two centimeters above the occipital protuberance. It is then carried forward toward the tip of the ear, high enough so as to avoid injury to the lateral (*transverse*) sinus. The flap is again broken over the ear, and should include at least one branch of the temporal artery. The occipital artery is usually sacrificed in the lower limb of the incision.

The **temporal lobe** comprises that portion of the lateral surface of the hemisphere of the cerebrum below the horizontal limb of the fissure of Sylvius (*lateral fissure*) and a line representing its continuation backward, and in front of the lower part of the line connecting the pre-occipital notch with the extremity of the lateral portion of the parieto-occipital fissure. Upon the inferior surface of the cerebral hemisphere it lies immediately behind the stem of the fissure of Sylvius (*lateral fissure*); it is not separated on this surface from the occipital lobe. A line drawn from the pre-occipital notch to the isthmus of the gyrus fornicatus, or limbic lobe, marks the line of union of the temporal and occipital lobes.

The **island of Reil** (**insula**), or the fifth lobe of the cerebrum, is described with the fissure of Sylvius (*lateral fissure*) at p. 115.

Secondary Fissures and Convolutions.—The arrangement of the principal fissures and the boundaries of the lobes of the cerebral hemispheres having been given, the description of the secondary fissures and convolutions naturally follows. Secondary convolutions frequently bridge these secondary fissures, making it difficult to trace them.

The frontal lobe (Plate XXIV), as already indicated, has three surfaces: a lateral, an inferior, or orbital, and a medial surface. The lateral surface has three secondary fissures: the superior and inferior frontal fissures, running horizontally, and the precentral, or transverse fissure (also known as the ascending frontal fissure), running vertically almost parallel with the lower half of the fissure of Rolando (*central sulcus*), and usually divided into a superior and inferior part. Frequently, a small medial frontal fissure is seen between the superior and inferior frontal fissures. It subdivides the middle frontal convolution, and ends anteriorly in a wide bifurcation. The lateral surface also has four main convolutions: the precentral, or ascending frontal (*anterior central*), the superior, or first frontal, the middle, or second frontal, and the inferior, or third frontal gyri. The anterior ascending, and the anterior horizontal limbs of the fissure of Sylvius (*lateral fissure*) are also in relation with it.

The **superior frontal fissure** commences a short distance in front of the fissure of Rolando (*central sulcus*), and runs forward and downward parallel with the longitudinal fissure, the gyrus included between the longitudinal fissure and superior frontal fissure being the superior, or first, frontal convolution.

The **inferior frontal fissure** usually commences in the precentral fissure, but sometimes in front of it, and runs forward and downward about midway between the superior frontal fissure and the lower border of the frontal lobe. Between the superior and the inferior frontal fissures lies the middle, or second, frontal convolution, and between the inferior frontal fissure and the lower margin of the frontal lobe is the inferior frontal convolution.

The **precentral fissure** lies in front of, and parallel with the fissure of Rolando (*central sulcus*), its lower end being between the latter fissure and the, ascending limb of the fissure of Sylvius (*lateral fissure*). The superior precentral fissure, as a rule, is continuous with the superior frontal fissure, and at times the inferior precentral fissure is continuous with the inferior frontal fissure.

The **ascending frontal (anterior central) convolution** is situated between the precentral fissure and the fissure of Rolando (*central sulcus*), and extends along the entire anterior border of the latter fissure. It is the only gyrus of the frontal lobe having a vertical direction. This convolution is continuous with the ascending parietal (*posterior central*) convolution around both ends of the fissure of Rolando (*central sulcus*), immediately behind which the latter convolution is situated.

The **superior, or first, frontal convolution** is continuous posteriorly with the precentral, or ascending frontal, medially with the marginal, and anteriorly, upon the basilar surface, with the gyrus rectus and the medial and anterior orbital convolutions, thus extending horizontally from the precentral sulcus to the frontal pole.

The **middle, or second, frontal convolution** extends from the precentral sulcus to the temporal pole, and is continuous in front with the anterior orbital convolution and the anterior extremities of the superior and inferior frontal convolutions. Posteriorly, it frequently bridges the precentral fissure, and joins the ascending frontal (*anterior central*) convolution.

The **inferior, or third, frontal convolution,** the shortest of the three frontal gyri, is continuous posteriorly with the ascending frontal (*anterior central*) convolution, and anteriorly, upon the basilar surface, with the anterior and posterior orbital convolutions. Through the medium of the anterior and ascending limbs of the fissure of Sylvius (*lateral fissure*), both of which extend into this

PLATE XXVII.

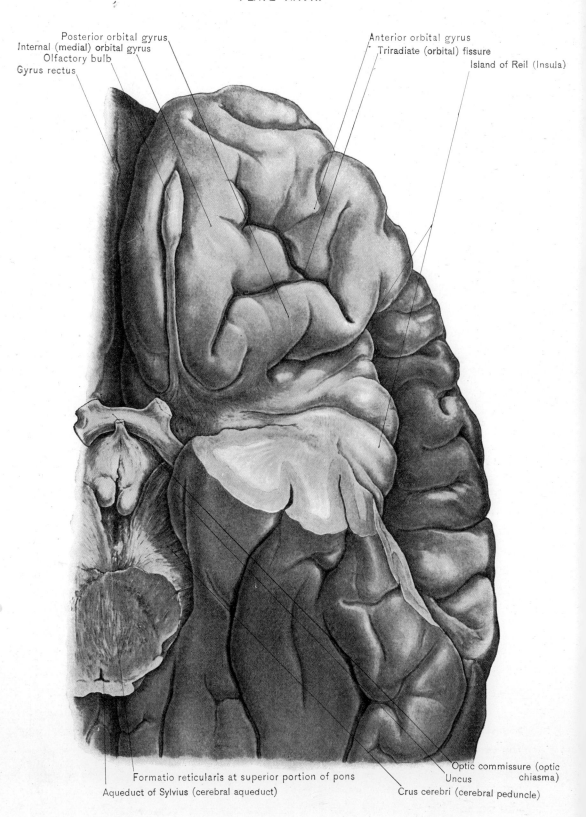

Posterior orbital gyrus
Internal (medial) orbital gyrus
Olfactory bulb
Gyrus rectus

Anterior orbital gyrus
Triradiate (orbital) fissure
Island of Reil (Insula)

Optic commissure (optic chiasma)
Uncus
Formatio reticularis at superior portion of pons
Aqueduct of Sylvius (cerebral aqueduct)
Crus cerebri (cerebral peduncle)

INFERIOR SURFACE OF FRONTAL LOBE.

convolution, it is divided into three parts: the pars orbitalis, in front of the anterior limb; the pars triangularis (base of triangle looks upward) between the anterior and the ascending limbs; and the pars basilaris behind the ascending limb. This convolution, as already mentioned, assists in the formation of the operculum. The posterior extremity of the inferior frontal gyrus, on the left side, is known as *Broca's convolution* (*parolfactory area*), and is believed to be the center for motor speech.

The **orbital,** or **inferior, surface** of the **frontal lobe** (Plate XXVII) is triangular in shape; the base, directed backward, is formed by the anterior perforated space (*substantia perforata*) and the main portion of the fissure of Sylvius (*lateral fissure*). The apex, directed forward, is formed by the curving of the convolutions in passing from the convex to the orbital surface, and the sides are formed by the longitudinal fissure and the lower border of the hemisphere. This surface has two secondary fissures, the olfactory and the orbital, and four main convolutions: lateral, anterior, posterior, and medial orbital.

The **olfactory fissure** runs parallel with, and a short distance lateral to the longitudinal fissure. It lodges the olfactory tract and bulb. It marks off a strip, the **gyrus rectus,** situated between the olfactory and longitudinal fissures, and corresponds to the orbital surface of the superior frontal convolution.

The **orbital,** or **triradiate, fissure** is situated at about the middle of that portion of the orbital surface, which lies lateral to the olfactory fissure. Typically, its arms represent the letter H or K, consisting of a main transverse portion, which is directed forward and runs nearly parallel with the olfactory fissure, and of two longitudinal branches, one directed backward and medialward, and the other lateralward.

The **anterior, posterior, lateral, and medial orbital gyri** are located between the branches of the triradiate fissure, and are named from their relation to the branches of the fissure. They are continuous with the first, second, and third frontal convolutions.

The **medial surface of the frontal lobe** has only one convolution, the superior frontal gyrus, or marginal gyrus. It has several *annectant convolutions,* or *gyri,* small convolutions which form bridges across fissures and connect neighboring convolutions.

The **superior frontal gyrus** (marginal gyrus) lies between the calloso-marginal fissure (*sulcus cinguli*) and the supero-anterior margin of the hemisphere of the cerebrum. This convolution commences below the rostrum of the corpus callosum at the anterior perforated space (*substantia perforata*), and extends upward and backward between the calloso-marginal fissure (*sulcus cinguli*) and the margin of the hemisphere, as far as a line which represents the continuation of the precentral fissure into the longitudinal fissure.   It is continuous along the margin of the hemisphere with the superior, or first, frontal convolution.   At its posterior end the superior frontal, or marginal gyrus is continuous with the two central convolutions on each side of the Rolandic fissure (*central sulcus*); but sometimes this posterior extremity is almost completely cut off from the rest of the gyrus by an ascending limb, the *paracentral sulcus*, the portion thus isolated being known as the *paracentral lobule*.

The **parietal lobe** is that portion of the hemisphere situated behind the fissure of Rolando (*central sulcus*), above the horizontal limb of the fissure of Sylvius (*lateral fissure*), and in front of the lateral limb of the parieto-occipital fissure.   The portion of the lobe below the lateral limb of the parieto-occipital fissure and beyond the termination of the horizontal limb of the fissure of Sylvius (*lateral fissure*) is continuous with the occipital lobe by means of annectant gyri. The limit of the parietal lobe posteriorly is represented by the lateral limb of the parieto-occipital fissure and a line, already described (p. 118), which extends from the end of that fissure to the pre-occipital notch.   It presents two surfaces, a lateral and a medial surface.

Upon the *lateral surface* are seen one, and sometimes two chief secondary fissures.   When but one fissure is present, it is the intraparietal (*interparietal sulcus*), and when two fissures are present, they are the intraparietal (*interparietal sulcus*) and the postcentral.

The **intraparietal fissure** (**interparietal sulcus**) commences above the horizontal limb of the fissure of Sylvius (*lateral fissure*), a short distance behind the fissure of Rolando (*central sulcus*), and runs upward, parallel to the lower portion of the latter fissure; it then turns backward, runs nearly parallel with the longitudinal fissure, and terminates in the occipital lobe, usually in the transverse occipital fissure.   The posterior portion of the horizontal part of the intraparietal fissure (*interparietal sulcus*) is often separated from the main fissure by an annectant convolution.

The **postcentral fissure,** when present, exists either as a continuation of the ascending limb of the intraparietal fissure (*interparietal sulcus*) beyond its junction of the ascending with the horizontal limb, thus making the intraparietal fissure (*interparietal sulcus*) T shaped; or it is entirely separated from the ascending limb of the intraparietal fissure (*interparietal sulcus*), the former being the more common arrangement.   The postcentral fissure runs parallel to the upper portion of the fissure of Rolando (*central sulcus*) almost to the longitudinal fissure.   It may be divided into an inferior and a superior portion.

PARIETAL CONVOLUTIONS.—Through the medium of the intraparietal fissure (*interparietal sulcus*) or the intraparietal (*interparietal sulcus*) and postcentral fissures, the lateral surface of the parietal lobe is divided into three principal convolutions: the postcentral, or ascending parietal, the superior parietal, and the inferior parietal gyrus. The inferior parietal convolution is further sub-divided into a supramarginal and an angular convolution, and sometimes a postparietal convolution.

The **postcentral,** or **ascending parietal, gyrus,** or **convolution,** lies immediately behind the fissure of Rolando (*central sulcus*), in front of the ascending limb of the intraparietal fissure (*interparietal sulcus*), hnd the postcentral fissure when present, and above the horizontal limb of the fissure of Sylvius (*lateral fissure*). It is continuous with the ascending frontal convolution (*anterior central gyrus*) around the ends of the fissure of Rolando (*central sulcus*), and with the superior parietal convolution. Its lower extremity extends to the horizontal limb of the fissure of Sylvius (*lateral fissure*), forming the posterior part of the operculum; its upper extremity is limited by the longitudinal fissure, and, with the corresponding end of the ascending frontal convolution (*anterior central gyrus*), forms the paracentral lobule on the medial aspect of the brain.

The **superior parietal convolution** lies behind the ascending parietal convolution (*postcentral gyrus*), with which it is continuous. It is situated between the longitudinal fissure and the horizontal limb of the intraparietal fissure (*interparietal sulcus*) and posteriorly it extends around the superior end of the parieto-occipital fissure into the cortex of the occipital lobe. On the mesial aspect of the hemisphere it is continuous with the quadrate lobule, or precuneus.

The **inferior parietal convolution** lies behind the ascending limb and below the horizontal limb of the intraparietal fissure (*interparietal sulcus*) and above the horizontal limb of the fissure of Sylvius (*lateral fissure*). Posteriorly, it is con-nected with the second occipital convolution by means of the second and third annectant gyri, and also with the superior temporal and the middle temporal convolutions. It is subdivided into two convolutions, the supramarginal and the angular, and sometimes into a third, the postparietal convolution.

The *supramarginal convolution* includes the anterior portion of the inferior parietal as far as the posterior extremity of the horizontal limb of the fissure of Sylvius (*lateral fissure*). It winds around this limb and becomes continuous inferiorly with the superior temporal convolution, and posteriorly with the angular convolution.

The *angular convolution* is the posterior portion of the inferior parietal convo-lution; it lies posterior to the terminal part of the horizontal limb of the fissure of Sylvius (*lateral fissure*) as it inclines upward. It winds around the posterior end of the superior temporal fissure, and becomes continuous with the second

9

occipital convolution through the medium of the second and third annectant gyri. It is also continuous with the middle temporal convolution.

The postparietal convolution forms a third subdivision of the inferior parietal convolution when, as sometimes happens, the middle temporal fissure terminates in the inferior parietal convolution, and with the fissure of Sylvius (*lateral fissure*) and the superior temporal, or parallel, fissure divides this convolution into three. It winds around the posterior extremity of the middle temporal fissure, and is continuous with the third occipital convolution.

Upon the mesial surface of the parietal lobe is seen the terminal part of the **calloso-marginal fissure (cingulate sulcus)** (Plate XXIV), one of the most important secondary fissures (mentioned in describing the fissure of Rolando (*central sulcus*). This fissure commences below the anterior extremity, or rostrum, of the corpus callosum, runs parallel to, and a short distance above the corpus callosum, from which it is separated by the convolution of the corpus callosum, or gyrus fornicatus, to nearly opposite the posterior extremity, or splenium of the corpus callosum. Here it turns upward and pursues a slightly backward course, terminating on the superior border of the hemisphere of the cerebrum, immediately posterior to the fissure of Rolando (*central sulcus*). The calloso-marginal fissure (*cingulate sulcus*), particularly its anterior part, is frequently bridged over by small convolutions.

The **subparietal fissure** is a much smaller fissure, which commences at the point where the terminal portion of the calloso-marginal fissure (*cingulate sulcus*) begins to turn upward. For all practical purposes it may be considered the continuation backward of the main portion of the calloso-marginal fissure (*cingulate sulcus*).

The **paracentral fissure** is an inconstant, small fissure running out of the main portion of the calloso-marginal (*cingulate sulcus*), on a line with the anterior limit of the medial end of the ascending frontal convolution. When present, it definitely marks the posterior limit of the marginal convolution.

MESIAL CONVOLUTIONS.—Through the medium of the calloso-marginal (*cingulate sulcus*) and the paracentral, subparietal, and parieto-occipital fissures the medial surface of the parietal lobe is divided into two lobules or convolutions: the precuneus, or quadrate, and the paracentral, the former being posterior to the latter.

The **precuneus,** or **quadrate lobule,** an irregularly quadrilateral area embracing the greater part of this surface, lies between the medial limb of the parieto-occipital and the terminal portion of the calloso-marginal fissure (*cingulate sulcus*) and above the subparietal fissure (Plate XXVIII).

PLATE XXVIII.

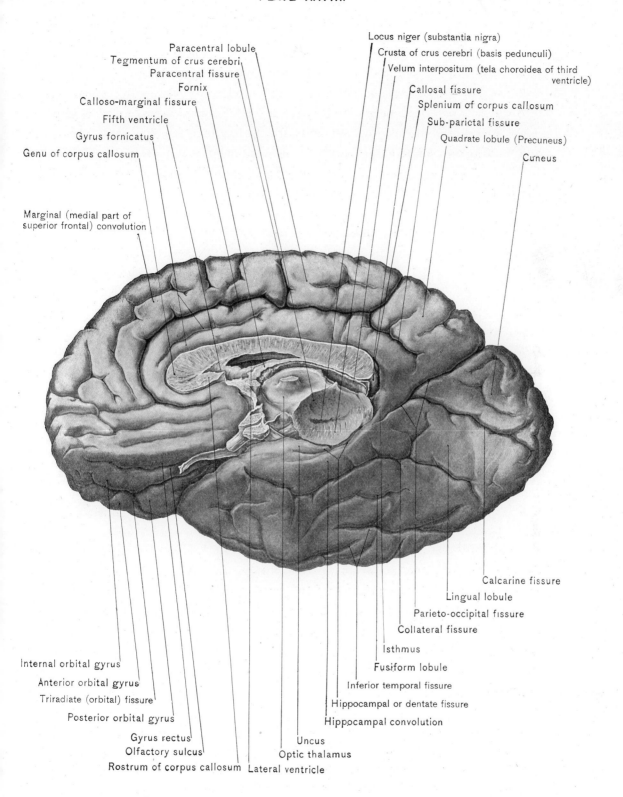

Locus niger (substantia nigra)
Crusta of crus cerebri (basis pedunculi)
Velum interpositum (tela choroidea of third ventricle)
Callosal fissure
Splenium of corpus callosum
Sub-parietal fissure
Quadrate lobule (Precuneus)
Cuneus

Paracentral lobule
Tegmentum of crus cerebri
Paracentral fissure
Fornix
Calloso-marginal fissure
Fifth ventricle
Gyrus fornicatus
Genu of corpus callosum

Marginal (medial part of superior frontal) convolution

Calcarine fissure
Lingual lobule
Parieto-occipital fissure
Collateral fissure
Isthmus
Fusiform lobule
Inferior temporal fissure
Hippocampal or dentate fissure
Hippocampal convolution

Internal orbital gyrus
Anterior orbital gyrus
Triradiate (orbital) fissure
Posterior orbital gyrus
Gyrus rectus
Olfactory sulcus
Rostrum of corpus callosum

Uncus
Optic thalamus
Lateral ventricle

MEDIAN AND INFERIOR SURFACES OF CEREBRUM.

The **paracentral convolution** includes the medial ends of the ascending parietal convolution (*postcentral gyrus*) and ascending frontal convolution (*anterior central gyrus*). It lies immediately in front of the terminal portion of the calloso-marginal fissure (*cingulate sulcus*), above the horizontal portion of this fissure, and behind the paracentral fissure, or a line representing the extension of the precentral fissure of the frontal lobe into the longitudinal fissure.

The **Occipital Lobe** (Plate XXVI) forms the posterior extremity of the hemisphere of the cerebrum, and next to the island of Reil (*insula*) is the smallest of the five divisions of the hemisphere of the cerebrum. It is triangular in shape, with its base directed forward and its apex, the occipital pole, backward; it fills the superior fossa of the occipital bone, and rests upon the tentorium cerebelli. Since it is represented on all the aspects of the hemisphere it has three surfaces: a lateral, a medial, and a tentorial, or basilar, surface. Owing to the absence of a distinct line of demarcation, the lateral surface of the occipital lobe is continuous with the corresponding surface of the parietal and temporal lobes, and its basilar surface is continuous with the corresponding surface of the temporal lobe. The medial surface of the occipital lobe is clearly marked off from the corresponding surface of the parietal lobe by the medial limb or main portion of the parieto-occipital fissure. Practically the anterior limit of the lobe can be marked off by a line drawn from the extremity of the lateral limb of the parieto-occipital fissure over the lateral surface of the hemisphere to the pre-occipital notch, and continued across the basilar surface along the collateral fissure to meet the end of the medial limb of this fissure.

In studying the convolutions comprising the different lobes of the cerebrum, those of the occipital are the most variable and, therefore, the most difficult to understand. Upon its lateral surface are three horizontal fissures: the superior, the lateral, and the inferior occipital, with sometimes a fourth vertical fissure, the transverse occipital fissure. The transverse and the superior occipital fissures are the least variable of the four and are the most important in tracing the convolutions of this surface.

The **transverse occipital fissure,** into which the intraparietal (*interparietal sulcus*) frequently opens, runs over the lateral surface of the lobe a short distance behind the terminal portion of the lateral limb of the parieto-occipital fissure.

The **superior occipital fissure** runs anteroposteriorly as though it were a continuation of the horizontal limb of the intraparietal fissure (*interparietal sulcus*).

The **lateral occipital fissure** is seldom well developed, and extends anteroposteriorly.

The **inferior occipital fissure** is frequently interrupted by bridging convolutions, and runs anteroposteriorly along the line of junction of the lateral and basilar surfaces of the lobe.

CONVOLUTIONS OF THE OCCIPITAL LOBE.—Through the medium of the superior, lateral, and inferior occipital fissures the lateral surface of the occipital lobe is divided into the superior, or first, the middle, or second, and the inferior, or third, occipital convolutions.

The **superior occipital convolution** lies between the longitudinal and superior occipital fissures, and commences at the posterior end of the superior parietal convolution, to which it is connected by the first annectant gyrus. It then winds around the extremity of the lateral limb of the parieto-occipital, and the medial end of the transverse occipital fissure, when present, and becomes continuous with the cuneus, a wedge-shaped lobule seen upon the medial surface of the lobe.

The **lateral occipital convolution** lies between the superior and middle occipital fissures, and commences at the lateral side of the intraparietal fissure (*interparietal sulcus*) and behind the angular gyrus, to which it is connected by the second and third annectant gyri.

The **inferior occipital convolution** lies between the middle and inferior occipital fissures, and is connected to the inferior, or third, temporal convolution by the fourth annectant gyrus.

The medial surface of the occipital lobe is bounded anteriorly by the medial part of the parieto-occipital fissure, and presents only one fissure, the calcarine, which divides this portion of the brain into the cuneus and the lingual gyrus (described below).

The **calcarine fissure,** the beginning of which usually consists of two branches close to the lower border of the posterior extremity of the hemisphere of the cerebrum, runs almost horizontally forward along the margin formed by the medial and basilar surfaces of the hemisphere, and joins the parieto-occipital fissure at an acute angle, postero-inferior to the posterior extremity of the corpus callosum. The anterior portion of this fissure is the deeper, completely invaginating the brain wall and thereby giving rise to a prominence, the calcar avis, or hippocampus minor, seen in the posterior horn of the lateral ventricle.

The **cuneus,** a triangular lobule situated between the medial limb, or main portion, of the parieto-occipital fissure and the calcarine fissure, forms the main portion of the medial surface of the occipital lobe. Its base is directed upward and backward, and is formed by the medial border of the superior occipital convolution; its apex is directed downward and forward, and corresponds to the angle of union of the calcarine and parieto-occipital fissures. The **lingual gyrus** is that portion of the brain bounded by the calcarine fissure superiorly, the collateral fissure inferiorly, and the inferior medial extremity of the parieto-occipital fissure anteriorly.

The fissures and convolutions of the basilar, or tentorial, surface of the occipital lobe are uninterruptedly continuous with those of the corresponding surface of the temporal lobe. The inferior surface of these two lobes will therefore be considered together with the lower occipito-temporal surface.

The **Temporal Lobe** (Plates XXII; XXVI), the irregular pyramidal-shaped part of the hemisphere of the cerebrum, the apex of which extends into the middle cranial fossa, and which, at its posterior portion, rests upon the tentorium cerebelli, lies behind the commencement of the basilar, or main, portion of the fissure of Sylvius (*lateral fissure*), in front of a line drawn over the lateral surface of the hemisphere of the cerebrum from the extremity of the lateral limb of the parieto-occipital fissure to the pre-occipital notch and below the horizontal limb of the fissure of Sylvius (*lateral fissure*), and a line representing its continuation backward. The posterior portion of this lobe is continuous with the parietal and occipital lobes (see the description of those lobes).

SURFACES.—The temporal lobe presents three surfaces: a lateral, an inferior, or basilar, and a superior, or opercular. The last-named is in relation with the horizontal limb of the fissure of Sylvius (*lateral fissure*). Upon the lateral surface are three secondary fissures which run horizontally: the superior temporal, or parallel, fissure, the middle temporal, and the inferior temporal fissure. Of these fissures, the superior temporal, or parallel, is the most constant, and lies entirely on the lateral surface; the middle and the inferior are variable. They are seldom clearly developed, and are frequently interrupted and bridged by convolutions. The middle temporal fissure lies almost entirely on the lateral surface, while the greater part of the inferior temporal fissure is on the inferior surface.

The **superior temporal,** or **parallel, fissure** commences near the anterior extremity, or apex, of the lobe. It then runs backward and upward, parallel with the horizontal limb of the fissure of Sylvius (*lateral fissure*) (hence the name of parallel fissure), and terminates in the inferior parietal convolution, its posterior extremity being surrounded by the angular convolution.

The **middle temporal fissure** commences on the inferior surface of the lobe, and runs upward and backward, parallel with the superior temporal fissure. It terminates in the inferior parietal convolution, its posterior extremity being surrounded by the postparietal convolution.

The **inferior temporal fissure** lies a short distance medial to the inferolateral margin of the hemisphere, and terminates posteriorly on the lateral surface. It separates the inferior temporal convolution from the lateral occipito-temporal gyrus, or fusiform lobule.

CONVOLUTIONS.—Through the medium of the superior and middle temporal fissures the lateral surface of the temporal lobe is divided into three convolutions: the superior temporal, the middle temporal, and the inferior temporal convolution.

The **superior temporal,** or **inframarginal, convolution** lies between the horizontal limb of the fissure of Sylvius (*lateral fissure*) and the parallel fissure; it is continuous at its posterior part with the supramarginal and angular convolutions of the parietal lobe.

The **middle temporal convolution** lies between the parallel and the middle temporal fissures, being clearly marked off above by the parallel fissure. Its lower boundary, not always so well marked, is frequently continuous with the inferior temporal convolution. It is continuous posteriorly with the angular and postparietal convolutions.

The **inferior temporal convolution** lies along the lateral margin of the hemisphere, between the middle and the inferior temporal fissures. It passes above the pre-occipital notch, and is continuous behind with the third occipital convolution. Upon the basilar surface of the lobe it is continuous with the lateral occipito-temporal convolution, or fusiform lobule.

The **superior,** or **Sylvian, surface of the temporal lobe** is in contact with the operculum, and is intimately related to the island of Reil (*insula*); it presents two or three transverse convolutions.

The fissures and convolutions presenting on the *basilar surface,* being continuous with those of the occipital lobe, will be described as part of the lower occipito-temporal surface.

Collateral Fissure.—The basilar surface of the temporal lobe contains the greater portion of the inferior temporal fissure (as described at p. 135). That portion of this surface which is continuous with the occipital lobe, and is designated as the inferior occipito-temporal surface, presents a constant and important secondary fissure, the inferior occipito-temporal, or collateral, fissure. This fissure commences at the posterior extremity of the occipital lobe; thence runs forward parallel to and below the calcarine fissure, nearly to the apex of the temporal lobe, extending almost as far as the beginning of the Sylvian (*lateral*) fissure. It is sometimes bridged over by a secondary convolution. The anterior portion of this fissure produces the eminentia collateralis, a prominence in the floor of the descending cornu of the lateral ventricle, seen at the point of divergence of the middle and posterior cornua of the ventricle. Through the medium of the collateral and hippocampal fissures, the **inferior occipito-temporal surface** (Plate XXVI) is divided into three convolutions: the fusiform lobule, the lingual lobule, and the hippocampal, or uncinate, convolution. The hippocampal convolution and the lingual lobule are in reality portions of the internal, or medial, occipito-temporal convolution.

The **lingual lobule** lies between the collateral fissure on the lateral side, and the calcarine fissure on the medial side. It occupies chiefly the occipital part of the lower occipito-temporal surface. It is wide behind and narrow in front.

The **hippocampal gyrus** lies between the collateral fissure on the lateral side, and the hippocampal on the medial side. It comprises the inferior part of the limbic lobe. It continues forward, bordering the hippocampal fissure and embracing the crura cerebri (*cerebral peduncles*), to terminate immediately behind the anterior perforated space (*substantia perforata*) by turning upward and backward upon itself in a rounded hook-like projection, the *uncus*. Between the uncus and the apex of the temporal lobe is the incisura temporalis.

The **lateral occipito-temporal convolution,** or **fusiform lobule,** belonging partly to the occipital and partly to the temporal lobe, lies between the collateral fissure on the medial side, and the inferior temporal fissure, when present, on the lateral side. When the inferior temporal fissure is wanting or is incomplete, the lateral boundary of this convolution is indistinct. It extends from the apex of the temporal lobe to the posterior extremity of the occipital lobe.

The **hippocampal,** or **dentate, fissure** (Plate XXVI), previously mentioned as being bordered by the hippocampal convolution, corresponds to the lateral portion of the transverse fissure of Bichat. It is situated in front of the calcarine fissure, between the crura cerebri (*cerebral peduncles*) and the hippocampal convolution, and extends lateralward, downward, and forward from the splenium of the corpus callosum to the uncus. It produces the cornu ammonis, or hippocampus major, a prominence forming part of the medial wall of the middle (*inferior*) cornu of the lateral ventricle. By drawing the hippocampal convolution away from the crus cerebri (*cerebral peduncle*), thus widening the hippocampal fissure, there will be seen a band of gray matter, the *fascia dentata*, or the *dentate convolution*, reaching from the splenium of the corpus callosum to the uncus. This is the free edge of the hippocampal convolution. Its notched appearance is produced by the choroid arteries, which with the pia mater pass through the fissure into the descending (*inferior*) horn of the lateral ventricle.

The remaining fissures seen on the medial surface of the hemisphere of the cerebrum are the calloso-marginal (*cingulate sulcus*) and the callosal, and the remaining convolution is the gyrus fornicatus.

The **calloso-marginal fissure** (**sulcus cinguli**), the terminal portion of which was mentioned when describing the location of the fissure of Rolando (*central sulcus*) (p. 115), commences below the rostrum of the corpus callosum, curves forward around the genu, and backward above the body of the corpus callosum. It runs about midway between the corpus callosum and the upper border of the hemisphere to a point opposite the splenium of the corpus callosum, where it turns upward and slightly backward to terminate on the upper border of the hemisphere of the cerebrum, immediately behind the commencement of the fissure of Rolando (*central sulcus*). From the point where the fissure turns upward to reach the margin of the hemisphere there is frequently found, following the original direction of the calloso-marginal fissure (*cingulate sulcus*), a small fissure which separates the quadrate lobule from the gyrus fornicatus. This, under the name of the *subparietal fissure*, is a branch of the calloso-marginal, as is also the paracentral fissure. The calloso-marginal fissure (*cingulate sulcus*) is frequently bridged over in places by secondary convolutions which connect the marginal gyrus with the gyrus fornicatus.

The **callosal fissure,** or ventricle of the corpus callosum, commences below the rostrum, follows the superior surface of the corpus callosum, and terminates behind the splenium of the corpus callosum in the hippocampal fissure.

The **gyrus fornicatus** lies between the calloso-marginal fissure (*cingulate sulcus*) and the callosal fissure. It is composed of two parts, an anterosuperior portion, the callosal gyrus, and an inferior portion, the hippocampal gyrus, connected by an isthmus. It commences in front of the anterior perforated space (*substantia perforata*), between the rostrum of the corpus callosum and the marginal convolution (*medial part of superior frontal convolution*), follows the superficial surface of the corpus callosum, and terminates below the splenium of the corpus callosum in a narrow extremity, the *isthmus*, which joins the hippocampal convolution.

The **limbic lobe** (frequently spoken of as the gyrus fornicatus) includes a number of convolutions arranged in a ring-like manner; some of the parts are quite rudimentary in the human brain, and are the representatives of more highly developed structures in some of the lower animals. The limbic lobe is made up of the gyrus fornicatus, hippocampal gyrus, the rudimentary gyrus supracallosus of Zuckerkandl (formed by the peduncles of the corpus callosum, fascia dentata, and the longitudinal striæ on the upper surface of the corpus callosum), together with half of the fornix and the corresponding lamina of the septum lucidum (*septum pellucidum*). This lobe is bounded by the calloso-marginal fissure (*cingulate sulcus*) and the collateral fissure, and each of its extremities is continuous with one of the roots of the olfactory tract.

CRANIO-CEREBRAL TOPOGRAPHY

Sensory and Motor Areas (Plate XXIX).—Having completed the study of the fissures, the lobes, and the convolutions of the hemisphere of the cerebrum,

PLATE XXIX.

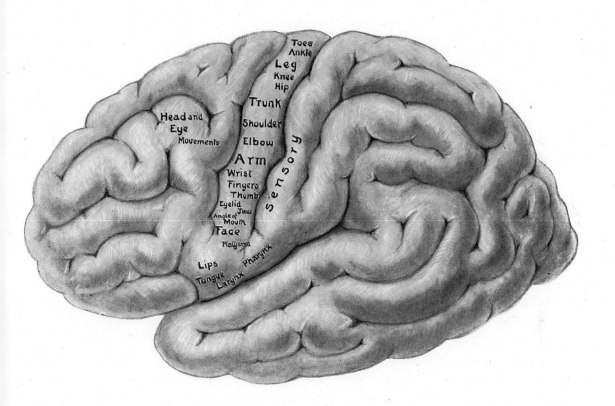

MOTOR AND SENSORY AREAS OF CEREBRUM.

we will consider the functions of the convolutions in certain areas of the surfaces of the cerebrum before commencing the dissection of that part of the brain. The two principal regions of the hemisphere are the motor and the sensory areas. The motor area comprises the posterior ends of the superior, middle, and inferior frontal convolutions, the ascending frontal convolution, the ascending parietal convolution, and the adjoining part of the superior parietal convolution. The sensory area of the surface of the cerebrum is less perfectly outlined on account of the greater difficulty attending its localization.

The Silent Region.—The anterior two-thirds of the superior, middle, and inferior frontal convolutions, or that portion of the frontal lobe which, with the brain in its natural position, practically lies in advance of the coronal suture, is the *prefrontal*, or *silent*, *region* of the brain. A lesion of this area does not give rise to any localizing symptoms. The prefrontal region may be severely injured in gunshot wounds or by abscess formation with entire absence of any paralytic symptoms. The function over which this region of the brain is believed to preside is that of the higher mental faculties, and in disease or injury of this region, particularly upon the left side, there is very apt to be more or less hebetude, dullness of intellect, and lack of self-control. There may also be present a tendency toward jocosity.

Motor Centers.—The motor area embraces the centers which preside over the movements of the opposite side of the body, and is conveniently divided into an upper, a middle, and a lower third. The *upper third* includes the centers which control the movements of the muscles of the lower extremity; the *middle third*, those which control the movements of the muscles of the upper extremity, and the *lower third*, those which control the movements of the muscles of the face, the mouth, and the tongue. In other words, the motor areas are inverted on the surface of the brain, the lower extremity being at the top of the fissure of Rolando (*sulcus centralis*), the arm at the middle, and the face at the bottom. It would seem that the centers for *tactile sensation* are located in the same area as that occupied by the motor centers, for some loss of tactile sense may accompany motor paralysis; hence the centers about to be described are at times referred to as the sensory-motor areas. There is some evidence in favor of locating the centers for *muscular sense* in the region just posterior to the motor area, in the neighborhood of the great longitudinal fissure. The following is a detailed description of the location of the individual centers of the motor and sensory areas (Ferrier): The centers which control the movements of the opposite leg and foot, such as are concerned, for example, in walking, are situated in the anterior part of the superior parietal convolution, at its junction with the ascending parietal, in the paracentral lobule and part of the quadrate lobule. The upper part of the ascending frontal convolution with the neighboring part of the base of the superior frontal convolution includes the centers which control the various complex movements of the arms and legs, such as climbing, swimming, etc. The posterior third of the superior frontal convolution anterior to the junction of its base with the ascending frontal includes the centers for the forward extension of the arm and hand, as in reaching forth the hand to touch something in front. The upper part of the middle third of the ascending frontal convolution includes the centers for those movements of the hand and forearm which call into action the biceps, as supination of the hand and flexion of the forearm. The ascending frontal convolution, at about the junction of its middle and lower thirds, includes the centers which control the action of the elevators and depressors of the angle of the mouth.

The base of the third frontal convolution and, to a slight degree, the lower end of the ascending frontal and ascending parietal convolutions include the centers for the movements of the lips and tongue in talking. This region is known as *Broca's region*, disease of which on the left side causes *aphasia*, or loss of the power of speech. The speech center, however, is not always in the left side of the brain. In left-handed persons it is located, as has been demonstrated clinically, in the base of the right third frontal convolution.

Aphasia may be *motor* or *sensory* in character. There are four centers in the brain concerned in this condition. Two are sensory, two are motor. The *Auditory Speech Center* (A) in the first left temporal convolution, known as Wernicke's zone, is the area devoted to the understanding of the spoken word (*hearing*), and the auditory memory centers lie close by in the temporal lobe. The *Visual Speech Center* (V) is in the angular and supramarginal gyri, is also sensory, and is the center for the understanding of the written word. The *Motor Speech Center* (S) lies in the third left frontal convolution, which region is also known as *Broca's* area. It is the center devoted to the expression of words by speech, and, it will be noted, lies close to the cortical area for movements of the tongue and larynx. The *Writing Center* (W) is situated in the second left frontal convolution, and thus close to the motor cortical areas for the hand. Although rare, discrete lesions may produce pure forms of these aphasias, however, in lesions of the motor speech area there is frequently an associated agraphia, or disturbance in writing, because of the proximity of the two centers. In lesions of the angular gyrus (*sensory visual area*) and the first temporal convolution (*sensory auditory area*), there may be disturbances of one or both functions due to their proximity. There may also be visual field defects because of the presence just below the cortex of the visual pathways in the temporal lobe, giving rise to a right homonymous field defect. Lesions which affect the pathways between

PLATE XXX.

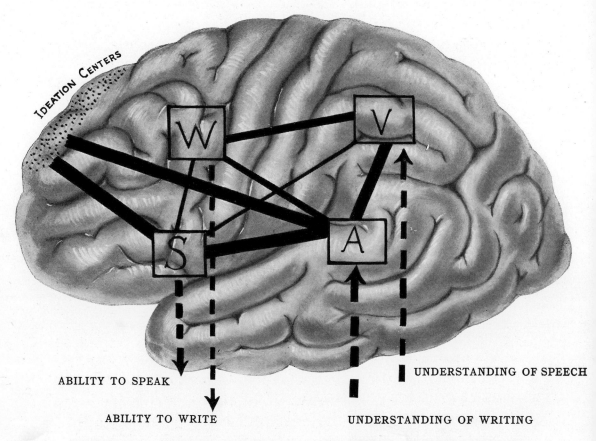

CORTICAL SPEECH CENTERS AND THEIR CONNECTIONS

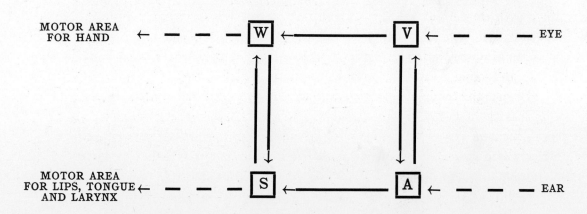

DIAGRAMATIC RELATIONS OF SPEECH CENTERS

these centers give rise to partial forms. This is especially true in lesions just anterior to the auditory-visual areas, producing what is known as jargon aphasia. The patient can speak but is unable to say the word that he desires, due to either a loss of this memory area or involvement of the connecting pathways to the motor speech center. Plate XXX may help to fix the relation of these centers in the reader's mind.

The lower third of the ascending parietal convolution, at its junction with the inferior parietal, includes the center which controls the movements of the platysma muscle in bringing about retraction of the angle of the mouth. The base of the middle frontal convolution includes the center for lateral movements of the head and eyes, with elevation of the eyelids and dilatation of the pupil. The middle third of the ascending parietal convolution includes the centers for the movements of the fingers and wrist.

The cortical centers for the different muscles and limbs overlap to a certain extent, so that while there is a more or less distinct focus of representation for a given set of muscles, adjacent parts of the cortex are also concerned in governing the muscles presided over by the focus; hence, total paralysis does not necessarily follow removal of a limited area of the cortex of the cerebrum.

The supramarginal and angular convolutions, in addition to the occipital lobe, include the *centers of vision;* these, taken together, have been termed by Ferrier the occipito-angular region. The posterior part of the superior temporal convolution includes the *centers of hearing.* The anterior extremity of the hippocampal convolution, or uncus, includes the *center of smell,* while in close proximity to the center of smell is the *center of taste.* The convolution of the corpus callosum and the posterior part of the hippocampal convolution include the *center of touch.*

Each occipital lobe receives visual impulses from one-half of each retina, so that a unilateral cerebral lesion may produce what is known as *hemianopsia,* a symmetric defect in the field of vision of the two eyes.

Disease of the Cortex of the Cerebrum.—Irritation of the motor area, as by a small meningeal hemorrhage, meningitis, or the application of a weak Faradic current, causes twitching or convulsive movements of the muscles of the opposite side. When the motor area is destroyed by disease or injury, there is complete paralysis of motion of the opposite side. If both the motor and the sensory areas are involved in the pathologic process, both sensation and motion of the opposite side will be affected. In trephining for focal, or Jacksonian, epilepsy it is customary when the brain cortex has been exposed to apply a weak Faradic current to that portion believed to include the centers which were concerned in the initial convulsive seizure; in other words, the convulsive movements which

10

the patient exhibited during the attacks are reproduced by the application of the current. In this manner the different centers presiding over the various movements of the opposite side can be located. It is hardly necessary to say that if a lesion, such as an enlarged Pacchionian body (*arachnoid granulation*), a cyst, a cicatrix, or a neoplasm is found, it should be excised. This operation therefore demonstrates the effect of both irritation and destruction of the motor area. In following up the cases of Jacksonian epilepsy treated by operation, it is interesting to note that the paralysis which follows any destruction of the cortex diminishes after a time.

Abolition of the function of certain groups of centers in the motor area of the cortex cerebri results in one or other of the following varieties of paralysis: if of the arm and leg, it is called brachio-crural paralysis, or hemiplegia; if of the leg alone, crural monoplegia; if of the arm alone, brachial monoplegia; if of the face alone, facial monoplegia. Facial monoplegia seldom occurs alone, and is most commonly associated with motor aphasia, owing to the close proximity of the facial and speech centers.

The centers of hearing, vision, smell, and taste may be irritated by various lesions, so that hallucinations of these senses, like motor disturbances, may arise from irritation of the sensory cortex, producing the so-called sensory equivalent of a Jacksonian convulsion. From the character of this attack deductions as to the location of the lesion may be drawn. In the case of visual hallucinations they may be divided into two groups: (a) the crude, composed of flashes of light or color, (b) the formed, wherein objects such as tables, horses, men etc. appear. The crude indicate the presence of a lesion in the occipital lobe or pathways connecting it with the thalamus. The formed hallucinations occur from irritation of lesions in the thalamus or the optic tracts between it and the eye.

DISSECTION.—Shave the scalp upon one side of the head, and upon the other turn its entire thickness down in one flap. Upon that side where the skull wall is exposed remove half of the calvaria with a saw or a chisel and mallet. Next reflect the dura mater in one flap and dissect off the arachnoid and pia mater to expose the fissures and convolutions.

A familiarity with certain of the cranial landmarks is essential in the study of cranio-cerebral topography. These include the glabella (a point between the eyebrows), the frontal eminence, the external angular (*zygomatic*) process of the frontal bone, the zygomatic arch, the pre-auricular fossa (the depression in front of the tragus on a level with the upper border of the external auditory meatus), the external auditory meatus, the mastoid process, the parietal eminence, and the external occipital protuberance, or inion.

PLATE XXXI.

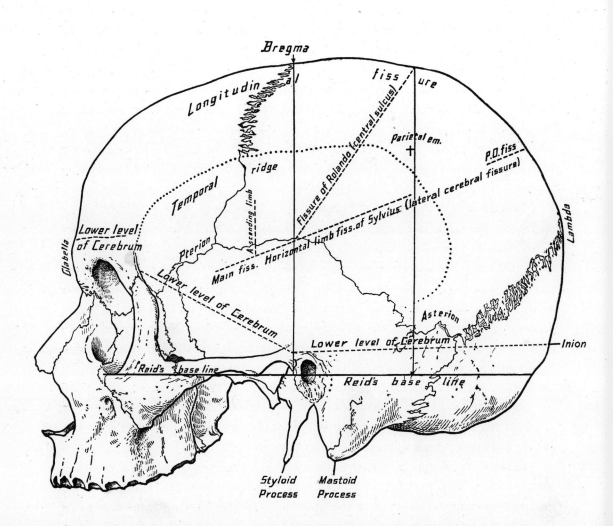

LINES FOR FISSURES; LOWER LEVEL OF CEREBRUM.

The Lower Level of the Cerebrum (Plate XXXI).—A line drawn horizontally across the forehead through the upper part of the glabella approximately corresponds to the lower level of the cerebrum in front. A line drawn from the external angular (*zygomatic*) process of the frontal bone through the pre-auricular fossa to the external occipital protuberance approximately corresponds to the lower level of the cerebrum at the sides and back. This is known as Reid's base line. The **cerebellum** lies below that portion of the last-mentioned line included between the posterior border of the mastoid process and the inion.

Longitudinal and Transverse Fissures.—A line drawn from the glabella over the vertex and along the median line to the inion corresponds to the position of the longitudinal fissure. A line drawn from the inion along the superior curved (*superior nuchal*) line of the occipital bone to a point two and a half centimeters above the external auditory meatus corresponds to the position of the transverse fissure.

Fissure of Sylvius (Lateral Fissure).—To indicate the position of the fissure of Sylvius (*lateral fissure*), draw a line from a point three centimeters (one and one-fourth inches) behind the external angular (*zygomatic*) process of the frontal bone to a point two centimeters (three-fourths of an inch) below the most prominent part of the parietal eminence. The first two centimeters of the line represent the main fissure; the remainder of the line, the horizontal limb of the fissure. The ascending limb of the fissure is represented by drawing a line, two and a half centimeters in length, vertically upward from the point of termination of the main fissure, that is, two centimeters from its commencement, or five centimeters behind the external angular (*zygomatic*) process of the frontal bone.

Reid's base line is drawn from the lower border of the orbit through the center of the external auditory meatus. This line is of assistance in locating the fissure of Rolando (*central sulcus*).

Fissure of Rolando (Central Sulcus).—To represent the position of the fissure of Rolando, first draw two perpendicular lines from the base line to the line representing the position of the great longitudinal fissure. The anterior of these lines passes through the pre-auricular fossa, and the posterior one passes along the posterior border of the mastoid process. From the point of intersection of the posterior perpendicular line with that of the great longitudinal fissure, to the point of intersection of the anterior perpendicular line with that of the horizontal limb of the fissure of Sylvius (*lateral fissure*), draw a third line, which represents the position of the fissure of Rolando (*central sulcus*). The fissure of Rolando (*central sulcus*) may also be located by drawing a line downward, lateralward, and forward from a point one centimeter behind a point midway between the glabella and the inion and at an angle of sixty-seven and one-half degrees with the anterior portion of the line for the longitudinal fissure. The angle formed by the fissure of Rolando (*central sulcus*) and the anterior portion of the longitudinal fissure varies, but, in many instances, the line for the fissure is merely an approximate guide. The fissure measures about eight and one-half centimeters (three and three-eighths inches) in length. Upon each side of, and running parallel with the fissure of Rolando (*central sulcus*) are the ascending frontal and ascending parietal convolutions, each of which occupies a space about two centimeters (three-fourths of an inch) in width.

Parieto-occipital fissure.—Extend the line indicating the horizontal limb of the fissure of Sylvius (*lateral fissure*) backward to that of the longitudinal fissure, and the lateral limb of the parieto-occipital fissure will be represented by about the posterior two and a half centimeters of this line. The lateral portion of the parieto-occipital fissure is also found from eight to nine centimeters (three to three and one-half inches) above the external occipital protuberance.

Frontal Lobe.—Through the medium of the lines indicating the course of the primary fissures of the hemisphere the lobes are mapped out. The frontal lobe lies lateral to the line of the longitudinal fissure, in front of the line of the fissure of Rolando (*central sulcus*), and above the lines for the lower level of the cerebrum and for the main and horizontal limbs of the fissure of Sylvius (*lateral fissure*). The course of the secondary fissures and the position of the convolutions of this lobe will be represented by the following lines: a line drawn from the supra-orbital notch backward and parallel with the line of the longitudinal fissure to within about two centimeters of the line of the fissure of Rolando (*central sulcus*) indicates the course of the superior frontal sulcus. A line drawn from the external angular (*zygomatic*) process of the frontal bone upward and backward along the temporal ridge to within about two centimeters of the line of the fissure of Rolando (*central sulcus*) indicates the course of the inferior frontal fissure. A line drawn two centimeters in front of, and parallel with the lower two-thirds of the line of the fissure of Rolando (*central sulcus*) indicates, approximately, the course of the precentral fissure. The superior frontal convolution corresponds to the interval between the lines of the longitudinal and superior frontal fissures. The middle frontal convolution corresponds to the interval between the lines of the superior and inferior frontal fissures. The inferior frontal convolution corresponds to the interval between the line of the inferior frontal fissure and the lines representing the fissure of Sylvius (*lateral fissure*) and the lower level of the cerebrum in front. The ascending frontal convolution corresponds to the interval between the lines of the fissure of Rolando (*central sulcus*) and the precentral fissure.

The **parietal lobe** lies between the lines of the longitudinal fissure and the horizontal limb of the fissure of Sylvius (*lateral fissure*), and between the line of the fissure of Rolando (*central sulcus*) and that of the lateral limb of the parieto-occipital fissure. The boundary between the parietal and occipital lobes is indicated, approximately, by a line drawn from the lateral limb of the parieto-occipital fissure to the posterior border of the base of the mastoid process. The course of the intraparietal fissure (*interparietal sulcus*) and the position of the convolutions of the parietal lobe are represented as follows: To indicate the course of the intraparietal fissure (*interparietal sulcus*) draw a line from a point one centimeter lateral to the end of the lateral limb of the parieto-occipital fissure to a point two centimeters behind the lower end of the fissure of Rolando (*central sulcus*), which is convex forward; the lower third of the line should run parallel with the fissure of Rolando (*central sulcus*). The interval bounded by this line and the lines of the fissure of Rolando (*central sulcus*), the longitudinal fissure, and the lateral limb of the parieto-occipital fissure will correspond to the ascending and superior parietal convolutions. The ascending parietal convolution runs parallel with the line of the fissure of Rolando (*central sulcus*), and corresponds to the space directly behind it to the extent of two centimeters, while the remaining portion of the space included in the above boundaries corresponds to the superior parietal convolution. The inferior parietal convolution, including the supramarginal and angular gyri, corresponds to the interval bounded by the line of the intraparietal fissure (*interparietal sulcus*), that of the horizontal limb of the fissure of Sylvius (*lateral fissure*), and the line drawn from the lateral limb of the parieto-occipital fissure to the posterior margin of the base of the mastoid process. The supramarginal gyrus lies under the most prominent part of the eminence.

The **occipital lobe** lies behind the line drawn from the lateral limb of the parieto-occipital fissure to the posterior margin of the base of the mastoid process.

The **temporal lobe** lies below the line of the horizontal limb of the fissure of Sylvius (*lateral fissure*) and above the upper border of the zygoma, and a line representing the continuation of the latter backward to a point slightly above the superior curved (*superior nuchal*) line of the occipital bone. The posterior boundary of this lobe corresponds, approximately, to a line drawn from the external portion of the parieto-occipital fissure to the posterior limit of the base or root of the mastoid process. This lobe in front reaches as far as the posterior superior border of the malar (*zygomatic*) bone. A line drawn parallel with, and two and one-half centimeters (one inch) below the line of the horizontal limb of the fissure of Sylvius (*lateral fissure*) indicates the course of the superior temporal fissure.

A line drawn parallel with, and two centimeters below the latter line indicates the course of the middle temporal fissure. The superior temporal convolution corresponds to the interval between the line of the horizontal limb of the fissure of Sylvius (*lateral fissure*) and the line of the superior temporal fissure. The middle temporal convolution corresponds to the interval between the lines of the superior and middle temporal fissures.

Individual Variations and How to Determine Them.—It should be borne in mind that the brain of one individual differs from that of another; therefore, there is no method which will in all instances represent the position of the fissures and convolutions with absolute correctness. After the brain cortex is exposed in an operation, the Faradic current can be applied to decide what portion of the motor area of the cortex has been exposed. It can be readily appreciated that through so small an opening as that made by the trephine it is scarcely possible to recognize special fissures and convolutions, especially in view of the difficulty often experienced in locating them in the dissection of the brain.

Indications for Trephining.—Excluding trephining for fracture of the skull, the cranial cavity is opened for one of several purposes: to expose the superior maxillary (*maxillary*) and inferior maxillary (*mandibular*) nerves for the purpose of excising one or both for trigeminal neuralgia, or section of the posterior root of the trigeminal nerve; to remove a blood clot; to control hemorrhage from one or both branches of the middle meningeal artery; to open the lateral (*transverse*) sinus in septic thrombosis due to middle ear disease; to remove a brain tumor or a foreign body; to evacuate an abscess; to relieve intracranial pressure; to tap the lateral ventricles, and for traumatic epilepsy, where localizing symptoms occur.

To Expose the Lateral (Transverse) Sinus.—In septic thrombosis of the lateral (*transverse*) sinus due to middle ear disease, that portion of the sinus in relation with the mastoid process, the sigmoid portion, is exposed. To reach this portion, first draw two lines, one vertical through the middle of the mastoid process, and a second on a level with the roof of the external auditory (*acoustic*) meatus and at a right angle to the first. At the point of junction of these two lines apply the center pin of a two and a half centimeter trephine. The most superficial portion of this sinus is not so deeply situated as the mastoid antrum, being, as a rule, about six millimeters (one-fourth of an inch) from the surface of the bone. Before removing the clot from the sigmoid sinus, the internal jugular vein should be ligated to control hemorrhage and prevent dissemination of emboli. As a thrombus of the sigmoid sinus seldom occurs except as a complication of disease of the mastoid antrum, the latter is usually opened first, and it is then desirable to expose the sinus on its anterior aspect by removing the bony tissue between the antrum and the sinus, which often contains the channels through which the sinus has become infected.

Localized Affections.—In operating for focal epilepsy, brain tumor, or blood clot the trephine is applied to the skull directly over the part of the brain believed to be the site of involvement, as determined by localizing symptoms. The lines which indicate the courses of the fissures are the principal guides.

Foreign Bodies.—In removing, or perhaps it would be better to say in attempting to remove a foreign body (as these are most commonly bullets and in the majority of cases located with difficulty), the cranial cavity is attacked at the wound of entrance. The operation of trephining in this class of cases increases the chance of finding the foreign body and establishes drainage. Where the bullet is located in a portion of the brain that is silent, or if the patient shows no irritative symptoms, it is wise to let the foreign body alone, as the damage due to exploration of a deep-seated object is greater than the presence of the foreign body.

Intracranial Abscess.—The most common locations for intracranial abscess, usually the result of middle ear disease, are the temporal, cerebellar, and extradural regions. In operating for *temporal abscess*, which is usually located in the posterior half of the lobe, first draw two parallel lines at right angles to Reid's base line, the anterior passing through the center of the external auditory (*acoustic*) meatus, and the other about three centimeters behind it. Apply the center pin of the trephine over a point three centimeters above Reid's base line and between the two vertical lines. In operating for *cerebellar abscess*, which is usually situated in the anterior and lateral part of the hemisphere of the cerebellum, apply the center pin of the trephine at a point four centimeters behind the center of the external auditory (*acoustic*) meatus, and two and one-half centimeters below Reid's base line. The point over which to trephine in *extradural* or *subdural abscess* must depend, to a great degree, upon the presence of localizing symptoms. The constitutional evidences of pus and the history of the case, together with circumscribed edema and localizing symptoms, such as spastic contraction or paresis of certain muscles, would constitute the most reliable guides. Septic meningitis, as far as the constitutional symptoms are concerned, frequently so closely simulates cerebral abscess that a differential diagnosis, in the absence of localizing symptoms, is impossible.

To Tap the Lateral Ventricles, and Ventriculograms.—By means of ventriculograms it is now possible to determine the size and shape of the ventricles. This is accomplished by introducing a cannula into the posterior cornu of the lateral ventricle and withdrawing its fluid content. Air is then injected to replace the fluid, and stereoscopic x-ray pictures taken of the head. These will definitely throw a shadow of the ventricular outline, so that it becomes possible to determine the presence of hydrocephalus or a distortion or deformity of the ventricles due to a deep-seated unlocalizable lesion of the brain. The operation is undertaken at a point three centimeters (one and one-fourth inches) from the midline and six centimeters (two and a half inches) above the occipital protuberance. A small skin incision is made large enough to permit a trephine opening, and the dura carefully incised. A Cotton cannula is then introduced through the occipital pole, on a plane on a level with the tip of the ear and passing forward and slightly lateralward. Normally, the posterior horn of the ventricle is usually encountered at about five and one-half centimeters from the skin surface.

The interpretation of the x-ray plates becomes most important, as frequently the distortion of the ventricle leads to definite localization in subcortical lesions. Lesions obstructing the aqueduct of Sylvius (*cerebral aqueduct*) produce intense internal hydrocephalus with dilatation of both the lateral and third ventricles. Lesions in one hemisphere usually produce a filling defect in the outline and a displacement and enlargement of the opposite ventricle.

THE INTERIOR OF THE CEREBRUM

Material.—In order to study the brain to the best advantage the dissector should have at least two brains at his disposal. One may be used for the study of the fissures, convolutions, and interior of the brain; and the other for making sections of the brain.

Dissection.—Having completed the study of the fissures and the convolutions, next examine the interior of the cerebrum. Place the brain on its base, and separate the hemispheres of the cerebrum, to widen the longitudinal fissure, thus exposing the bottom of the fissure. This is formed in great part by a mass of white matter, the corpus callosum, or the great transverse commissure of the cerebrum, while in front of, and behind the corpus callosum the fissure extends without interruption to the base of the brain. Make a horizontal section of one or both hemispheres on a level with the floor of the longitudinal fissure. When both hemispheres are sliced away to the level of the floor of the longitudinal fissure, the upper surface of the corpus callosum is well exposed. The corpus callosum can now be studied from two points of view: from above in the present dissection, and from the side by looking at its sagittal section, seen in the preparation previously made by severing the two halves of the brain in the line of the longitudinal fissure.

The **Corpus Callosum** (Plate XXXII), the great transverse commissure of the cerebrum, is a transverse band of white matter which spans the longitudinal

PLATE XXXII.

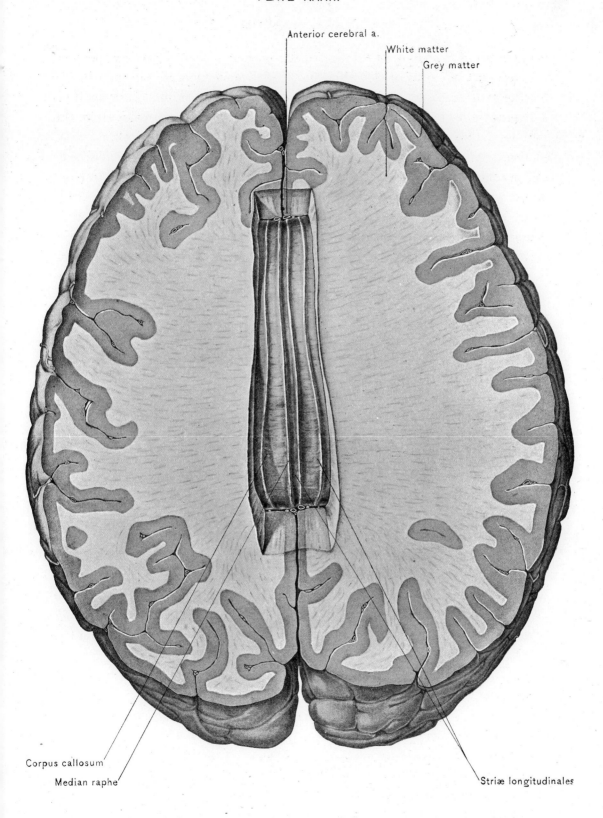

Anterior cerebral a.

White matter

Grey matter

Corpus callosum

Median raphe

Striæ longitudinales

CORPUS CALLOSUM AND HORIZONTAL SECTION OF CEREBRUM.

fissure and connects the hemispheres of the cerebrum for nearly half their length. The *falx cerebri* touches the posterior portion of the corpus callosum; the greater part of the body of the corpus callosum and its anterior extremity are separated for a considerable distance from the falx cerebri. The corpus callosum is slightly convex from before backward on the upper surface; it is from seven to ten centimeters (three to four inches) in length, and extends nearer to the anterior than to the posterior end of the cerebrum. It is wider posteriorly, where it measures about two and one-half centimeters, and is thicker at each end, especially at the posterior extremity, than in the middle. It forms the roof of the lateral ventricles, which are cavities located within the hemispheres of the cerebrum. On its dorsal surface, extending along its middle line, a linear depression exists, the **raphe.** On each side of the raphe, and running parallel with it, are two slightly elevated longitudinal bands, the **striæ longitudinales,** or **nerves of Lancisi.** External to these are the faintly marked **striæ longitudinales laterales,** or **tæniæ tectæ,** which, with the brain intact, underlie the convolutions of the corpus callosum, or gyri fornicati. The tæniæ tectæ are separated bundles of a group of fibers known as the **cingulum,** which forms part of the callosal and hippocampal gyri. The fibers proper of the corpus callosum run transversely, as its name, the great transverse commissure, implies. The corpus callosum consists of a main portion, or body, seen best on longitudinal section, and of two extremities, the anterior and the posterior.

The **anterior extremity,** or **genu,** is formed by the downward and backward bend of the corpus callosum; from this bend it is continued to the base of the brain as the beak, or *rostrum,* which is the reflected portion of the genu, and is thin and narrow. Within the concavity of the genu is situated the septum lucidum (*septum pellucidum*), between the layers of which is the fifth ventricle. The rostrum of the corpus callosum has been described with the base of the brain (p. 93); it is connected to the tuber cinereum by the lamina cinerea (*lamina terminalis*). It gives off two bands of white substance, which are continuations of the nerves of Lancisi (*striæ longitudinales*) and form the peduncles of the corpus callosum. These peduncles then diverge from each other and run backward and lateralward across the anterior perforated space (*substantia perforata anterior*) to the tips of the temporal lobes, meeting the inner roots of the olfactory tracts. The fibers from the genu of the corpus callosum pass lateralward and forward and then medialward, into the prefrontal region, forming the *forceps minor.*

The **posterior extremity of the corpus callosum,** or **splenium,** is formed by a bending of the corpus callosum downward and forward upon itself, thus making a free, thickened, rounded border. This border forms the upper boundary of the central part of the transverse fissure, and beneath it passes the process of the pia mater known as the *velum interpositum* (*tela choroidea of the third ventricle*). The splenium is connected anteriorly with the fornix. The fibers of the splenium which curve lateralward and backward over the posterior horn of the lateral ventricle constitute the *forceps major;* some of these fibers form a long, rounded elevation, the bulb of the posterior cornu of the lateral ventricle.

The under surface of the body of the corpus callosum is connected along the middle line with the fornix and the septum lucidum (*septum pellucidum*), while laterally it forms the roof of the lateral ventricles.

DISSECTION.—Make two sagittal incisions from before backward through the corpus callosum, one centimeter to each side of the median line; this will open the lateral ventricles—cavities which occupy the interior of the hemispheres of the cerebrum. To expose the interior of one or both lateral ventricles so as fully to disclose the contained structures, cut away with a pair of scissors as much of the corpus callosum on each side of the incision as may be necessary. This dissection will not open the inferior or descending, cornu; to accomplish this a section of the lateral portion of the hemisphere (temporal lobe) must be removed. This can be done either from without inward or from within outward by following the course of the cornu with the scalpel.

The **Lateral Ventricles** (Plates XXXIII; XXXIV; XXXV) are two irregularly shaped cavities, one of which is situated in each hemisphere of the cerebrum. They communicate with the third ventricle by way of the foramina of Monro (*interventricular foramina*) and through the third ventricle with the fourth ventricle by way of the aqueduct of Sylvius (*aqueduct of the cerebrum*), or *iter a tertio ad quartum ventriculum.* They are lined by a membrane, the ependyma, whose function is to secrete part of the cerebro-spinal fluid. Each of the ventricles, which are separated in front by a vertical partition, the *septum lucidum* (*septum pellucidum*), consists of four parts: a body, or central, portion and three horns, or cornua. The cornua are designated anterior, inferior, or descending, and posterior; they extend respectively, into the frontal, the temporal, and the occipital lobe of the cerebrum.

The **body of the lateral ventricle (pars centralis)**, in a coronal section, is triangular in shape, its anteroposterior diameter being the longest, and its vertical diameter the shortest. It extends from the foramen of Monro (*interventricular foramen*) to the splenium of the corpus callosum. It is bounded *above* by the corpus callosum; *medially*, by the posterior narrow portion of the septum lucidum (*septum pellucidum*) and the attachment of the corpus callosum to the fornix, and *laterally*, by the merging angle formed by the corpus callosum and the white substance of the hemisphere. Its *floor* is formed by the following parts,

PLATE XXXIII.

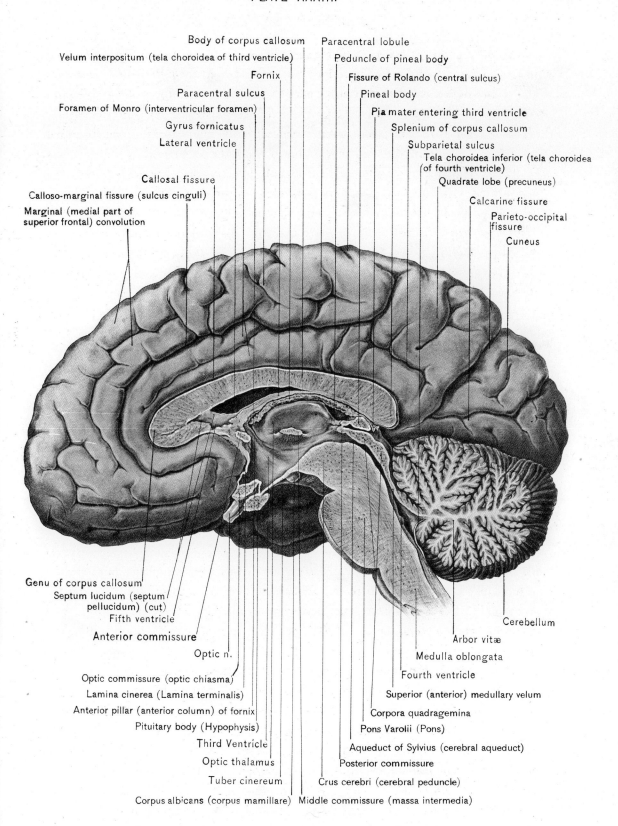

Body of corpus callosum
Velum interpositum (tela choroidea of third ventricle)
Fornix
Paracentral sulcus
Foramen of Monro (interventricular foramen)
Gyrus fornicatus
Lateral ventricle
Callosal fissure
Calloso-marginal fissure (sulcus cinguli)
Marginal (medial part of superior frontal) convolution

Paracentral lobule
Peduncle of pineal body
Fissure of Rolando (central sulcus)
Pineal body
Pia mater entering third ventricle
Splenium of corpus callosum
Subparietal sulcus
Tela choroidea inferior (tela choroidea of fourth ventricle)
Quadrate lobe (precuneus)
Calcarine fissure
Parieto-occipital fissure
Cuneus

Genu of corpus callosum
Septum lucidum (septum pellucidum) (cut)
Fifth ventricle
Anterior commissure
Optic n.
Optic commissure (optic chiasma)
Lamina cinerea (Lamina terminalis)
Anterior pillar (anterior column) of fornix
Pituitary body (Hypophysis)
Third Ventricle
Optic thalamus
Tuber cinereum
Corpus albicans (corpus mamillare)

Cerebellum
Arbor vitæ
Medulla oblongata
Fourth ventricle
Superior (anterior) medullary velum
Corpora quadragemina
Pons Varolii (Pons)
Aqueduct of Sylvius (cerebral aqueduct)
Posterior commissure
Crus cerebri (cerebral peduncle)
Middle commissure (massa intermedia)

MEDIAL SURFACE OF CEREBRUM AND SECTION OF VENTRICLES OF BRAIN.

PLATE XXXIV.

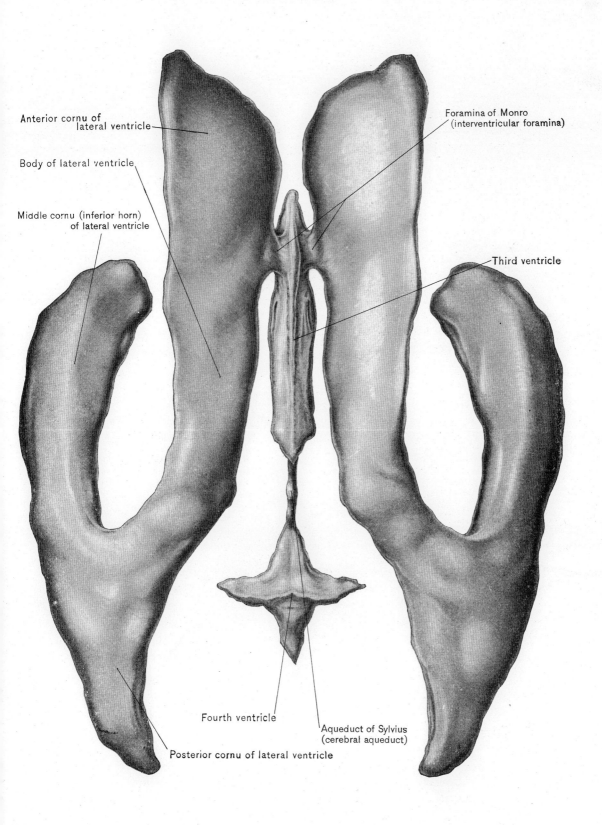

Anterior cornu of
lateral ventricle

Body of lateral ventricle

Middle cornu (inferior horn)
of lateral ventricle

Foramina of Monro
(interventricular foramina)

Third ventricle

Fourth ventricle

Aqueduct of Sylvius
(cerebral aqueduct)

Posterior cornu of lateral ventricle

DIAGRAM OF THE VENTRICLES—SUPERIOR VIEW.

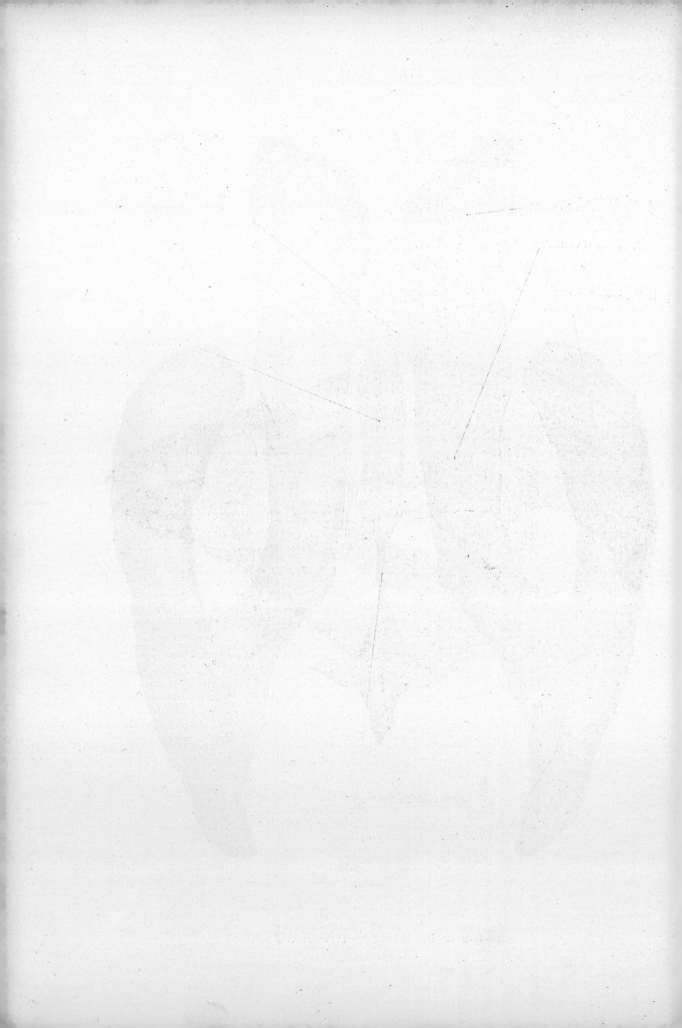

PLATE XXXV.

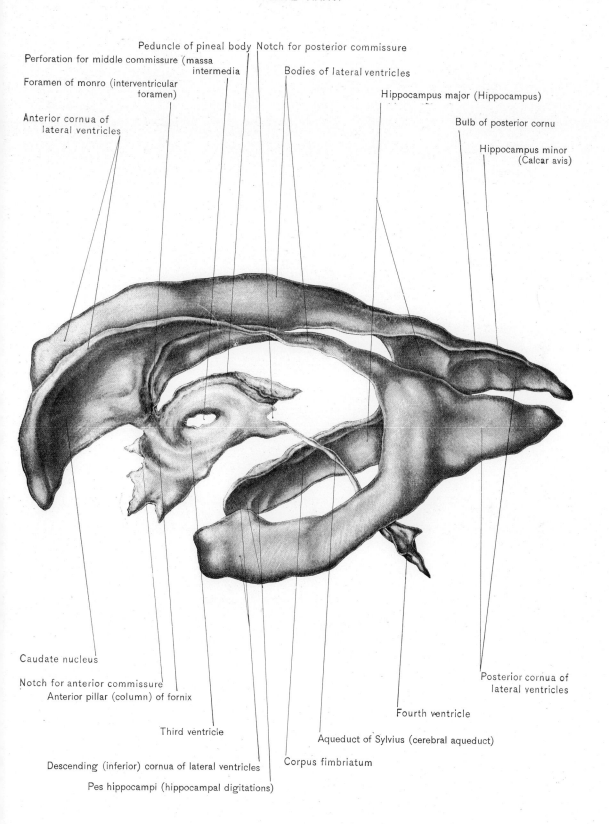

Peduncle of pineal body Notch for posterior commissure

Perforation for middle commissure (massa intermedia)

Foramen of monro (interventricular foramen)

Bodies of lateral ventricles

Hippocampus major (Hippocampus)

Anterior cornua of lateral ventricles

Bulb of posterior cornu

Hippocampus minor (Calcar avis)

Caudate nucleus

Notch for anterior commissure

Anterior pillar (column) of fornix

Posterior cornua of lateral ventricles

Fourth ventricle

Third ventricle

Aqueduct of Sylvius (cerebral aqueduct)

Descending (inferior) cornua of lateral ventricles

Corpus fimbriatum

Pes hippocampi (hippocampal digitations)

DIAGRAM OF THE VENTRICLES—LATERAL VIEW.

PLATE XXXV.

PLATE XXXVI.

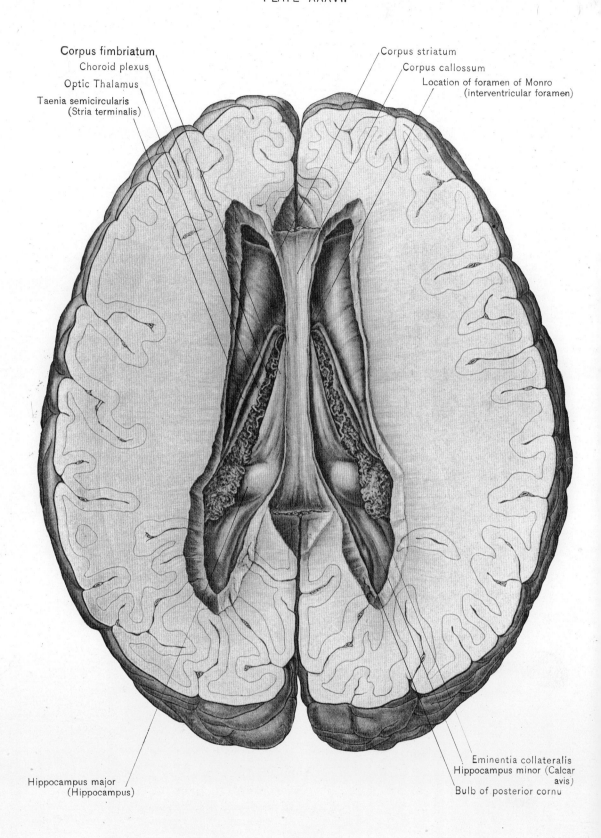

Corpus fimbriatum

Choroid plexus

Optic Thalamus

Taenia semicircularis
(Stria terminalis)

Corpus striatum

Corpus callossum

Location of foramen of Monro
(interventricular foramen)

Eminentia collateralis

Hippocampus minor (Calcar avis)

Bulb of posterior cornu

Hippocampus major
(Hippocampus)

BODIES, ANTERIOR CORNUA, AND POSTERIOR CORNUA OF LATERAL VENTRICLES.

named in their order from without inward: the intraventricular portion of the corpus striatum, or tail of the *caudate nucleus,* the *tænia semicircularis* and the *vein of the striate body,* a small vein of the corpus striatum contained in an oblique groove, the optic thalamus, the choroid plexus, half of the body of the fornix, with its lateral edge, or *corpus fimbriatum.*

The **anterior cornu of the lateral ventricle** (Plate XXXVI), in coronal sections of the brain, is triangular in shape. It extends forward, downward, and lateral-ward into the frontal lobe. It curves around the anterior end of the corpus striatum, and diverges from the anterior cornu of the lateral ventricle of the other side as it passes forward. It is bounded *above* by the fibers of the corpus callosum (forceps minor), which curve lateralward and forward; *medially,* by the septum lucidum (*septum pellucidum*), which separates it from the corresponding cornu of the opposite ventricle; *anteriorly,* by the genu of the corpus callosum, and laterally, by the caudate nucleus. Its *floor* is formed in great part by the cau-date nucleus, which projects into it, and to a slight extent by the rostrum of the corpus callosum.

The **posterior cornu of the lateral ventricle,** the smallest of the three cornua, commences in the body of the ventricle opposite the splenium of the corpus callo-sum, and at the same point as the middle cornu. It extends horizontally back-ward, lateralward, and then medialward into the occipital lobe. Its *roof* is formed by those fibers of the splenium of the corpus callosum (forceps major) which pass backward and lateralward and become continuous with the white matter of the occipital lobe. On its *medial wall* is seen the hippocampus minor, or calcar avis, produced by the calcarine fissure; above this is a smaller promi-nence, the *bulb of the cornu,* produced by the bulging of the fibers of the forceps major into the cavity above and medial to the hippocampus minor. On the *floor* is seen a slight elevation, produced by the fasciculus longitudinalis inferior, which passes from the occipital to the temporal lobe. At the point where the lateral and posterior cornua meet, a triangular, smooth surface is seen, called by Schwalbe the trigonum ventriculi (*trigonum collaterale*).

The **inferior,** or **descending, cornu of the lateral ventricle,** the longest of the three cornua, may be considered the continuation of the cavity of the ventricle into the temporal lobe. It commences opposite the splenium of the corpus callosum, in the body of the ventricle, at the same point at which the posterior cornu begins. It extends backward and lateralward around the posterior extrem-ity of the optic thalamus, and then runs downward, forward, and medialward to reach the base of the brain, terminating about two and one-half centimeters, from the tip of the temporal lobe. Its *roof* is formed by those fibers of the body of the corpus callosum (tapetum) which pass lateralward and become continuous with the white matter of the temporal lobe, and by the tail of the caudate nucleus, the tænia semicircularis, and the amygdaloid tubercle. The *floor* is formed in great part by the *eminentia collateralis*. Upon the *medial wall* are seen the following structures, named from without inward: the hippocampus major and pes hippocampi (*hippocampal digitations*), the corpus fimbriatum, the choroid plexus, and the fascia dentata, or dentate convolution.

DISSECTION.—Make a transverse section of the remaining portion of the body of the corpus callosum at about its middle, and dissect one half forward and the other half backward. If carefully executed, this dissection exposes the fornix and the septum lucidum (*septum pellucidum*).

The **Fornix** (Plate XXXVII), the longitudinal commissure of the cerebrum, is a triangular mass of white matter situated beneath the corpus callosum, and is continuous posteriorly with the splenium of the corpus callosum. It overlies the velum interpositum (*tela choroidea of the third ventricle*), which separates it from the third ventricle and the optic thalamus. It consists of a main portion, or body, and anterior and posterior crura, or pillars.

The **body of the fornix** is triangular in shape, the apex of the triangle being directed anteriorly. The fornix is adherent posteriorly to the splenium of the corpus callosum, and is attached superiorly and anteriorly to the septum lucidum (*septum pellucidum*), and superiorly and posteriorly to the corpus callosum; inferiorly, it rests upon the velum interpositum (*tela choroidea of the third ventricle*), and lies above the third ventricle. The sides of the body of the fornix project into the lateral ventricles, overlapping the medial portion of the optic thalami and choroid plexuses. Owing to their arrangement, the fibers of the under surface of the fornix posteriorly are sometimes called *the lyra Davidis, or psalterium*.

The **anterior crura,** or **pillars of the fornix,** are two cylindrical bundles of nerve-fibers which are given off from the anterior extremity, or apex, of the body of the fornix, whence they diverge and descend in front of the optic thalami and the foramina of Monro (*interventricular foramina*) and then through the gray matter in the sides of the third ventricle to the base of the brain, where they form the white matter of the corpora albicantia or mamillary eminences. Fibers pass from the corpora albicantia (*corpora mamillaria*) to the optic thalami; these fibers constitute the bundles of Vicq d'Azyr (*fasciculi mamillo-thalamici*), and are probably not directly continuous with the fibers of the fornix. In their descent the anterior pillars are joined by the tæniæ semicirculares (*striæ terminales*) and by fibers from the septum lucidum (*septum pellucidum*) and peduncles of the pineal gland. Between the anterior crura and the anterior extremities of the optic thalami are the oval openings of communication between the lateral ventricles and the third ventricle, the foramina of Monro (*interventricular formina*).

PLATE XXXVII.

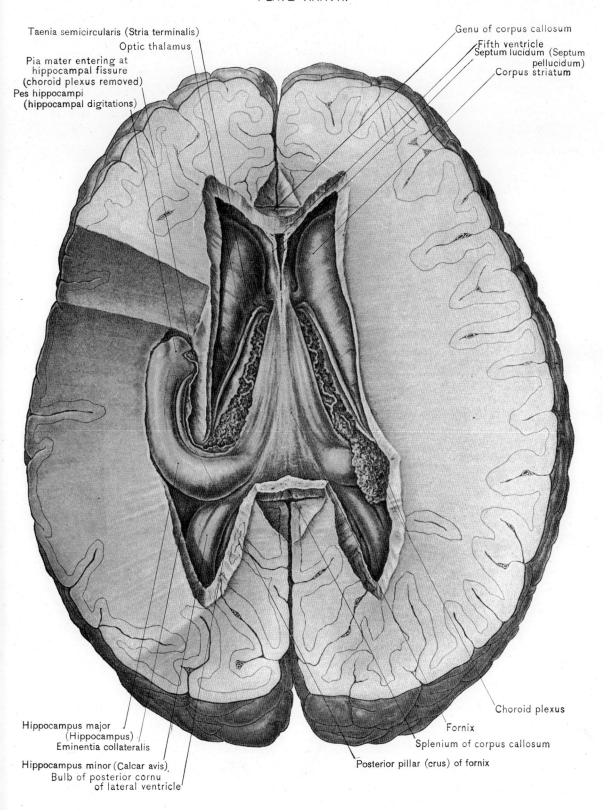

Taenia semicircularis (Stria terminalis)

Optic thalamus

Pia mater entering at
hippocampal fissure
(choroid plexus removed)

Pes hippocampi
(hippocampal digitations)

Genu of corpus callosum

Fifth ventricle
Septum lucidum (Septum
pellucidum)
Corpus striatum

Hippocampus major
(Hippocampus)
Eminentia collateralis

Hippocampus minor (Calcar avis)
Bulb of posterior cornu
of lateral ventricle

Posterior pillar (crus) of fornix

Choroid plexus

Fornix

Splenium of corpus callosum

FORNIX AND LATERAL VENTRICLES, AND DESCENDING (INFERIOR) CORNU OF LEFT LATERAL VENTRICLE.

The **posterior crura,** or **pillars of the fornix,** arise posteriorly from each side of the body of the fornix, hence they diverge and descend into the inferior, or descending, cornua of the lateral ventricles. Here each crus lies within the concavity of the curve described by the hippocampus major as far as the pes hippocampi (*hippocampal digitations*). The lateral borders of the posterior crura of the fornix are known as **corpora fimbriata,** or **tæniæ hippocampi.**

The **septum lucidum** (**septum pellucidum**) is a triangular, vertical partition situated between the anterior portion of the bodies of the two lateral ventricles and between the anterior cornua of those ventricles. The base of the triangle is directed downward and forward, and the apex backward, into the narrow interval between the anterior part of the body of the fornix below, and the corpus callosum above. The septum lucidum (*septum pellucidum*) is attached above to the under surface of the body of the corpus callosum; anteriorly, to the concavity of the genu of the corpus callosum, and below, to the rostrum of the corpus callosum and to the body and anterior crura of the fornix. It is composed of two laminæ, between which is the cleft-like interval known as the fifth ventricle.

The **fifth,** or **Sylvian, ventricle** differs from the other ventricles in its mode of development; it is a portion of the great longitudinal fissure which has become inclosed by the formation of the corpus callosum and fornix. It is thus a completely inclosed space not provided with an outlet. Each of the laminæ of the septum lucidum (*septum pellucidum*), which bound this ventricle laterally, consists of a medial gray layer, a middle white layer, and a lateral layer of ependyma which is part of the ependyma that lines the lateral ventricles.

DISSECTION.—With a pair of scissors slice away a horizontal section from the superior portion of the septum lucidum (*septum pellucidum*), when, with a little care, the laminæ can be pushed apart and the fifth ventricle opened. Should the ventricle contain more than the usual quantity of fluid, it can be more readily seen than in the normal state.

Before reflecting the fornix examine the structures seen within the lateral ventricle, commencing with the corpora striata, which project into the anterior cornua.

Corpus Striatum (Plate XXXVII).—The corpora striata, or anterior cerebral ganglia, are the anterior pair of basal ganglia. The portion seen within the anterior cornu of the lateral ventricle is known as the intraventricular portion, or caudate nucleus, in contradistinction to the larger extraventricular portion, or lenticular (*lentiform*) nucleus, which occupies the white substance of the hemisphere of the cerebrum. To expose both the lenticular (*lentiform*) nucleus and the caudate nucleus in one dissection it is necessary to make horizontal sections of the hemisphere; these sections will be described later.

The **caudate nucleus** is a pear-shaped mass of gray matter having its broad extremity, or head, directed forward into the forepart of the body and the anterior cornu of the lateral ventricle, and its narrow extremity, or tail, directed lateralward and backward. It lies to the lateral side of the optic thalamus, and is prolonged into the roof of the inferior, or descending, horn of the lateral ventricle as far as its anterior extremity, where it terminates in the *amygdaloid tubercle*. Crossing the surface of the caudate nucleus are numerous small veins emptying into the vein of the corpus striatum, which lies in the groove between the caudate nucleus and the optic thalamus. (Plates XXXVII; XLVIII.)

The **tænia semicircularis**, or **stria terminalis**, is a very narrow, longitudinal band of white fibers, which lies in the groove between the caudate nucleus and the optic thalamus, and conceals from view the vein of the corpus striatum. It extends from the anterior crus of the fornix, with which it is continuous in front, backward through the floor of the body of the ventricle, and into and along the roof of the descending (*inferior*) cornu as far as the amygdaloid tubercle, where it ends. A part of the surface of the anterior portion of the tænia semicircularis (*stria terminalis*) is more transparent and less dense than elsewhere and was called by Tarinus the "horny band."

The **optic thalami**, the posterior pair of basal ganglia, cannot be seen to advantage at this stage of the dissection without disarranging the parts overlying them and until the fornix and the velum interpositum (*tela choroidea of the third ventricle*) have been removed; their description, therefore, will be deferred. It is sufficient to say here that the optic thalamus is an oblong mass of white and gray matter lying to the medial side of the caudate nucleus and the tænia semicircularis (*stria terminalis*), part of the upper surface of which is hidden by the choroid plexus, the corpus fimbriatum, and the lateral portion of the body of the fornix.

The **choroid plexus** is a red, convoluted, vascular fringe, formed in the free margin of the velum interpositum (*tela choroidea of the third ventricle*), extending from the foramen of Monro (*interventricular foramen*) backward over the optic thalamus into the descending (*inferior*) cornu of the lateral ventricle, where it lies on the hippocampus major and extends to the end of this cornu of the ventricle. It is covered throughout by the ventricular epithelium, or ependyma, which passes from the corpus fimbriatum to the tænia semcircularis (*stria terminalis*) and optic thalamus; the ependyma thus separates the plexus from the cavity of the ventricle. Behind and between the foramina of Monro (*interventricular foramina*) the choroid plexus of one lateral ventricle becomes continuous with that of the other, and from the point of junction the choroid plexuses of the ventricle extend backward.

PLATE XXXVIII.

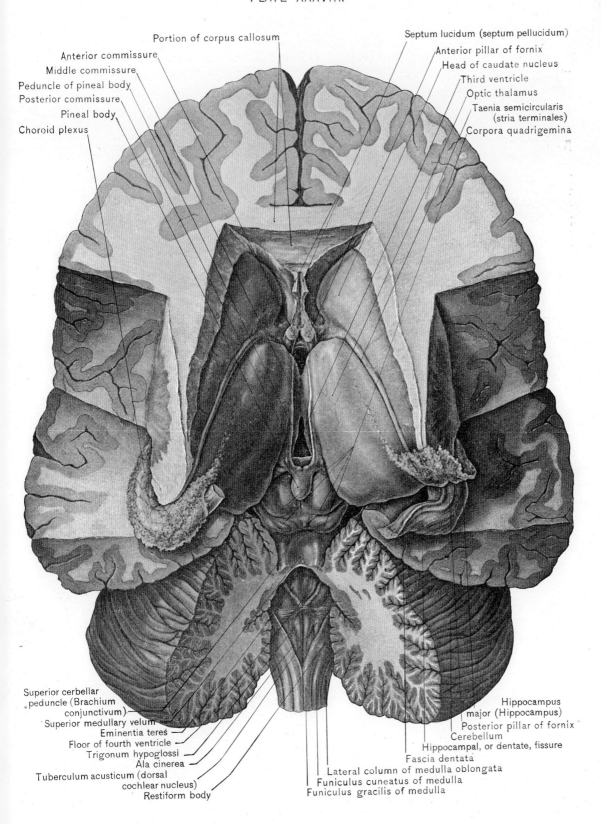

Portion of corpus callosum

Anterior commissure
Middle commissure
Peduncle of pineal body
Posterior commissure
Pineal body
Choroid plexus

Septum lucidum (septum pellucidum)
Anterior pillar of fornix
Head of caudate nucleus
Third ventricle
Optic thalamus
Taenia semicircularis
(stria terminales)
Corpora quadrigemina

Superior cerbellar
peduncle (Brachium
conjunctivum)
Superior medullary velum
Eminentia teres
Floor of fourth ventricle
Trigonum hypoglossi
Ala cinerea
Tuberculum acusticum (dorsal
cochlear nucleus)
Restiform body

Hippocampus
major (Hippocampus)
Posterior pillar of fornix
Cerebellum
Hippocampal, or dentate, fissure
Fascia dentata
Lateral column of medulla oblongata
Funiculus cuneatus of medulla
Funiculus gracilis of medulla

VENTRICLES AND NUCLEI OF THE BRAIN.
173

The **corpus fimbriatum, tænia hippocampi,** or **fimbria,** a narrow band of white matter, is the edge of the posterior crus of the fornix, which rests upon the posterior end of the optic thalamus, the choroid plexus intervening, and is continued into the descending (*inferior*) cornu of the lateral ventricle. Here it rests between the concave margin of the hippocampus major and the pia mater, which passes through the hippocampal fissure. It extends as far as the uncus of the hippocampal gyrus.

The **hippocampus major,** or **cornu ammonis,** is the prominent convex, white eminence which forms part of the floor and medial wall of the descending (*inferior*) cornu of the lateral ventricle, and extends throughout the entire length of this cornu. It is produced by extension of the hippocampal fissure into the descending (*inferior*) cornu of the lateral ventricle. Along its anterosuperior, or concave, margin is the corpus fimbriatum. Its anterior extremity, the *pes hippocampi (hippocampal digitations)*, is enlarged, and presents two or more grooves, somewhat resembling the paw of an animal.

DISSECTION.—Carefully separate the medial border of the corpus fimbriatum from the choroid plexus of the descending (*inferior*) cornu of the lateral ventricle, thus breaking through the epithelial lining of the ventricle; displace the choroid plexus medialward, and slightly depress the corpus fimbriatum and hippocampus major. This exposes the fascia dentata, and separates the margins of the hippocampal fissure.

The **fascia dentata,** or **dentate convolution,** a serrated band of gray matter, is the margin of the hippocampal convolution in relation with the hippocampal fissure. The serrations or indentations of the fascia dentata are produced by the vessels of the pia mater, which project through the hippocampal fissure into the descending (*inferior*) cornu of the lateral ventricle. The fascia dentata extends from near the splenium of the corpus callosum to the anterior extremity of the descending (*inferior*) cornu of the lateral ventricle. As the epithelial lining of the ventricle must be divided in order to expose the fascia dentata, that convolution is external to the wall of the ventricular cavity.

The **hippocampus minor (calcar avis)** is a small, convex, white eminence which occupies the floor and medial wall of the posterior cornu of the lateral ventricle. It is produced by the calcarine fissure, and is at times only faintly marked.

The **eminentia collateralis,** or **pes accessorius,** may be recognized at its commencement as a smooth, white eminence fitting into the angle of divergence of the hippocampus major and hippocampus minor (*calcar avis*), at the junction of the descending (*inferior*) and posterior cornua of the lateral ventricle. It extends forward as the floor of the descending (*inferior*) cornu of the lateral ventricle almost to the extremity of this cornu. It is produced by the collateral fissure.

DISSECTION.—Next divide the fornix transversely at about its middle, and reflect the one half forward and the other backward, thus exposing the greater part of that process of pia mater—the velum interpositum (*tela choroidea of the third ventricle*)—which lies above the epithelial roof of the third ventricle. To expose the entire velum interpositum (*tela choroidea of the third ventricle*), especially that part of it which occupies the central portion of the transverse fissure, make a longitudinal incision through the posterior part of the fornix and corpus callosum; then reflect these flaps laterally.

The **velum interpositum (tela choroidea of the third ventricle)** (Plate XXXIX) is that process of the pia mater which reaches the interior of the brain by way of the horizontal portion of the transverse fissure, passing between the splenium of the corpus callosum and the corpora quadrigemina. It is a double layer of pia mater, and like the fornix is triangular in shape. It lies beneath the fornix and the corpus callosum, and covers the quadrigeminal bodies, the pineal body, the third ventricle, and part of the optic thalami. Its borders contain the choroid plexuses of the lateral ventricles, while in its under surface are situated the two choroid plexuses of the third ventricle. The latter plexuses are continuous with the choroid plexuses of the lateral ventricles just behind the foramina of Monro (*interventricular foramina*). Running, one on each side of the median line of the velum interpositum (*tela choroidea of the third ventricle*), between its two layers, are the two veins of Galen (*internal cerebral veins*), formed by the union of the veins of the corpora striata and the choroid veins, in addition to small twigs from surrounding structures. They unite posteriorly to form a single trunk, which joins the inferior longitudinal (*inferior sagittal*) sinus to form the straight sinus at the junction of the inferior margin of the falx cerebri with the anterior margin of the tentorium cerebelli.

DISSECTION.—Raise the velum interpositum (*tela choroidea of the third ventricle*) and the choroid plexuses and turn them backward. Especial care is necessary in raising the posterior part of the velum interpositum (*tela choroidea of the third ventricle*) so as not to raise the pineal gland with it, as the gland is closely invested by the lower layer of pia mater entering the velum. This dissection exposes the third ventricle, with its three commissures, the anterior crura of the fornix, the optic thalami, the pineal body and its peduncles, and the quadrigeminal body. In making the dissection it frequently happens that the middle commissure of the third ventricle is broken, and the dissector, if not familiar with this fact, might conclude that it was absent in the brain under examination.

PLATE XXXIX.

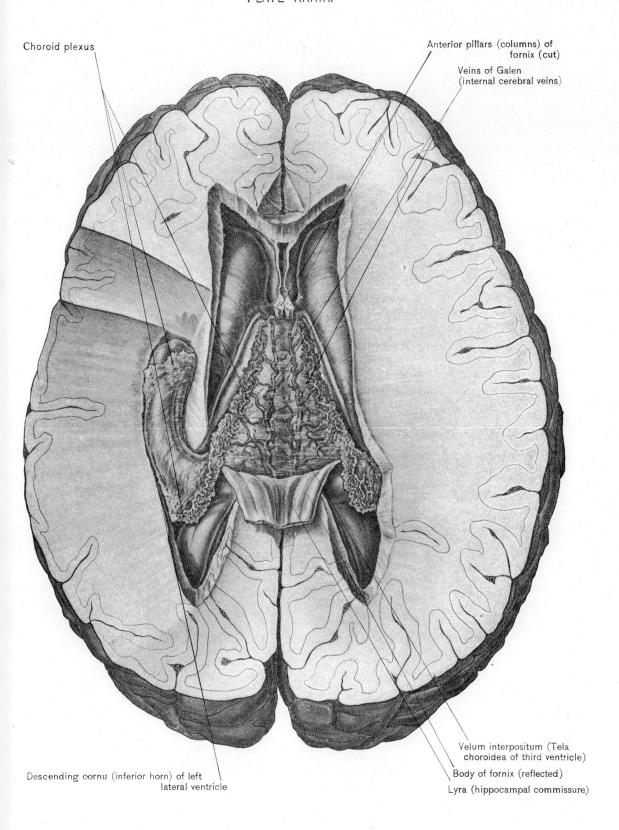

Choroid plexus

Anterior pillars (columns) of
fornix (cut)

Veins of Galen
(internal cerebral veins)

Velum interpositum (Tela
choroidea of third ventricle)

Body of fornix (reflected)

Lyra (hippocampal commissure)

Descending cornu (inferior horn) of left
lateral ventricle

VELUM INTERPOSITUM (TELA CHOROIDEA OF THIRD VENTRICLE) AND CHOROID PLEXUS

PLATE XL.

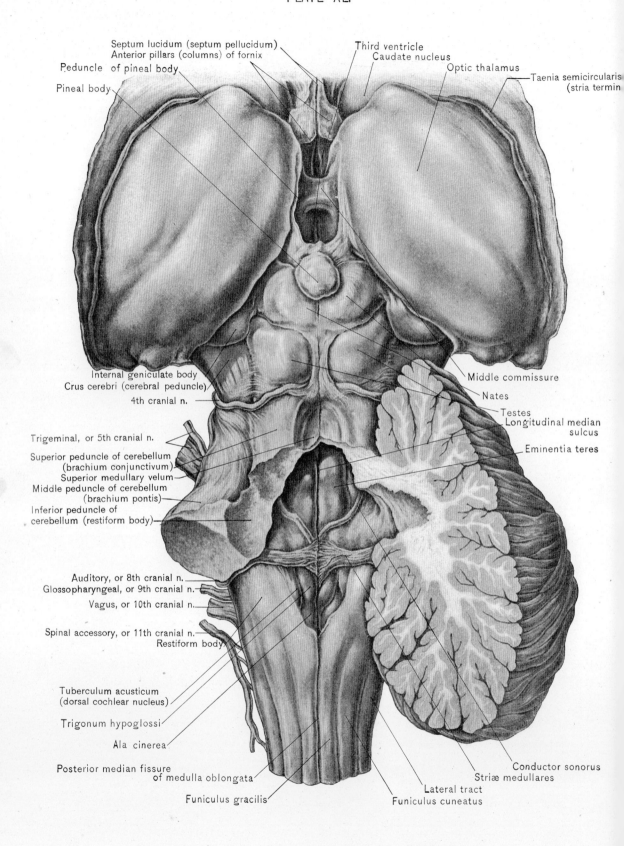

Septum lucidum (septum pellucidum)
Anterior pillars (columns) of fornix
Peduncle of pineal body
Pineal body

Third ventricle
Caudate nucleus
Optic thalamus
Taenia semicircularis
(stria termin

Internal geniculate body
Crus cerebri (cerebral peduncle)
4th cranial n.

Middle commissure
Nates
Testes
Longitudinal median
sulcus
Eminentia teres

Trigeminal, or 5th cranial n.
Superior peduncle of cerebellum
(brachium conjunctivum)
Superior medullary velum
Middle peduncle of cerebellum
(brachium pontis)
Inferior peduncle of
cerebellum (restiform body)

Auditory, or 8th cranial n.
Glossopharyngeal, or 9th cranial n.
Vagus, or 10th cranial n.

Spinal accessory, or 11th cranial n.
Restiform body

Tuberculum acusticum
(dorsal cochlear nucleus)
Trigonum hypoglossi
Ala cinerea

Posterior median fissure
of medulla oblongata
Funiculus gracilis

Conductor sonorus
Striæ medullares

Lateral tract
Funiculus cuneatus

THIRD AND FOURTH VENTRICLES AND CORPORA QUADRIGEMINA.

Transverse Fissure, or **Fissure of Bichat.**—Before describing the parts exposed by the removal of the velhm interpositum (*tela choroidea of the third ventricle*), the great transverse fissure of the brain, or fissure of Bichat, which is now opened up throughout, should be carefully observed. This can best be done by removing the velum interpositum (*tela choroidea of the third ventricle*) and the choroid plexuses of the lateral and third ventricles with the adherent epithelium. The central horizontal, or transverse, portion of this fissure, through which the velum interpositum (*tela choroidea of the third ventricle*) passes, is the continuation of the interspace between the cerebrum and the cerebellum seen in the undissected brain with the pia mater removed. This central portion is continuous with the lateral portions, or hippocampal fissures, which are seen in the dissection of the descending (*inferior*) cornua of the lateral ventricles, thus making the fissure, as a whole, horseshoe-shaped.

The **Third Ventricle** (Plates XXXVIII and XL) is a narrow, oblong cavity situated in the middle line of the cerebrum, between the optic thalami and the peduncles of the pineal body, and reaching to the base of the brain. It is wider and shallower posteriorly than anteriorly. It is bounded *superiorly* by the velum interpositum (*tela choroidea of the third ventricle*), although its immediate roof is formed by a thin epithelial layer which is continuous with the lining epithelium, or ependyma, of the ventricle; *laterally,* by the optic thalami and the peduncles of the pineal body; *anteriorly,* by the anterior commissure and the anterior pillars of the fornix, and *posteriorly,* by the posterior commissure, the orifice of the aqueduct of Sylvius (*aqueduct of cerebrum*), and the pia mater, passing from the superior surface of the pineal body to the inferior layer of the velum interpositum (*tela choroidea of the third ventricle*). Its *floor* is formed by the bodies which fill the interpeduncular space of the base of the brain and the superior surface of the crura cerebri (*cerebral peduncles*) at their origin from the pons. The structures in the interpeduncular space, named from before backward are: the lamina cinerea (*lamina terminalis*), the tuber cinereum, the infundibulum, the corpora albicantia, or corpora mamillaria, and the posterior perforated space (*substantia perforata posterior*).

Commissures (Plate XXXVIII).—Stretching across the ventricle are the anterior, middle, and posterior commissures. The *anterior commissure* is situated in front of the anterior pillars of the fornix. It is composed of white matter and connects the two temporal lobes of the cerebrum. The *middle commissure,* composed almost entirely of gray matter, is the largest, and is about twelve millimeters (one-half inch) in width. It connects the optic thalami, and, as has been observed, is frequently torn across in the dissection of the brain. The *posterior commissure,* the smallest of the three, is situated in front of, and beneath the pineal body, and above the anterior opening of the aqueduct of Sylvius (*aqueduct of cerebrum*). It is composed of white matter, connects the optic thalami, and probably contains decussating fibers derived from various sources.

The **foramina of Monro** (**interventricular foramina**) are the orifices of communication between the lateral ventricles and the third ventricle. Each foramen is bounded anteriorly by the corresponding anterior crus of the fornix, posteriorly, by the optic thalamus and choroid plexus, superiorly, by the anterior crus of the fornix, and inferiorly, by the ependyma reflected from the optic thalamus to the anterior crus of the fornix. The two foramina have a common orifice in the third ventricle, thus forming a Y-shaped passage, called the *foramen commune anterius*, through which cerebro-spinal fluid in one lateral ventricle may enter the other lateral ventricle. (Plate XXXIV.)

Aqueduct of Sylvius (**Aqueduct of the Cerebrum**).—At the posterior extremity of the third ventricle, and beneath the posterior commissure, is seen the anterior orifice of the aqueduct of Sylvius (*aqueduct of cerebrum*), *or iter a tertio ad quartum ventriculum.* This is a narrow passageway about two centimeters (three-fourths of an inch) in length, and passes beneath the quadrigeminal body to establish a communication between the third and fourth ventricles. It is lined with ependyma which is continuous with, and similar to that lining the ventricles which it connects. Its *roof* is formed by the lamina quadrigemina, a plate of gray matter which supports the corpora quadrigemina. Its *floor* is formed by the tegmental portions of the crura cerebri (*cerebral peduncles*). The gray matter in its floor contains the nuclei which give origin to the oculomotor, or third cranial, and trochlear, or fourth cranial, nerves.

The **optic thalami,** the posterior pair of cerebral ganglia, are two oval masses of white and gray matter. They are convex anteroposteriorly, and slightly so laterally, and have their long axis directed obliquely anteroposteriorly and mediolaterally. They lie one upon each side of the third ventricle, between the tails of the caudate nuclei, and rest upon the crura cerebri (*cerebral peduncles*). Each optic thalamus forms a large portion of the floor of the body of the lateral ventricle, while its posterior end projects into the descending (*inferior*) cornu of that ventricle. Each optic thalamus consists of two extremities: an anterior, called the **anterior tubercle,** which forms the posterior boundary of the foramen of Monro (*interventricular foramen*), and a posterior, called the **pulvinar,** or **posterior tubercle.** The upper surface of each is partly free and partly covered by the choroid plexus of the lateral ventricle, the velum interpositum (*tela choroidea of the third ventricle*), and the lateral border of the body of the fornix. On its superior surface is situated an anteroposterior groove, called the **sulcus choroideus,** for the attachment of the velum interpositum (*tela choroidea of the third*

PLATE XLI.

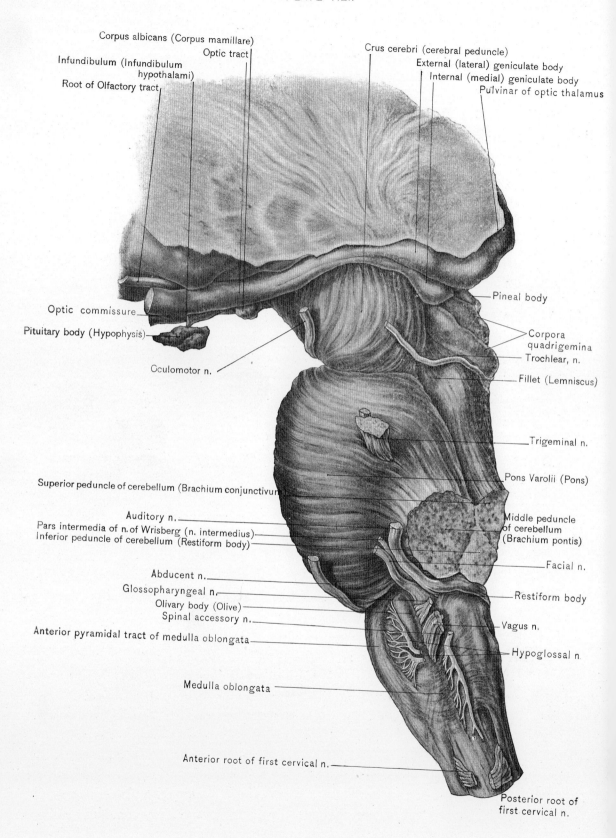

Corpus albicans (Corpus mamillare)

Optic tract

Infundibulum (Infundibulum
hypothalami)

Root of Olfactory tract

Crus cerebri (cerebral peduncle)

External (lateral) geniculate body

Internal (medial) geniculate body

Pulvinar of optic thalamus

Optic commissure

Pituitary body (Hypophysis)

Oculomotor n.

Pineal body

Corpora
quadrigemina

Trochlear, n.

Fillet (Lemniscus)

Trigeminal n.

Pons Varolii (Pons)

Superior peduncle of cerebellum (Brachium conjunctivum)

Auditory n.

Pars intermedia of n. of Wrisberg (n. intermedius)

Inferior peduncle of cerebellum (Restiform body)

Middle peduncle
of cerebellum
(Brachium pontis)

Facial n.

Abducent n.

Glossopharyngeal n.

Olivary body (Olive)

Spinal accessory n.

Anterior pyramidal tract of medulla oblongata

Restiform body

Vagus n.

Hypoglossal n.

Medulla oblongata

Anterior root of first cervical n.

Posterior root of
first cervical n.

LATERAL VIEW OF CORPORA QUADRIGEMINA, PONS, AND MEDULLA.

ventricle). In the groove between the caudate nucleus and the optic thalamus lies the tænia semicircularis (*stria terminalis*). The optic thalami are connected by the middle and posterior commissures of the third ventricle. Running along the superior border of each optic thalamus postero-anteriorly are the peduncles of the pineal body.

Geniculate Bodies.—The inferior surface of the posterior extremity of each optic thalamus, which forms part of the roof of the descending (*inferior*) cornu of the lateral ventricle, presents two small gray eminences, the **medial** and **lateral geniculate bodies.** To see these bodies satisfactorily, turn the brain on its side and raise the posterior extremity of the optic thalamus. The medial geniculate bodies are connected medially with the anterior pair of corpora quadrigemina through the medium of the brachia, and laterally, are directly continuous with the optic tract.

The **pineal body, conarium,** or **epiphysis cerebri,** is a small, reddish-gray, oval body, about six millimeters (one-fourth of an inch) in length. It is directed forward and upward, and rests upon the groove between the anterior pair of corpora quadrigemina and above the posterior commissure of the third ventricle. From the base of the pineal body a white crus, or peduncle, passes forward upon each side of the third ventricle and along the superior and medial surface of the optic thalami to the anterior crura of the fornix, with which the peduncles become continuous. Posteriorly, they are joined together in front of the base of the pineal body, and are connected with the posterior commissure of the third ventricle.

The **corpora quadrigemina** (Plate XLI), or **optic lobes,** are situated immediately behind the third ventricle, and are composed of four eminences. These are arranged in two pairs: an anterior or upper, the larger of the two, and called the nates, and a posterior or lower, the testes. They are situated upon a layer of gray matter known as the **lamina quadrigemina,** which overlies the aqueduct of Sylvius (*aqueduct of the cerebrum*). Anteriorly, they give off four bands, or brachia, which are composed of white matter externally and gray matter internally. The superior brachia, or *brachia of the nates*, pass under the medial geniculate bodies into the optic tracts. The inferior brachia, or *brachia of the testes*, pass below and lateral to the brachia of the nates, and leave the surface below the medial geniculate bodies. The posterior quadrigeminal bodies, or testes, are each connected with the hemisphere of the cerebellum by a broad band of white matter, the superior peduncle of the cerebellum (*brachium conjunctivum*).

DISSECTION.—In order to see the superior cerebellar peduncles (*brachia conjunctiva*) more clearly, the anterior extremity of the middle lobe of the cerebellum should be lifted slightly and pushed backward, or better, a longitudinal incision should be carried through the middle of this lobe, and each half displaced laterally. This will expose these peduncles clearly and also show the fillet and the valve of Vieussens (*anterior medullary velum*).

The **superior peduncle of the cerebellum** (**brachium conjunctivum**) connects the hemisphere of the cerebellum with the opposite hemisphere of the cerebrum. It passes upward, forward, and inward along the side of the anterior part of the fourth ventricle, and beneath the corpora quadrigemina, where the fibers of the two peduncles decussate; beyond the corpora quadrigemina, along with the tegmental fibers of the crura cerebri (*cerebral peduncles*), the fibers of each peduncle are continued to the optic thalamus and the lenticular (*lentiform*) nucleus of the opposite hemisphere of the cerebrum.

The **valve of Vieussens** (**anterior medullary velum**), the anterior or superior medullary velum, is a triangular layer of white matter, narrow anteriorly and broad posteriorly, stretched between the superior peduncles of the cerebellum (*brachia conjunctiva*), and extending from the anterior extremity or nodule of the inferior vermiform process (*vermis*) of the cerebellum to the corpora quadrigemina. It forms a portion of the roof of the fourth ventricle. Along the middle line of the upper surface is a longitudinal ridge, the *frenulum*. The lower half is over lapped by the *lingula*, a corrugated lobule of gray matter prolonged from the anterior extremity of the superior vermiform process. The trochlear nerves decussate within it, and emerge from its dorsal surface, just behind the inferior quadrigeminal bodies.

The **fillet,** or **medial lemniscus,** is a small, flat band or bundle of nerve fibers situated below and lateral to the superior peduncle of the cerebellum (*brachium conjunctivum*). It emerges from the pons at the upper limit of its posterior region, and appears as a triangular band which is situated above the crus cerebri (*cerebral peduncle*) and disappears under the testis (*inferior quadrigeminal body*) and brachium of the testis.

DISSECTION.—If the superior and inferior vermiform processes (*vermis*) of the cerebellum were not divided longitudinally when exposing the valve of Vieussens (*anterior medullary velum*), they should be divided now, and each half reflected laterally to expose the fourth ventricle.

The **Fourth Ventricle** (Plate XL) is a quadrangular, lozenge-shaped space, situated between the cerebellum and the posterior surface of the medulla oblongata and pons.

The *roof* is formed anteriorly by the valve of Vieussens (*anterior medullary velum*), and the superior peduncles of the cerebellum (*brachia conjunctiva*), and posteriorly by the inferior medullary velum, the inferior vermiform process (*vermis*) of the cerebellum, the choroid plexus, and the tela choroidea inferior. The *floor* is formed by the posterior surface of the medulla oblongata and pons. It is bounded laterally by the superior peduncles of the cerebellum (*brachia conjunctiva*) above, and the inferior peduncles of the cerebellum (*restiform bodies*) below. The ventricle is lined by the ependyma, or epithelial wall of the ventricles of the brain. The ventricle presents four angles, a superior, an inferior, and two lateral (also called the lateral recesses of the ventricle). The widest part of the ventricle corresponds to the interval between the lateral angles, which are at about its middle.

The **tela choroidea inferior** is that part of the pia mater on the posterior surface of the medulla oblongata which completes the posterior part of the roof of the fourth ventricle. It contains three perforations: the foramen of Magendie (*median aperture of fourth ventricle*), and the foramina of Key-Retzius, or Luschka (*lateral apertures of the fourth ventricle*).

The foramen of Magendie (*median aperture of fourth ventricle*) is located in the median line near the inferior angle of the fourth ventricle. The foramina of Key-Retzius, or Luschka (*lateral apertures of the fourth ventricles*) are located at the lateral recesses of the ventricle. By way of these openings the ventricle communicates with the general subarachnoid space.

The two **choroid plexuses** of the fourth ventricle are also derived from the pia mater by the intrusion of its folded edge into the roof of that cavity. They extend forward from the posterior angle of the fourth ventricle near the median line for a short distance, and then diverge to reach the lateral recesses of the ventricle.

The fourth ventricle communicates with the third ventricle by way of the aqueduct of Sylvius (*aqueduct of cerebrum*), and with the central canal of the spinal cord through the *ventricle of Arantius*, a dilated opening in the inferior angle.

The floor of the fourth ventricle is its most important part, since it contains the nuclei of most of the cranial nerves. It is composed chiefly of gray matter continuous with the gray matter of the spinal cord. Occupying the median line of the floor of the fourth ventricle is the **median longitudinal fissure.** It extends from the posterior orifice of the aqueduct of Sylvius (*aqueduct of cerebrum*) to the posterior, or inferior, angle of the ventricle, which is at the point of divergence of the restiform bodies of the medulla. This fissure is continuous below with the central canal of the spinal cord. This portion of the fourth ventricle has received the name of **calamus scriptorius** because of the resemblance of the longitudinal fissure and the diverging posterior pyramids and restiform bodies to the point of a pen. Immediately to each side of the median furrow is a longitudinal ridge, the **eminentia teres** (**eminentia medialis**). Crossing this eminence in the lower half of the ventricle are bands of white matter, the auditory striæ, or **striæ acusticæ** (**striæ medullares**). To the lateral side of the eminentia teres (*eminentia medialis*) and anterior to the auditory striæ (*striæ medullares*) is a depressed area, the *superior fovea*, while behind the auditory striæ (*striæ medullares*), and to the lateral side of the eminentia teres (*eminentia medialis*), are two furrows so united as to form an inverted V, the *inferior fovea;* the floor of the inferior fovea is known as the **ala cinerea.**

The **trigonum hypoglossi** is the area of the floor of the fourth ventricle bounded by the longitudinal fissure, striæ acusticæ (*striæ medullares*) and inferior fovea, and covers the nucleus of the hypoglossal nerve. The **tuberculum acusticum** (**dorsal cochlear nucleus**) is the triangular area situated between the inferior fovea and the clava of the funiculus gracilis, and extending forward under the striæ acusticæ (*striæ medullares*).

In front of the superior fovea and external to the eminentia teres (*eminentia medialis*) is a small eminence of dark gray matter, the **locus cæruleus.** Prolonged forward from the locus cæruleus, at the side of the eminentia teres (*eminentia medialis*) and extending to the upper end of the floor of the ventricle, is a thin streak of dark gray matter, the **tænia violacea.** The locus cæruleus and tænia violacea are produced by the substantia ferruginea, whose dark color is seen through the overlying white matter. The **substantia ferruginea** is the dark, pigmented mass seen in sections of the upper part of the floor of the fourth ventricle. The ependyma lining the fourth ventricle is continuous through the aqueduct of Sylvius (*cerebral aqueduct*) with that lining the third ventricle.

DISSECTION.—Next complete the dissection of the cerebrum by making horizontal sections of the corpora striata and optic thalami, carrying the incisions through to the lateral surface of the hemisphere. This will expose the caudate nucleus, the internal capsule, the lenticular (*lentiform*) nucleus, the external capsule, the claustrum, and the island of Reil (*insula*) from within outward in the order named.

The **caudate nucleus,** or intraventricular portion of the corpus striatum, is the more anterior of the gray basal ganglia. It has been described at p. 172.

The **internal capsule** lies lateral to and behind the caudate nucleus, and separates the caudate from the lenticular (*lentiform*) nucleus, and the latter from the optic thalamus. The internal capsule, composed of white matter and somewhat crescentic or angular in shape, consists of a genu and two limbs, an anterior and a posterior. The *anterior limb*, named by Spitzka the caudo-lenticular portion, intervenes between the caudate and lenticular (*lentiform*) nuclei. The *posterior limb*, named by the same author the thalamo-lenticular portion, intervenes between the optic thalamus and the lenticular (*lentiform*) nucleus. The *genu*, the point where the capsule presents the greatest angularity, is opposite the interval between the caudate nucleus and the optic thalamus

Through the internal capsule the nerve fibers pass in their course from the gray matter of the cortex of the cerebrum and the caudate and lenticular (*lentiform*) nuclei to the crus cerebri (*cerebral peduncle*), which transmits these fibers from the cerebrum to the pons, the medulla oblongata, and the spinal cord. In addition to these fibers the internal capsule contains fibers from the cerebral cortex to the optic thalamus.

The anterior third of the interna capsule contains the fibers from the cortex of the prefrontal lobe, or silent region; the middle third, the fibers from the motor, or Rolandic, area of the cortex of the cerebrum, and the posterior third, the sensory fibers from the occipital and temporal lobes.

Destruction of the anterior two-thirds of the posterior segment of the internal capsule, which occurs in many cases of apoplexy, results in motor paralysis of the opposite side of the body. This paralysis is diffuse, and not confined to a group of muscles, as in lesions of the cerebral cortex, while destruction of the posterior part of the posterior limb of the internal capsule results in loss of sensation of the opposite side of the body. A small hemorrhage in the capsule will cause paralysis of that part of the opposite side of the body supplied by the fibers compressed by the clot of blood.

The **Lenticular (Lentiform) Nucleus,** or extraventricular portion of the corpus striatum, is larger than the caudate nucleus, is oval in form, and lies behind and lateral to the caudate nucleus. It is separated from the latter by the anterior limb and genu of the internal capsule, and from the optic thalamus by the posterior limb of the internal capsule.

The **external capsule** is a band of white matter which lies lateral to the lenticular (*lentiform*) nucleus, and joins the internal capsule below that nucleus.

The **claustrum** is a thin layer of gray matter, lying lateral to the external capsule.

The **island of Reil (insula)**, previously described, is lateral to the claustrum, and separated from it by a layer of white matter.

White Matter of Cerebrum.—In the dissection of the cerebrum, which will be completed when the crura cerebri (*cerebral peduncles*) have been traced from the upper border of the pons to each hemisphere, it should be noted that the white matter of the cerebrum is composed of three systems, or sets, of medullated nerve fibers: the ascending, or peduncular, the transverse commissural, and the longitudinal commissural. The *ascending*, or *peduncular, fibers* are those fibers of the crura cerebri (*cerebral peduncles*) which, in diverging to reach the nerve cells of the cerebral cortex, form the *corona radiata*, so called on account of the crown-like radiation of its fibers. The *transverse commissural fibers* include the fibers of the corpus callosum and the anterior and posterior commissures of the third ventricle. The *longitudinal commissural fibers* include the fibers of the fornix, the striæ longitudinales of the corpus callosum, the tænia semicircularis (*stria terminalis*), fibers in the gyrus fornicatus and gyrus hippocampi, and the peduncles of the pineal body. They also include the associating fibers which connect the cells of neighboring and of more distant convolutions.

THE PONS VAROLII (PONS). (Plate XLII)

DISSECTION.—Having completed the dissection of the cerebrum, excepting the tracing of the crura cerebri (*cerebral peduncles*), turn the brain so as to expose the base, and study the pons, then the medulla oblongata, and lastly the cerebellum.

The **Pons,** or **Tuber Annulare,** is that division of the brain through the medium of which its three divisions are united. It is connected with the cerebrum, above, by the crura cerebri (*peduncles of the cerebrum*); with the cerebellum, behind, by the middle peduncles of the cerebellum (*brachia pontis*), and with the medulla, below, by the fibers of the pyramidal tract of the medulla oblongata (*cerebro-spinal fasciculus*). It is situated behind the crura cerebri (*cerebral peduncles*), in front of the medulla oblongata, between and below the hemispheres of the cerebellum, and between the posterior portions of the temporal lobes of the cerebrum. In the cranial cavity it lies below the level of the superior occipital foramen of the tentorium cerebelli, and rests upon the basilar process of the occipital bone and the posterior surface of the body of the sphenoidal bone. It is quadrangular in shape, and is composed chiefly of white matter, the fibers of which are arranged transversely and longitudinally. It presents an anterior and a posterior surface. The *anterior surface* is markedly convex laterally, and slightly so anteroposteriorly; it measures transversely about four centimeters (one and one-half inches), and is about two and a half centimeters (one inch) in length. The anterior surface is marked along the middle line by a groove which lodges the basilar artery. The anterior surface presents two borders, a superior and an inferior border. The *superior border,* the longer, is convex, and arches beneath the crura cerebri (*cerebral peduncles*). The *inferior border* is almost straight, and is separated from the medulla oblongata by a transverse groove. The *posterior surface* is slightly concave laterally, and forms part of the floor of the fourth ventricle. From the side of the pons the trigeminal, or fifth cranial, nerve is seen emerging.

In coronal sections the pons can be divided into an anterior or ventral, and a posterior, or tegmental, region. The *anterior region of the pons* is composed

PLATE XLII.

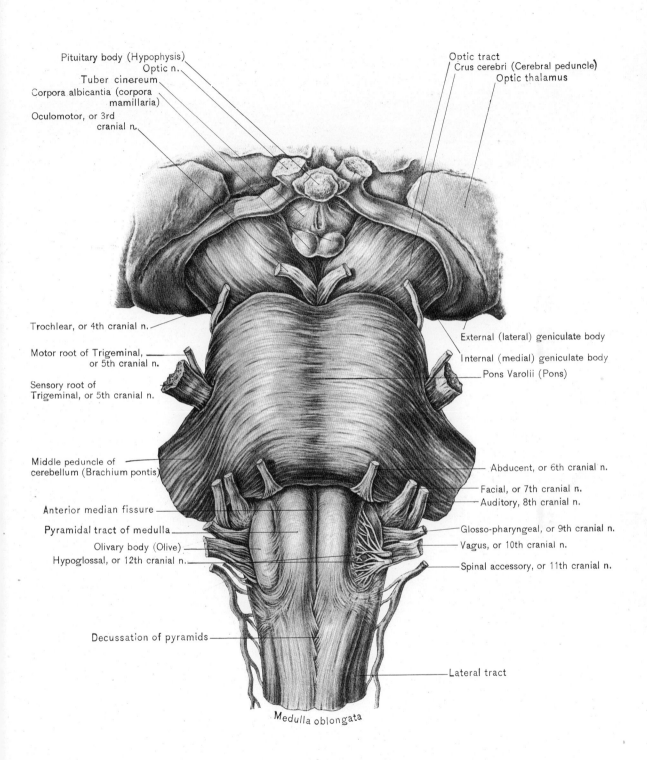

Pituitary body (Hypophysis)
Optic n.
Tuber cinereum
Corpora albicantia (corpora mamillaria)
Oculomotor, or 3rd cranial n.

Optic tract
Crus cerebri (Cerebral peduncle)
Optic thalamus

Trochlear, or 4th cranial n.

External (lateral) geniculate body

Motor root of Trigeminal, or 5th cranial n.

Internal (medial) geniculate body
Pons Varolii (Pons)

Sensory root of Trigeminal, or 5th cranial n.

Middle peduncle of cerebellum (Brachium pontis)

Abducent, or 6th cranial n.
Facial, or 7th cranial n.
Auditory, 8th cranial n.

Anterior median fissure

Pyramidal tract of medulla

Glosso-pharyngeal, or 9th cranial n.
Vagus, or 10th cranial n.

Olivary body (Olive)

Hypoglossal, or 12th cranial n.

Spinal accessory, or 11th cranial n.

Decussation of pyramids

Lateral tract

Medulla oblongata

PONS, MEDULLA, AND SUPERFICIAL ORIGINS OF CRANIAL NERVES.

of transverse and longitudinal fibers.   The *superficial transverse fibers* of the anterior region of the pons pass obliquely lateralward and backward to the hemispheres of the cerebellum, forming the middle peduncles of the cerebellum (*brachia pontis*). The *deep transverse fibers* of the anterior region of the pons are decussating fibers, which cross in the pons in passing from the cerebellar hemisphere of one side to that of the opposite side.   The *longitudinal fibers* are more deeply situated than the superficial transverse fibers, and are separated into bundles by the deep transverse fibers.   They are the fibers of the pyramidal tracts of the medulla oblongata (*cerebro-spinal fasciculi*), passing upward to enter the crustæ (*bases*) of the crura cerebri (*cerebral peduncles*).

In the *posterior, or tegmental, region of the pons* the chief structures observed are: the tract of the fillet, which is seen nearest the anterior region, the formatio reticularis, the posterior (*medial*) longitudinal bundle, and the superior olivary nucleus.   This region of the pons also contains the nuclei of the abducent and facial nerves, and a part of the nucleus of the auditory (*acoustic*) nerve.   These nuclei are not macroscopically visible.   Their importance has been clearly proven by clinical experience in cases of paralysis caused by hemorrhage occurring within the substance of the pons, as well as by microscopic investigation.

Hemorrhage into the pons is usually followed by coma and sudden death, particularly if the hemorrhage is extensive, or if the blood escapes into the fourth ventricle.   The decussation of the trigeminal and the facial nerves takes place within the pons; if, therefore, a lesion as, for example, a small hemorrhage occurs above the point of the crossing of the fibers of the facial nerve, paralysis of the face and body on the side opposite the lesion will occur; while if the lesion is immediately below the point of crossing, the paralysis of the face will be upon the side of the lesion and the hemiplegia upon the side opposite to the lesion, thus giving rise to the condition known as *crossed hemiplegia*.   Nerve fibers from the motor cortical area for speech run through the pons, and may be involved in a lesion of the pons, thus giving rise to a dysarthria and not an aphasia.

The **crura cerebri (peduncles of the cerebrum)** are two large round bodies of white matter, about two centimeters (three-fourths of an inch) in length, and broader anteriorly than posteriorly.   They emerge from the superior border of the pons, whence they pass lateralward and forward to enter the inferior part of the hemispheres of the cerebrum.   They pass through the superior occipital foramen in company with the superior peduncles of the cerebellum (*brachia conjunctiva*), the basilar artery, and the oculomotor and trochlear nerves.   Crossing the inferior surface of the crura just before they enter the hemispheres of the cerebrum, and adherent to them, are the optic tracts, while in relation with their

13

medial borders are the oculomotor nerves, and with their lateral margins, the trochlear nerves.

DISSECTION.—Divide one of the crura cerebri (*cerebral peduncles*) transversely, and a nucleus of gray matter—the *locus niger*, or substantia nigra—will be seen in the interior of the crus. Through the medium of this nucleus the crus cerebri (*cerebral peduncle*) is divided into an upper, or posterior, portion, known as the tegmentum, and a lower, or anterior, portion, the crusta (*basis pedunculi*).

The **tegmentum of the crus cerebri** (**cerebral peduncle**) is composed largely of the longitudinal fibers of the tegmental region of the pons, which proceed from the lateral tract and the posterior pyramids of the medulla oblongata; it also receives the fibers of the superior peduncle of the cerebellum (*brachium conjunctivum*). The tegmental fibers of the crus cerebri (*cerebral peduncle*) are sensory, and enter the hemisphere of the cerebrum below and through the optic thalamus, beyond which they form part of the corona radiata. The tegmentum contains two nuclei, the *subthalamic body* (*nucleus hypothalamicus*) and the *tegmental*, or *red, nucleus*. The admixture of gray and white matter of the tegmentum forms the *formatio reticularis*.

The **crusta** (*basis pedunculi*) is composed chiefly of the longitudinal fibers of the anterior region of the pons which proceed from the anterior pyramids of the medulla. The fibers of the crusta (*basis pedunculi*) are motor, and enter the hemisphere through the internal capsule, beyond which they form a part of the corona radiata. The medial one-fifth of the crusta (*basis pedunculi*) contains fibers which pass to the pons from the prefrontal lobe.

THE MEDULLA OBLONGATA (Plate XLII)

The **Medulla Oblongata,** or **Bulb,** the upper continuation of the spinal cord, begins at the decussation of the pyramids or the upper border of the atlas, and extends to the lower border of the pons, being not quite three and a half centimeters (one and a half inches) in length. It increases in width from below upward, and just below the pons it is about two centimeters (three-fourths of an inch) wide. Its anterior, or ventral, surface rests partly upon the basilar portion of the occipital bone, and its posterior, or dorsal, surface is directed toward the vallecula of the cerebellum, which lodges part of the medulla. In its median line the anterior surface presents the *anterior median fissure*, which is the continuation upward of the anterior median fissure of the spinal cord, but interrupted by white fibers crossing from one side to the other and forming the decussation of the pyramids. On its posterior aspect, for one-half the length of the medulla, is the *posterior median fissure*, or sulcus, also the continuation of the corresponding fissure of the spinal cord.

The medulla oblongata, like the spinal cord, is divided into an anterior, a lateral, and a posterior area. The *anterior area* is occupied by the anterior pyramids, the *lateral area* by the olivary body (*olive*) and the lateral column. The *posterior area* contains the funiculus of Rolando (*spinal tract of the fifth nerve*), funiculus cuneatus, and funiculus gracilis, and in its upper portion, the restiform body.

The **anterior pyramids (pyramids) of the medulla oblongata** are situated between the anterior median and the anterolateral fissures. They are larger above, but are somewhat constricted and rounded where they disappear beneath the superficial transverse fibers of the pons. On separating the pyramids below, bundles of fibers will be seen decussating across the anterior median fissure. This decussation is produced by the medial fibers of the pyramids, which contribute to the lateral, or crossed, pyramidal tracts (*lateral cerebro-spinal fasciculi*) of the spinal cord. The lateral fibers, which form the smaller number of fibers of the pyramid, continue downward without decussating as the direct pyramidal tract (*anterior cerebro-spinal fasciculus*) of the spinal cord; they then decussate in the anterior, or white, commissure of the spinal cord. The decussation of the pyramids of the medulla explains the fact that in disease or injury of the motor cortex of the brain the paralysis is found on the side of the body opposite to the lesion in the brain.

The continuation of the anterior ground bundle (*fasciculus proprius anterior*) of the spinal cord is not seen in the anterior area of the medulla oblongata, as the fibers of that tract are depressed from the surface by the decussating bundles of the crossed pyramidal tract (*lateral cerebro-spinal fasciculus*).

The **olivary body (olive)** is an oval prominence on the medulla oblongata, situated lateral to the anterior pyramid, from which it is separated by a narrow longitudinal groove, the hypoglossal sulcus, or *anterolateral furrow* of the medulla, which is continuous with the anterolateral fissure of the spinal cord. The olivary body (*olive*) is limited posteriorly by the *postolivary sulcus*. Like the pyramid, it is broader above than below. It is separated from the pons by a deep groove, and is about twelve to fifteen millimeters (one-half inch) in length. Emerging from the hypoglossal sulcus, or anterolateral furrow, are the roots of the hypoglossal nerve. Arching below and over the olivary body (*olive*) and emerging from the anterior median and the anterolateral fissures, several white bundles are seen, the **arcuate fibers**, which enter the restiform body of the same side. An oblique incision carried through the olivary body (*olive*) will reveal, in its interior, a nucleus of gray matter, the **corpus dentatum** of the olivary body (*olive*). This nucleus is arranged in the form of a hollow capsule, and presents a convoluted outline partly incomplete at its medial side. Through this open part of the capsule passes a bundle of white fibers, the **peduncle of the olivary body** (olive).

The **lateral tract,** or **region, of the medulla oblongata** is continuous with the lateral column of the spinal cord. It does not contain the crossed pyramidal tract (*lateral cerebro-spinal fasciculus*) of the cord, which enters the pyramidal tract of the medulla oblongata. The direct cerebellar tract of Flechsig (*posterior spino-cerebellar fasciculus*) of the cord leaves the medulla as a constituent of the restiform body. The lateral region of the medulla is bounded anteriorly by the anterolateral furrow, and posteriorly by the posterolateral furrow. Emerging from the anterolateral furrow, or hypoglossal sulcus, are the roots of the hypoglossal nerve, and from the posterolateral furrow the roots of the glosso-pharyngeal, vagus, and spinal accessory (*accessory*) nerves. As it ascends, the lateral tract of the medulla becomes less marked, the greater portion of it passing beneath the olivary body (*olive*).

DISSECTION.—The remaining portion of the medulla oblongata can be most satisfactorily examined by lifting it from the interval between the hemispheres of the cerebellum, and displacing it forward, thus exposing the posterior surface of the medulla, as well as that portion of the floor of the fourth ventricle formed by the medulla.

The **funiculus of Rolando** (**spinal tract of the fifth nerve**) which lies posterior to the lateral tract and on the lateral side of the funiculus cuneatus, is the upward continuation of a mass of gray matter, the substantia gelatinosa, which caps the posterior cornu of the gray matter of the spinal cord. This funiculus presents an enlargement on a level with the lower end of the olivary body (*olive*), called the **tubercle of Rolando** (*tuberculum cinereum*).

The **funiculus cuneatus,** the upward prolongation of Burdach's column (*fasciculus cuneatus*), lies between the funiculus of Rolando (*spinal tract of the fifth nerve*) and the funiculus gracilis, or posterior pyramid. It is the widest and thickest of the columns of the medulla. Opposite the clava of the funiculus gracilis it forms a prominence called the **cuneate tubercle.**

The **funiculus gracilis,** or **posterior pyramid,** the upward continuation of the posterior median column of Goll (*fasciculus gracilis*) of the spinal cord, lies immediately lateral to the posterior median fissure. At the lower end of the fourth ventricle it swells out and forms a prominence, called the **clava.** The cuneate tubercle and the clava are produced by accumulations of gray matter known, respectively, as the *nucleus cuneatus and nucleus gracilis;* almost all the fibers of the funiculus cuneatus and funiculus gracilis terminate in these nuclei.

The **inferior cerebellar peduncle,** or **restiform body,** contains fibers which come from the spinal cord and the medulla oblongata and pass to the cere-

bellum. The tracts ascending to the cerebellum from the spinal cord and the
medulla are its principal constituents. However, additional paths are contrib-
uted by the fiber bundles from the vestibular nerve and its end nucleus. By
the divergence of the restiform bodies the lateral boundaries of the lower part of
the fourth ventricle are formed, while the apex of the lower triangle of the
ventricle is situated at the point of separation of the two clavæ. This divergence
exposes the gray matter of the interior of the medulla, which forms the floor of
the lower portion of the fourth ventricle, and is continuous with the gray matter
of the spinal cord. Each restiform body contains a lateral and a medial division.
The lateral division is formed by the following fasciculi: (1) the direct cerebellar
(*posterior spino-cerebellar*) tract, which ends mainly in the superior vermiform
process (*vermis*); (2) the fibers from the nuclei cuneatus and gracilis of the same
and opposite sides; (3) fibers from the inferior olivary nucleus (*olivo-cerebellar
fibers*); (4) fibers from the arcuate or pyramidal nuclei; (5) fibers from the
lateral column nuclei. The medial division is formed by: (1) the direct sensory
cerebellar tract of Edinger, which consists of sensory root fibers of certain
cerebral nerves, such as the trigeminal and vestibular nerves; (2) other fibers
which connect the nuclei of the sensory cerebral nerves with the cerebellum.
The termination of both sets of fibers is in the roof nucleus (*nucleus fastigii*) of
the cerebellum. Fibers (cerebello-bulbar) also pass from the roof nucleus
(*nucleus fastigii*) and probably from the dentate nucleus of the same and opposite sides, and are said to end in Deiters' (*lateral vestibular*) nucleus and in the
formatio reticularis of the medulla. These bundles, which bring the nuclei of the
sensory cerebral nerves into relation with the cerebellum, form the nucleo-
cerebellar fasciculus, or indirect sensory cerebellar tract.

RECAPITULATION.—Review the parts seen in studying the medulla anteroposteriorly. They are: the anterior median fissure, the anterior pyramid, the
hypoglossal, or anterolateral, fissure with the roots of the hypoglossal nerve,
the olivary body (*olive*), containing the corpus dentatum (*inferior olivary
nucleus*), the postolivary sulcus, the lateral tract, the posterolateral fissure
with the roots of the glossopharyngeal, vagus, and spinal accessory (*accessory*)
nerves, the funiculus of Rolando (*spinal tract of the fifth nerve*) and its tubercle
(*tuberculum cinereum*). the funiculus cuneatus with the cuneate tubercle, the
funiculus gracilis with the clava, and the posterior median fissure.

FUNCTION.—The medulla is described by Ranney as "the true nerve center
of animal life." Several of the cranial nerves have their primary, deep, or
central origin wholly or in part in the medulla. Some of the centers contained
within the medulla are the respiratory, the vaso-motor, the cardio-inhibitory,
and the vomiting centers.

THE CEREBELLUM (Plate XLIII)

Position, Size, and Connections.—The cerebellum, or small brain, lies beneath the occipital lobes of the cerebrum, behind the pons and the corpora quadrigemina, and above and upon both sides of the medulla oblongata. It occupies the inferior occipital fossæ, and lies beneath the tentorium cerebelli, which separates it from the cerebrum.

The surface of the cerebellum, like that of the cerebrum, is composed of gray matter, which in the cerebellum is darker in color, and is arranged in *laminæ* instead of in convolutions. The cerebellum measures from nine to ten centimeters (three and a half to four inches) in its transverse diameter, from five to six centimeters (two to two and a half inches) in its anteroposterior diameter, and about five centimeters (two inches) in its vertical diameter at the thickest part. It is attached to the cerebrum by the superior peduncles (*brachia conjunctiva*), to the pons by the middle peduncles (*brachia pontis*), and to the medulla oblongata by the inferior peduncles (*restiform bodies*) of the cerebellum.

Lobes.—The cerebellum consists of two hemispheres and a central lobe, the vermiform process, or worm (*vermis*), through the medium of which the hemispheres are united. The hemispheres are separated inferiorly by a comparatively wide and deep median groove, the **vallecula,** or valley, which is occupied in great part by the medulla oblongata; the inferior vermiform process (*vermis*) of the cerebellum also projects into the valley. The hemispheres are separated anteriorly by a notch, the **incisura cerebelli anterior,** which lodges the inferior pair of corpora quadrigemina and the superior cerebellar peduncles (*brachia conjunctiva*); and posteriorly by another notch, the **incisura cerebelli posterior,** or **incisura marsupialis,** which is the posterior extremity of the valley and lodges the falx cerebelli. The **central lobe,** or **vermiform process** (**vermis**), presents two aspects: a superior, seen as a slight elevation in the middle of the superior surface of the cerebellum, and called the superior vermiform process (*superior vermis*), and an inferior, which is called the inferior vermiform process (*inferior vermis*). Passing along the free border of each hemisphere is the **great horizontal fissure of the cerebellum** (*horizontal sulcus*) which commences at the point where the middle peduncle of the cerebellum (*brachium pontis*) enters the hemisphere, and extends backward and around to the other middle peduncle of the cerebellum (*brachium pontis*). The horizontal fissure separates the superior from the inferior surface of the hemisphere.

DISSECTION.—Before proceeding further with the study of the cerebellum, remove what remains of the cerebrum by carrying an incision through the optic thalami and the crura cerebri (*cerebral peduncles*), and detach the pia mater from the cerebellum.

PLATE XLIII.

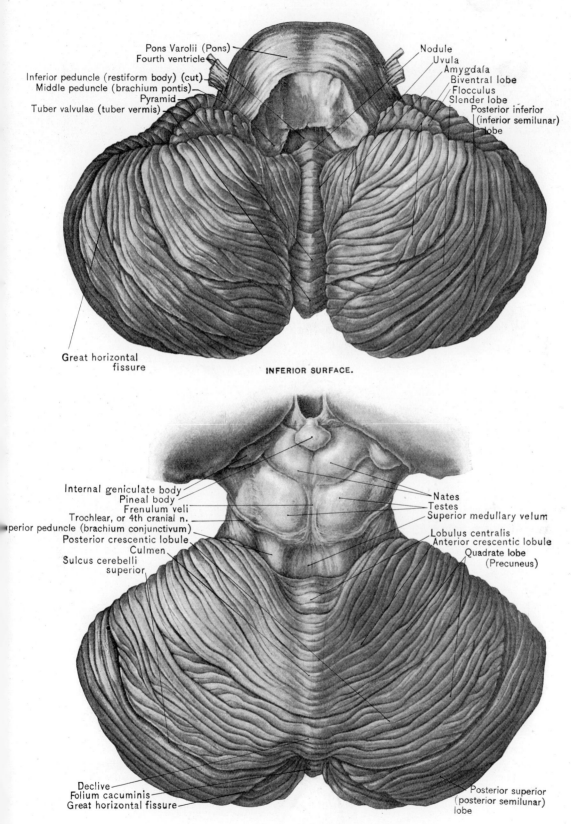

Pons Varolii (Pons)
Fourth ventricle
Inferior peduncle (restiform body) (cut)
Middle peduncle (brachium pontis)
Pyramid
Tuber valvulae (tuber vermis)

Nodule
Uvula
Amygdala
Biventral lobe
Flocculus
Slender lobe
Posterior inferior
(inferior semilunar)
lobe

Great horizontal
fissure

INFERIOR SURFACE.

Internal geniculate body
Pineal body
Frenulum veli
Trochlear, or 4th cranial n.
uperior peduncle (brachium conjunctivum)
Posterior crescentic lobule
Culmen
Sulcus cerebelli
superior

Nates
Testes
Superior medullary velum
Lobulus centralis
Anterior crescentic lobule
Quadrate lobe
(Precuneus)

Declive
Folium cacuminis
Great horizontal fissure

Posterior superior
(posterior semilunar)
lobe

SUPERIOR SURFACE.

INFERIOR AND SUPERIOR SURFACE OF CEREBELLUM.

The **superior vermiform process** (**superior vermis**) is the superior surface of the vermiform process, or middle lobe of the cerebellum, and is raised above the level of the superior surface of its hemispheres. It is divided into the following lobes: lingula, lobulus centralis, monticulus cerebelli, and folium cacuminis (*folium vermis*). The **lingula** overlies the posterior part of the superior (*anterior*) medullary velum and is adherent to it. It is attached at its base to the lobulus centralis. The **lobulus centralis** lies immediately posterior to and below the corpora quadrigemina; it spreads out laterally into the *alæ lobuli centralis*. The **monticulus cerebelli** is divided into two parts, the *culmen* and the *declive*, the latter being a sloping part; it is connected on each side to the quadrate lobe. The culmen joins the anterior semilunar division of the quadrate (*quadrangular*) lobe, and the declive joins the posterior semilunar division. The **folium cacuminis** (**folium vermis**), which connects the posterior superior lobes of the hemispheres, is posterior to the declive.

The **upper surface of each hemisphere of the cerebellum** slopes lateralward and backward from the superior vermiform process (*superior vermis*), and is divided into two lobes, the quadrate (*quadrangular*) and the posterior superior lobe (*superior semilunar lobule*), by the **posterior superior sulcus of the cerebellum**, which passes from the commencement of the transverse fissure toward the incisura cerebelli posterior. The **quadrate** (**quadrangular**) **lobe** is situated anterior to the sulcus cerebelli superior posterior, and extends nearly to the posterior end of the vermiform process (*vermis*), its laminæ passing without interruption through the monticulus cerebelli into the corresponding lobe of the opposite side. The quadrate lobe is divided by a small fissure, sulcus superior anterior, into an *anterior semilunar* and a *posterior semilunar lobule*. The **posterior superior** (*superior semilunar*) **lobe** is situated posterior to the sulcus cerebelli superior posterior and along the posterior border of the hemisphere, and is joined to the posterior superior (*superior semilunar*) lobe of the opposite side by the folium cacuminis (*folium vermis*).

DISSECTION.—Displace the medulla oblongata forward, and expose the inferior vermiform process (*inferior vermis*) at the bottom of the vallecula.

The **inferior vermiform process** (**inferior vermis**) is divided into four lobes, which, anteroposteriorly, are: the nodule, the uvula, the pyramid, and the tuber valvulæ. The **nodule,** designated by Malacarne the **laminated tubercle,** is the anterior extremity of the inferior vermiform process (*inferior vermis*), and projects into the fourth ventricle, forming a part of the roof of that ventricle. It is closely associated with the **posterior medullary velum,** a thin white sheet that is continuous laterally with the peduncles of the flocculus. The **uvula,** situated directly behind the nodule, is an elongated lobe compressed laterally, and is connected on each side to the tonsil, or amygdaloid lobe, by an indented strip of gray matter, the **furrowed band.** The **pyramid,** situated behind the uvula, is the largest of the divisions of the process, and connects with the biventral lobes of the hemispheres. The **tuber valvulæ,** the posterior extremity of the inferior vermiform process (*inferior vermis*), is continuous with the folia of the two inferior posterior (*inferior semilunar*) lobes of the hemispheres.

The **inferior surface of each hemisphere** of the cerebellum, which is convex and conforms to the occipital fossa in which it rests, is divided into four lobes, which, anteroposteriorly, are: the flocculus, the amygdala, or tonsil, the digastric, or biventral, lobe, and the posterior inferior (*inferior semilunar*) lobe. The **flocculus,** the smallest lobe, is situated at the anterior part of the hemisphere, between the digastric, or biventral, lobe and the middle peduncle of the cerebellum (*brachium pontis*), in the line of the great horizontal fissure of the cerebellum. The **amygdala,** or **tonsil,** is situated to the medial side of the digastric, or biventral, lobe and between that lobe and the vallecula. It is connected with the uvula by the furrowed band. The **digastric,** or **biventral,** the largest lobe, lies behind the flocculus, and lateral to the amygdala, or tonsil, and the pyramid; it is connected with the biventral lobe of the other hemisphere by the pyramid. The **posterior inferior (inferior semilunar) lobe** lies between the posterior border of the hemisphere and the biventral lobe and lateral to the tuber valvulæ. Frequently it is divided into two or three slender lobes by two of its curved sulci which appear deeper than the other sulci.

DISSECTION.—Cut away the amygdala, or tonsil, on one side, or slice off the digastric lobe until the amygdala, or tonsil, can be turned out; this will expose the furrowed band, the posterior medullary velum and the fossa, known as the "swallow's nest," or nidus hirundinis (*nidus avis*), which is indented by the posterior medullary velum, the nodule, and the uvula.

The **Peduncles of the Cerebellum** consist of three pairs: the superior, the middle, and the inferior.

The *superior peduncle* of the cerebellum (*brachium conjunctivum*) connects the cerebellum with the cerebrum, and passes forward, forming the lateral boundary of the superior portion of the fourth ventricle. Under the floor of the aqueduct of Sylvius (*cerebral aqueduct*) the two superior peduncles (*brachia conjunctiva*) decussate; each peduncle then enters the opposite subthalamic region of the cerebrum, to reach the red nucleus. The cells of the red nucleus, about which the fibers of the peduncle terminate, send axones into the rubrospinal tract of the cord and to the thalamus and internal capsule. The *middle peduncle (brachium pontis)* connects the cerebellum with the pons. The *inferior peduncle* or *restiform body* connects the cerebellum with the medulla oblongata and spinal cord.

Cerebellar Tumors.—Tumors of the cerebellum and cerebello-pontile angle are characterized by definite disturbances of gait, nystagmus, diminution of reflexes on the side of the lesion, and occasionally cranial nerve palsies, depending upon the situation of the tumor, associated with extreme choking of the discs. Occipital headache is frequently localized and severe; ataxia, dysmetria, Bárány test, tests for hearing, facial weakness, and eighth cranial, or auditory, nerve involvement are important determinations in localization.

Operative Procedure.—The operation for cerebellar tumor consists of a cross-bow incision extending from the base of one mastoid to the base of the other, the upper curve of the incision reaching a point about four centimeters above the occipital protuberance in the midline. From this point the incision is carried down the neck over the spinous processes to about the sixth cervical spinous process, the muscles being carefully separated in the midline down to the occipital bone and over the spinous processes. After this step the muscles are separated from their attachment on the occipital bone and divided on each side, allowing enough to remain along the superior occipital ridge (*superior nuchal line*), so that reconstruction is possible when closing up. In order effectively to cut the muscles far enough below the attachment, it is necessary to dissect back the skin flaps until they may fold lateralward along a line drawn from the tip of the mastoid process to the spinous process of the sixth cervical vertebra. The next step in the operation consists of opening the occipital region of the skull. This opening is made as high as the transverse (*lateral*) sinus and down to and including the foramen magnum. Laterally, the exposure is carried out to the base of the mastoid. The dura having been exposed, the occipital sinus is ligated. Two parallel incisions are made along the sinus, and mosquito forceps introduced to clamp it on each side of the point of division. The sinus is then severed and a mattress stitch is placed so as to tie each end securely; the dura is opened over both hemispheres. The cerebellum may then be explored and even the cerebello-pontile angle. Extreme care must be taken to avoid any pressure on the medulla, as this will cause serious respiratory symptoms. The ventricle should always be tapped preliminary to a suboccipital craniectomy to insure ample freedom for exploration. This is done by introducing a Cotton cannula six centimeters (two and four-tenths inches) above the occipital protuberance and three centimeters (one and one-fifth inches) from the mid-line. The cannula is advanced along a plane with the tip of the ear and parallel to the sagittal sinus. The posterior horn of the ventricle should be encountered at a depth of about five and one-half centimeters (two and one-fifth inches).

DISSECTION.—Carry a vertical incision through the center of the hemisphere of the cerebellum, to expose the white matter and gray nucleus.

INTERIOR ARRANGEMENT.—In the interior of the white matter of the cerebellum are four nuclei, each of which is paired. Those of each pair are opposite each other on either side of the mid-line. The white matter sends processes into the laminæ of the gray matter which forms the surface of the cerebellum, and give rise to the appearance that has been termed the *arbor vitæ*. The **nucleus dentatus of the cerebellum** is the largest of the nuclei. Its cells give rise to most of the fibers forming the superior cerebellar peduncles (*brachia conjunctiva*); the **nucleus emboliformis** is a smaller mass of gray substance lying close to the medial side of the nucleus dentatus; the **nucleus globosus** is an elongated mass on the medial side of the nucleus emboliformis, and the **roof nucleus** (**nucleus fastigii, or tegmenti**), somewhat larger than the other two, lies close to the mid-line immediately over the roof of the fourth ventricle.

SECTIONS OF THE BRAIN (Plates XLIV; XLV; XLVI; XLVII)

Having reviewed the topography of the encephalon, together with its intraventricular aspect, in the study of which some of its parts were seen in horizontal sections, it will now be well to study coronal and sagittal sections, so as to obtain a more accurate knowledge of the relations of the various parts of the encephalon.

A **sagittal section** lies in a vertical longitudinal plane, running anteroposteriorly, as if through the entire length of the brain through or parallel with the sagittal suture; a section of this kind is not, however, limited to the median line.

A **coronal section** lies in a vertical transverse plane, running from side to side, at right angles to a sagittal plane; this is also called a frontal section.

A coronal section through the brain at the tips of the temporal lobes will traverse the anterior end of the lenticular (*lentiform*) nucleus of the corpus striatum, and one a short distance beyond this will pass through the anterior end of the caudate nucleus. A section passing through the optic commissure, or just behind it, will include the front of the optic thalami. A frontal section must, therefore, be made back of the optic commissure if it is to include both sets of basal ganglia.

A coronal section about midway between the optic commissure and the tips of the temporal lobes will not include the optic thalami. It will expose, from within outward: the septum lucidum (*septum pellucidum*), the lateral ventricle with the corpus callosum above it, the caudate nucleus, the internal capsule, the lenticular (*lentiform*) nucleus, the external capsule, the claustrum, the white matter, the island of Reil (*insula*), and the fissure of Sylvius (*lateral fissure*).

PLATE XLIV.

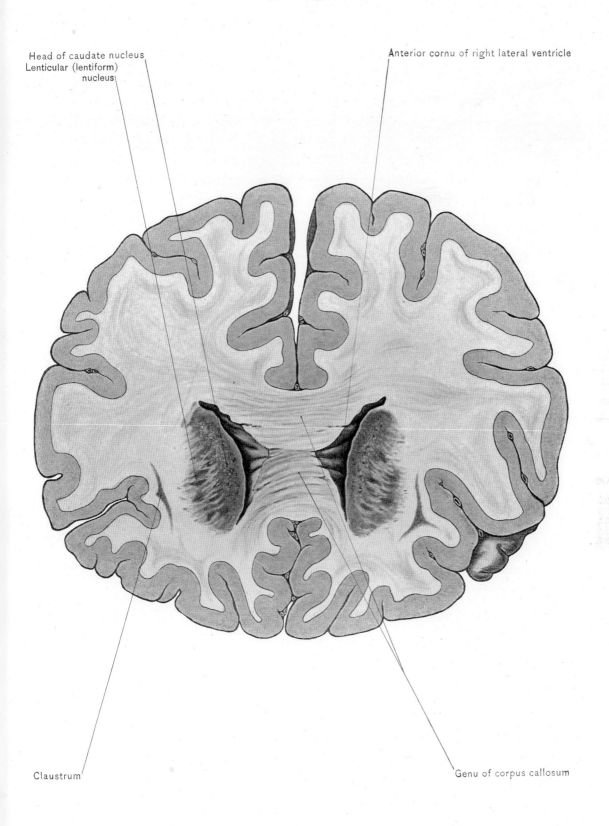

Head of caudate nucleus
Lenticular (lentiform) nucleus

Anterior cornu of right lateral ventricle

Claustrum

Genu of corpus callosum

CORONAL SECTION OF CEREBRUM.

205

PLATE XLV.

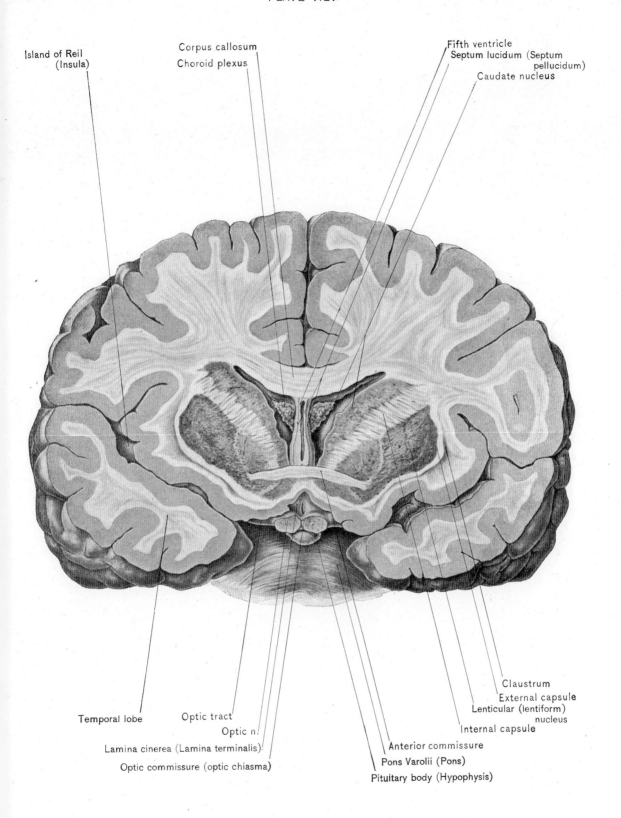

Island of Reil (Insula)

Corpus callosum
Choroid plexus

Fifth ventricle
Septum lucidum (Septum pellucidum)
Caudate nucleus

Claustrum
External capsule
Lenticular (lentiform) nucleus
Internal capsule

Temporal lobe

Optic tract

Optic n.

Lamina cinerea (Lamina terminalis)

Optic commissure (optic chiasma)

Anterior commissure

Pons Varolii (Pons)

Pituitary body (Hypophysis)

CORONAL SECTION OF CEREBRUM JUST ANTERIOR TO OPTIC CHIASMA.

PLATE XLVI.

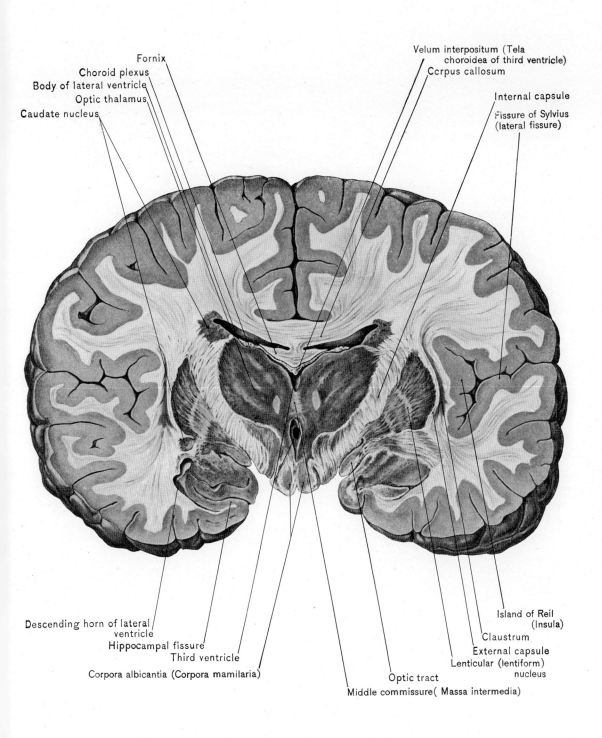

Fornix

Choroid plexus

Body of lateral ventricle

Optic thalamus

Caudate nucleus

Velum interpositum (Tela choroidea of third ventricle)

Corpus callosum

Internal capsule

Fissure of Sylvius (lateral fissure)

Descending horn of lateral ventricle

Hippocampal fissure

Third ventricle

Corpora albicantia (Corpora mamilaria)

Optic tract

Middle commissure(Massa intermedia)

Island of Reil (Insula)

Claustrum

External capsule

Lenticular (lentiform) nucleus

CORONAL SECTION OF CEREBRUM THROUGH CORPORA ALBICANTIA (CORPORA MAMILLARIA) AND MIDDLE COMMISSURE (MASSA INTERMEDIA).

PLATE XLVII.

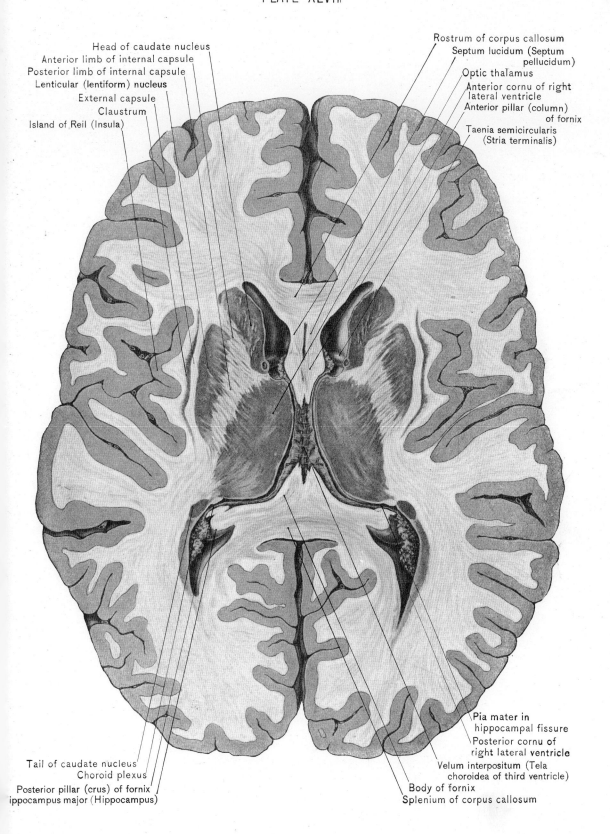

Head of caudate nucleus
Anterior limb of internal capsule
Posterior limb of internal capsule
Lenticular (lentiform) nucleus
External capsule
Claustrum
Island of Reil (Insula)

Rostrum of corpus callosum
Septum lucidum (Septum pellucidum)
Optic thalamus
Anterior cornu of right lateral ventricle
Anterior pillar (column) of fornix
Taenia semicircularis (Stria terminalis)

Tail of caudate nucleus
Choroid plexus
Posterior pillar (crus) of fornix
Hippocampus major (Hippocampus)

Pia mater in hippocampal fissure
Posterior cornu of right lateral ventricle
Velum interpositum (Tela choroidea of third ventricle)
Body of fornix
Splenium of corpus callosum

TRANSVERSE SECTION OF CEREBRUM.

PLATE XLVII.

PLATE XLVIII.

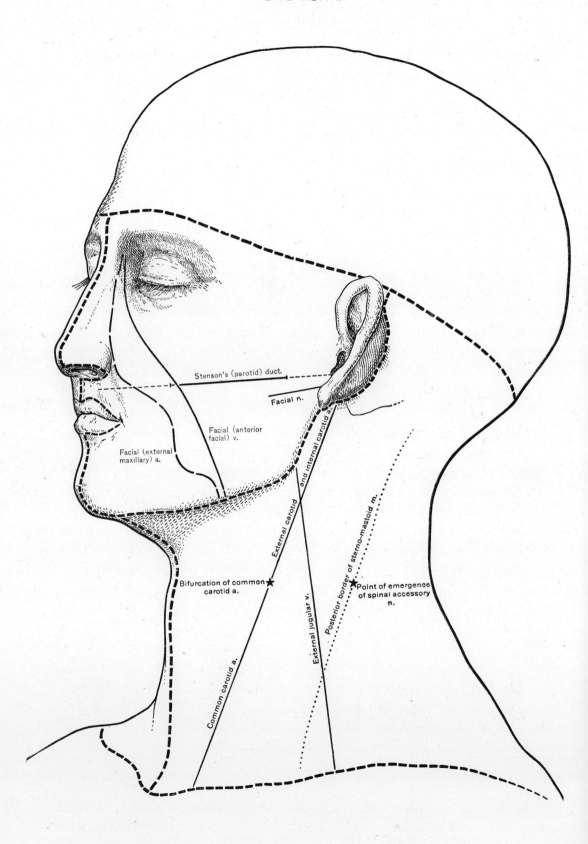

Stenson's (parotid) duct.

Facial n.

Facial (anterior facial) v.

Facial (external maxillary) a.

and internal carotid a.

External carotid

Posterior border of sterno-mastoid m.

Bifurcation of common carotid a.

Point of emergence of spinal accessory n.

Common carotid a.

External jugular v.

INCISIONS FOR DISSECTION AND LINES FOR VESSELS AND NERVES.

The wedge shape of the lateral ventricle is plainly shown in this section, as is also the formation of its lateral wall and part of its floor by the sloping caudate nucleus. The lenticular (*lentiform*) nucleus is clearly separated into three portions, defined by fine white curved lines extending between them.

When these sections are made further back, the anterior parts become smaller and finally disappear, while the more posterior ones gradually increase in size; the caudate nucleus grows smaller and recedes toward the superolateral angle of the lateral ventricle, while the optic thalamus occupies an increasing amount of the inferolateral wall of the lateral ventricle. Notable changes in the median line also occur: the fifth ventricle and the septum lucidum (*septum pellucidum*) vanish, and the fornix and third ventricle appear instead, while the infundibulum (*infundibulum hypothalami*), the mamillary bodies, and the posterior perforated spaces (*substantia perforata posterior*) successively appear at the base. The crura cerebri (*cerebral peduncles*) at first appear to be separated, gradually coming closer, until they merge. The substantia nigra is distinctly visible, as are also the two adjacent divisions of the crura cerebri (*cerebral peduncles*). The upper, or anterior, end of the pons comes into view, and at its upper edge the aqueduct of Sylvius (*aqueduct of the cerebrum*) appears. The velum interpositum (*tela choroidea of the third ventricle*) containing the choroid plexuses becomes wider as the sections pass backward. The tæniæ semicirculares (*striæ terminales*), the dentate fasciæ, the hippocampal gyri, and the descending (*inferior*) cornua of the lateral ventricles are also seen in these sections.

No study of the cerebrum is complete without a careful consideration of these sections, as they portray exactly the relarions of the cortex and the intra-encephalic parts to one another.

Sagittal sections do not offer so wide a field for the study of these relations because of the rapid loss of important structures as the median line is departed from, though the length of the basal ganglia, and particularly of the caudate nucleus, is better shown in these sections than in any other way.

THE FACE

DISSECTION. (Plate XLVIII).—For the dissection of the face which now follows, the head should be placed in the same position as for the dissection of the scalp, but slightly lower, and turned so that the side of the face to be dissected is upward. The cheeks and nostrils should be distended with cotton or oakum. The muscles and vessels should be dissected on one side of the face and the nerves on the other. The incisions are made as follows: the first incision is made from the nasal eminence along the median line of the nose, around the aperture of the nostril, along the median line of the upper lip, around the mouth along the line where the skin joins the mucous membrane to the median line of the lower lip, and thence to the point of the chin A second incision is carried along the lower border of the mandible to the angle of the mandible, then upward to the lobe of the ear. Reflect the skin lateralward, being careful not to remove the facial muscles (muscles of expression) which are inserted partly into the skin.

The **skin of the face** is remarkably thin and vascular, and its cellular tissue is loose, except over the chin and lower third of the nose where the skin is dense and closely adherent to the parts beneath. On account of the free blood supply it is a common site of nevi. It is very freely supplied with sebaceous and sudoriferous glands, and hence is commonly the site of acne and eruptions which especially involve the sebaceous follicles; it is also the site of sebaceous tumors. Because of the vascularity and lax subcutaneous tissue sloughing is rare, edema is marked, when present, and cellulitis tends to spread. Facial abscesses usually point quickly and seldom attain a large size. Infections in the chin or lower third of the nose are very painful because of the density of tissue. Epithelioma is common, and the face is often the site of lupus.

The **superficial fascia,** or the cellular tissue layer of the face, is closely related to, and intermingled with the facial muscles. It contains a considerable amount of fat, except in the eyelids, over the bridge of the nose, and in the upper lip. The laxity of the cellular tissue favors the spread of infiltrations, so that the cheeks and other parts of the face may become greatly swollen. In general dropsy the face soon becomes puffy, the edema generally first appearing in the lax areolar tissue of the lower eyelids. The soft tissues of the cheek favor the spread of destructive processes. In necrotic processes involving the loose cellular and fatty tissue, such as cancrum oris, or noma, the whole cheek may be lost in a few days Great contraction is apt to follow loss of substance, so that the mandible may be firmly closed in some cases, as is seen after recovery from deep ulceration. The mobility of the tissues of the face renders this region especially amenable to plastic operations, their vascularity insuring prompt union. Notwithstanding the fact that there is a large quantity of fat in the subcutaneous tissue, fatty tumors are rarely seen in this region.

DISSECTION.—Remove the superficial fascia in the same manner as the skin, taking care not to disturb the muscles. Since the superficial fascia is not easily removed in a continuous layer, and also in order to avoid dividing the bloodvessels and nerves of the face, the dissection is made in sections in the line of the muscle fibers. This exposes the muscles, the vessels, and the nerves.

The **Muscles of the Face** (muscles of expression) (Plate XLIX) are divided into three groups: those of the nose, of the eyebrows and eyelids, and of the mouth.

PLATE XLIX.

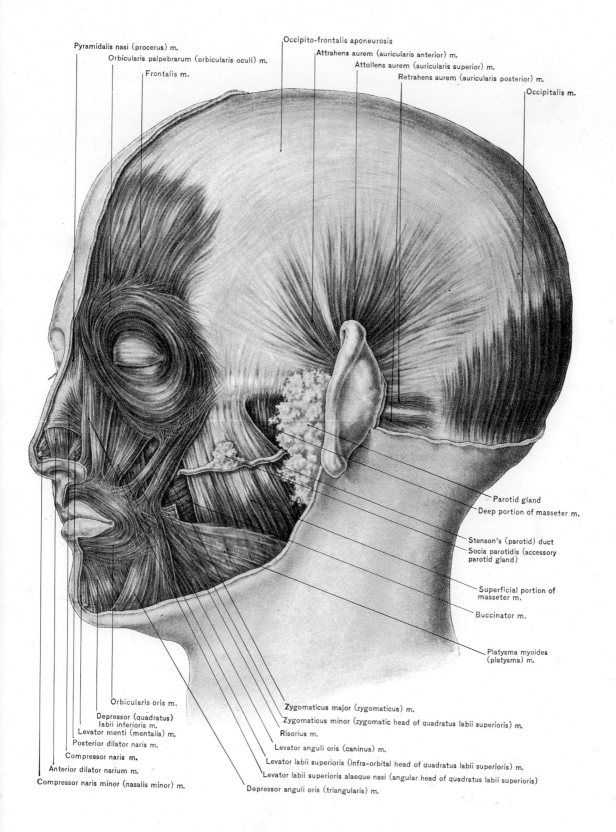

Pyramidalis nasi (procerus) m.

Orbicularis palpebrarum (orbicularis oculi) m.

Frontalis m.

Occipito-frontalis aponeurosis

Attrahens aurem (auricularis anterior) m.

Attollens aurem (auricularis superior) m.

Retrahens aurem (auricularis posterior) m.

Occipitalis m.

Parotid gland

Deep portion of masseter m.

Stenson's (parotid) duct

Socia parotidis (accessory parotid gland)

Superficial portion of masseter m.

Buccinator m.

Platysma myoides (platysma) m.

Orbicularis oris m.

Depressor (quadratus) labii inferioris m.

Levator menti (mentalis) m.

Posterior dilator naris m.

Compressor naris m.

Anterior dilator narium m.

Compressor naris minor (nasalis minor) m.

Zygomaticus major (zygomaticus) m.

Zygomaticus minor (zygomatic head of quadratus labii superioris) m.

Risorius m.

Levator anguli oris (caninus) m.

Levator labii superioris (infra-orbital head of quadratus labii superioris) m.

Levator labii superioris alaeque nasi (angular head of quadratus labii superioris)

Depressor anguli oris (triangularis) m.

MUSCLES OF FACE AND SCALP.

217

The **Muscles of the Nose** are five in number: the pyramidalis nasi (*procerus*), the compressor naris, the levator labii superioris alæque nasi (*angular head of quadratus labii superioris*), the dilator naris, and the depressor alæ nasi.

The **pyramidalis nasi (procerus) muscle** covers the nasal bone, and is continuous above with the frontalis muscle, where it is attached to the deep surface of the intersuperciliary integument. It *inserts* into the aponeurosis over the cartilage of the nose, where it joins the inferior edge of the nasal bone and the compressor naris muscle.

NERVE SUPPLY.—From the infra-orbital branch of the temporo-facial division of the facial nerve.

ACTION.—It draws the skin between the eyebrows downward, thus forming the transverse crease at the root of the nose.

The **compressor naris muscle,** triangular in shape, *arises* by its apex from the canine fossa of the superior maxillary bone (*maxilla*), and *inserts* into the aponeurosis covering the cartilaginous part of the nose, blending with the corresponding muscle of the opposite side, under cover of the levator labii superioris alæque nasi (*angular head of quadratus labii superioris*) muscle.

NERVE SUPPLY.—From the infra-orbital branch of the upper division of the facial nerve.

ACTION.—It draws the ala nasi downward and compresses the cartilaginous part of the nose.

When the compressor naris muscle is reflected from the median line lateralward, the superficial (*naso-labial*) branch of the nasal nerve, which becomes subcutaneous between the nasal bone and the lateral nasal cartilage, will be seen running downward to the tip of the nose.

The **levator labii superioris alæque nasi (angular head of quadratus labii superioris) muscle** passes along the side of the nose, overlapping the origin of the compressor naris muscle. It *arises* from the root of the frontal process of the superior maxilla (*maxilla*), and descending, divides into two portions: the median and smaller part being inserted into the medial side of the ala nasi, and the lateral part into the upper lip at the sulcus naso-labialis, blending with the orbicularis oris muscle. It is partially overlapped near its origin by the orbicularis palpebrarum (*orbicularis oculi*) muscle.

NERVE SUPPLY.—From the infra-orbital branch of the facial nerve.

ACTION.—It raises the upper lip and draws upward and lateralward the ala of the nose, thus dilating the anterior naris and deepening the naso-labial fold.

The **dilator naris muscle** consists of two feeble muscular slips: an anterior and a posterior. The *anterior* portion is a thin fasciculus which passes from the

lower edge of the cartilage of the ala to the integument over the margin of
the nostril; the *posterior* portion *arises* from the margin of the nasal notch of the
superior maxilla (*maxilla*) and from the lateral surface of the sesamoid cartilages
of the nose, and is *inserted* into the skin near the margin of the nose.

NERVE SUPPLY.—From the infra-orbital branch of the facial nerve.

ACTION.—It raises the lateral edge of the nostril, thus widening the nasal
orifice.

The **depressor alæ nasi** is a short, flat muscle which can be exposed when the
upper lip is everted and the mucous membrane removed from the side of the labial
frenulum. It *arises* from the incisor fossa of the superior maxilla (*maxilla*),
whence its fibers ascend to be *inserted* into the septum nasi and the postero-inferior
part of the ala of the nose.

NERVE SUPPLY.—From the buccal branch of the cervico-facial division
of the facial nerve.

ACTION.—It draws downward and inverts the edge of the nasal
cartilages.

The **Muscles of the Eyelids and Eyebrows** are four: the orbicularis palpebrarum (*orbicularis oculi*), the corrugator supercilii, the levator palpebræ superioris (*infra-orbital head of quadratus labii superioris*), and the tensor tarsi (*lacrimal
part of the orbicularis oculi*).

Tendo oculi (medial palpebral ligament).—Before examining the orbicularis
palpebrarum (*orbicularis oculi*), the tendo oculi (*medial palpebral ligament*) should
be noted. It is a short tendon, about four millimeters (one-sixth of an inch) in
length, by two millimeters (one-twelfth of an inch) in breadth, and can readily be
felt at the medial angle of the eye after drawing the eyelids lateralward. It is
attached to the frontal process of the superior maxilla (*maxilla*) in front of the
lacrimal groove, passes transversely lateralward in front of the lacrimal sac, and
divides into two portions, separated by the caruncula lacrimalis. The superior
portion is attached to the medial extremity of the superior, and the inferior
portion to the medial extremity of the inferior tarsal (*palpebral*) cartilage. As the
tendon crosses the lacrimal sac it gives off a strong aponeurotic lamina, which
covers the sac and is attached to the margin of the lacrimal groove. This expansion will be seen on reflecting that portion of the orbicularis palpebrarum (*orbicularis oculi*) muscle which covers the lacrimal sac. To puncture the lacrimal sac,
a knife is inserted below the tendo oculi (*medial palpebral ligament*) in a downward
and slightly backward direction, dividing the skin, the orbicularis palpebrarum
(*orbicularis oculi*) muscle, and the fibrous expansion derived from the tendo oculi
(*medial palpebral ligament*). The angular artery and vein are situated on the
medial side of the incision.

PLATE L.

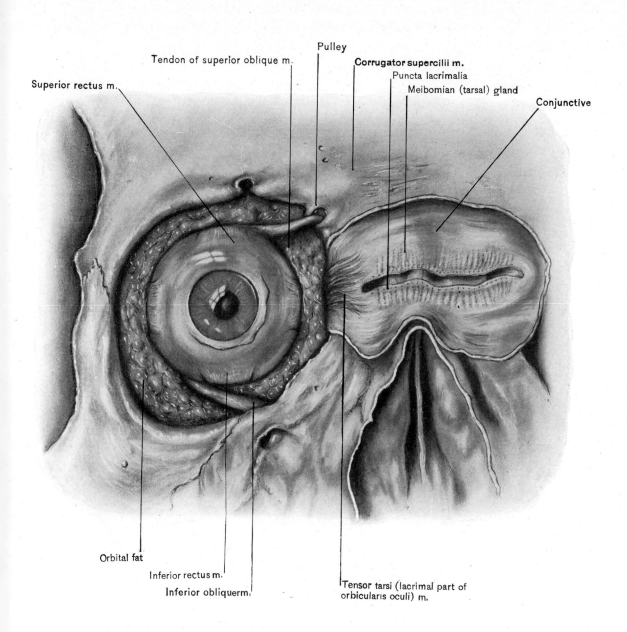

Pulley

Tendon of superior oblique m.

Corrugator supercilii m.

Puncta lacrimalia

Meibomian (tarsal) gland

Superior rectus m.

Conjunctive

Orbital fat

Inferior rectus m.

Inferior obliquerm.

Tensor tarsi (lacrimal part of orbicularis oculi) m.

TENSOR TARSI AND CORRUGATOR SUPERCILII MUSCLES.

The **external tarsal ligament** (**lateral palpebral raphe**) extends undivided, transversely medialward, from the edge of the frontal process of the malar (*zygomatic*) bone to the adjacent lateral extremities of the two tarsal (*palpebral*) cartilages.

The **orbicularis palpebrarum** (**orbicularis oculi**) is a thin, broad muscle which surrounds the margin of the orbit and the eyelids, forming a sphincter; it is continuous above with the fibers of the frontalis muscle. It *arises* from the internal angular process of the frontal bone, the nasal process of the superior maxilla (*maxilla*), the tendo oculi (*medial palpebral ligament*), and the inferior margin of the orbit. From this origin the fibers are directed lateralward, forming a series of oval curves which cover the eyelids, surround the margin of the orbit, and spread over the forehead, temple, and cheek. The central fibers, occupying the eyelids and connected medially with the tendo oculi (*medial palpebral ligament*) and laterally with the external tarsal ligament (*lateral palpebral raphe*) and the malar (*zygomatic*) bone, constitute the *palpebral portion* of the muscle. The fibers of this portion which extend along the margins of the lids are called the ciliary bundle. More peripheral fibers constitute the *orbital portion* of the muscle. The latter *arise* from the internal angular process of the frontal bone and from the nasal process of the superior maxillary bone (*maxilla*), and are distributed around the margin of the orbit.

NERVE SUPPLY.—From the temporal and malar (*zygomatic*) branches of the temporo-facial division of the facial nerve; hence, in paralysis of this nerve the eyelids on the paralyzed side cannot be closed.

ACTION.—The orbicularis palpebrarum (*orbicularis oculi*) muscle closes the eyelids and protects the eye. The attachment of the orbital portion to the skin draws the eyebrow downward and the skin of the cheek upward to form a fold around the orbit, thus giving additional protection to the eyeball. The palpebral portion of the muscle contracts during winking. Contraction of the orbital portion presses the eyeball backward into the orbit, and draws the soft parts covering the margin of the orbit around the eyeball, thus protecting it from injury. While this cushion of tissue may be severely bruised, as is seen in a "black" eye, the eyeball itself is rarely injured. As the outer portion of the orbicularis mingles with the fibers of the frontalis muscle and the elevators of the upper lip and nose, slight depression of the eyebrow and elevation of the upper lip and of the wing of the nose follow contraction of this portion. Contraction of the palpebral portion of the muscle, following that of the orbicular portion, tends to draw the lids medialward, thus directing the tears to the medial angle of the fissure between the eyelids, near which are situated the puncta lacrimalia.

The **tensor tarsi** (**lacrimal part of orbicularis oculi**), or Horner's muscle, (Plate L) is a small muscle, really a deep portion of the orbicularis palpebrarum (*orbicularis oculi*), situated at the medial angle of the orbit behind the tendo-oculi (*medial palpebral ligament*).   To expose it, cut perpendicularly through the middle of the superior and inferior eyelids, reflect the nasal half of each lid medialward, and remove the mucous membrane.   The muscle will be seen to *arise* from the ridge on the lacrimal bone.   It passes lateralward behind the lacrimal sac, and divides into two portions which cover the posterior aspect of the canaliculi.   The two portions terminate in the medial ends of the superior and inferior tarsal cartilages near the puncta lacrimalia.

NERVE SUPPLY.—From the infra-orbital branch of the temporo-facial division of the facial nerve.

ACTION.—It compresses the lacrimal sac.

DISSECTION.—The nasal half of the orbicularis palpebrarum (*orbicularis oculi*) and a small part of the frontalis muscle having been reflected medialward, the corrugator supercilii is exposed.

The **corrugator supercilii muscle** *arises* from the medial end of the superciliary ridge of the frontal bone.   Its fibers are directed lateralward and a little upward to the under surface of the orbicularis palpebrarum (*orbicularis oculi*) and frontalis muscles, to be *inserted* into the former over the medial portion of the supra-orbital arch.   This muscle may also be considered as part of the orbital portion of the orbicularis palpebrarum (*orbicularis oculi*).

NERVE SUPPLY.—From the temporal branch of the temporo-facial division of the facial nerve.

ACTION.—It draws the eyebrow downward and medialward, thus making the vertical wrinkle of the forehead at the medial extremity of the eyebrow.

The **levator palpebræ superioris muscle.**—By reflecting the lateral as well as the nasal half of the orbicularis palpebrarum (*orbicularis oculi*) muscle and detaching the orbito-tarsal ligament from the superior orbital margin and reflecting the ligament downward, the *insertion* of the *levator palpebræ superioris muscle* by a broad aponeurosis into the superior border of the tarsal cartilage of the upper eyelid can be seen.   (This muscle is described at p. 417).

The **Muscles of the Mouth** are all bilaterally placed except the orbicularis. They are: the orbicularis oris, risorius, levator labii superioris (*infra-orbital head of quadratus labii superioris*), levator anguli oris (*caninus*), depressor labii inferioris (*quadratus labii inferioris*), depressor anguli oris (*triangularis*), levator menti (*mentalis*), zygomaticus, and the buccinator.

The **risorius muscle,** or Santorini's muscle, a part of the platysma, consists of a thin bundle of fibers which *arises* from the fascia covering the masseter muscle and parotid gland.   It passes horizontally forward to the angle of the mouth, where it joins the fibers of the orbicularis oris and depressor anguli oris (*tri-angularis*) muscles; some of its fibers are *inserted* into the skin at the angle of the mouth.

NERVE SUPPLY.—From the buccal branch of the lower division of the facial nerve, which enters it from beneath.

ACTION.—It retracts the corner of the mouth. Its contraction during certain conditions, such as tetanus, causes the "risus sardonicus."

The **orbicularis oris muscle,** or sphincter oris, about two and a half centimeters (one inch) in breadth, is the sphincter muscle surrounding the lips, uniting at its periphery with the other muscles which act upon the mouth. The lower fibers are continued laterally into the buccinator and levator anguli oris (*caninus*) muscles, and the upper fibers into the buccinator and depressor anguli oris (*triangularis*). It consists of a medial, or labial, part, and a lateral, peripheral, or facial part, the two differing in appearance and in the arrangement of their fibers. The medial, or *labial*, portion consists of pale, thin fibers, fine in texture. It corresponds in position with the red margin of the lips, and has no bony attachment, but is continuous around the angles of the mouth from one lip to the other. The peripheral, or *facial*, portion is thinner and wider than the labial. It has a bony attachment and is also connected with the adjacent muscles. In the upper lip the orbicularis oris muscle is attached at each side of the middle line to the lower part of the septum nasi by the *naso-labial slip*, and to the alveolar border of the maxilla opposite the incisor teeth by the *superior incisive bundle;* in the lower lip it is attached to the alveolar border of the mandible opposite the canine teeth by a single fasciculus, the *inferior incisive bundle*. The cutaneous surface of the muscle is intimately connected with the skin of the lips and surrounding parts. The intimacy of this union is so great in some instances that the mouth is surrounded by radiating wrinkles, especially marked in the upper lips of women. The labial integument of the male probably contains fewer wrinkles on account of the presence of large hair-bulbs. The deep surface of the orbicularis oris is covered by mucous membrane, between which and the muscle, in the submucous tissue, are the coronary (*labial*) arteries and the labial glands.

NERVE SUPPLY.—From the buccal and supramandibular (*mandibular*) branches of the cervico-facial division of the facial nerve.

ACTION.—When the facial and labial portions act conjointly they press together and project the lips. The labial fibers acting alone bring the lips and the angles of the mouth together and invert the lips. The facial fibers acting alone press the lips against the alveolar borders of the maxillæ, and at the same time evert the lips. The orbicularis oris is the antagonist of all those muscles which converge to the lips from the various parts of the face.

15

The **depressor labii superioris** (**quadratus labii superioris**) is a thin quadrangular muscle having three heads—angular, infra-orbital, zygomatic—all of which are *inserted* into the skin and the musculature of the upper lip.

The levator labii superioris alæque nasi, the *angular head*, has already been described.

The *zygomatic head* is described with the zygomatic muscles (p. 227).

The **levator labii superioris** (**the infra-orbital head of the quadratus labii superioris**) *arises* from the superior maxilla (*maxilla*) above the infra-orbital foramen, and is *inserted* into the upper lip, its fibers blending with the orbicularis oris muscle. At its origin it is overlapped by the orbicularis palpebrarum (*orbicularis oculi*), and covers the infra-orbital vessels and nerves. It is a landmark in exposing the infra-orbital nerve.

NERVE SUPPLY.—From the infra-orbital (*zygomatic*) branch of the upper division of the facial nerve.

ACTION.—It raises the upper lip.

DISSECTION.—Reflect the levator labii superioris (*infra-orbital head of the quadratus labii superioris*) muscle downward from its origin, and expose the levator anguli oris (*caninus*), the infra-orbital plexus of nerves, and the infra-orbital vessels.

The **levator anguli oris** (**caninus**) **muscle** *arises* from the canine fossa of the superior maxilla (*maxilla*) below the infra-orbital foramen, and is *inserted* into the angle of the mouth, superficial to the buccinator muscle, its fibers blending with the orbicularis oris, the zygomaticus, and the depressor anguli oris (*triangularis*) muscles.

NERVE SUPPLY.—From the infra-orbital (*zygomatic*) branch of the upper division of the facial nerve.

ACTION.—It raises and draws the angle of the mouth medialward.

The **depressor labii inferioris** (**quadratus labii inferioris**) **muscle** *arises* from the oblique line of the mandible by a wide origin, extending from a point below the mental foramen almost to the symphysis. Its fibers are associated with those of the muscle of the opposite side, ascend, and are *inserted* into the integument of the lower lip, blending with the orbicularis oris. Its origin is covered by the depressor anguli oris (*triangularis*) muscle.

NERVE SUPPLY.—From the supramandibular (*mandibular*) branch of the cervico-facial division of the facial nerve.

ACTION.—It depresses and everts the lower lip.

The **depressor anguli oris** (**triangularis**) **muscle** *arises* from the oblique line of the mandible lateral to the depressor labii inferioris (*quadratus labii inferioris*) muscle, and is continuous with the platysma. Its fibers ascend to be *inserted* into the angle of the mouth, intermingling with the zygomaticus, the levator anguli oris (*caninus*), the risorius, and the orbicularis oris muscles. Its lateral border overlaps the anterior part of the buccinator muscle.

NERVE SUPPLY.—From the supramandibular (*mandibular*) branch of the cervico-facial division of the facial nerve.

ACTION.—It draws the angle of the mouth downward and lateralward, producing an expression of sorrow.

The **levator menti** (**mentalis**) is a small muscle, seen by everting the lip and dissecting off the mucous membrane on each side of the labial frenulum. It *arises* from the fossa below the incisor teeth near the symphysis, and is *inserted* into the integument of the chin.

NERVE SUPPLY.—From the supramandibular (*mandibular*) branch of the cervico-facial division of the facial nerve.

ACTION.—It assists in raising the lower lip, at the same time wrinkling the integument of the chin over the point of its insertion, as in pouting.

The **zygomatic muscles** pass obliquely from the zygomatic arch to the upper lip and the angle of the mouth. The **zygomaticus major** (**zygomaticus**) *arises* from the lateral part of the malar (*zygomatic*) bone, in front of the suture between it and the zygoma; its fibers pass obliquely downward and medialward to be *inserted* into the angle of the mouth, blending with the fibers of the orbicularis oris and depressor anguli oris (*triangularis*) muscles.

NERVE SUPPLY.—From the infra-orbital branch of the temporo-facial division of the facial nerve.

ACTION.—The zygomaticus major draws the corner of the mouth upward and backward, as in smiling; the zygomaticus minor assists the levator labii superioris (*infra-orbital head of quadratus labii superioris*) muscle in raising the upper lip.

Bucco-pharyngeal fascia.—Before making a dissection of the buccinator muscle study the bucco-pharyngeal fascia, the thin layer of fascia which covers and adheres closely to its surface. It is attached to the alveolar borders of the superior maxilla (*maxilla*) and inferior maxilla (*mandible*), and posteriorly, where it is thickest and forms the pterygo-maxillary ligament (*pterygo-mandibular raphe*), it is continuous with the fascia over the constrictors of the pharynx. The bucco-pharyngeal fascia supports and strengthens the walls of the pharynx and the mouth; its density acts as a barrier to the escape of pus into the mouth or pharynx from an abscess in the cheek.

The **buccinator** muscle is a quadrangular, thin, flat muscle which occupies the interval between the superior maxilla (*maxilla*) and the mandible at the side of the face. It *arises* from the lateral surface of the alveolar borders opposite the middle and posterior molar teeth of the superior maxilla (*maxilla*), and the mandible; posteriorly, from the pterygo-maxillary ligament (*pterygo-mandibular raphe*). The *pterygo-maxillary ligament* (*pterygo-mandibular raphe*) is a fibrous band extending from the apex (hamular process) of the medial pterygoid plate (*lamina*) of the pterygoid process of the sphenoidal bone to the posterior extremity of the mylo-hyoid ridge of the mandible; it separates the buccinator muscle from the superior constrictor of the pharynx. The fibers of the buccinator pass forward, to be *inserted* into the orbicularis oris muscle at the angle of the mouth. The central fibers intersect one another, while the upper fibers pass to the upper lip and the lower fibers to the lower lip. In relation with the superficial surface of the buccinator muscle is a large mass of fat (*corpus adiposum buccæ, or buccal fat pad*), which separates it from: the ramus of the mandible, the masseter muscle, a small portion of the temporal muscle, and the muscles converging toward the angle of the mouth. Absorption of the fat overlying the muscle is followed by sinking of the cheek, as is seen in persons who are emaciated. The duct of the parotid gland, *Stenson's* (*parotid*) *duct*, which pierces the buccinator muscle opposite the second molar tooth of the superior maxilla (*maxilla*), crosses the upper part of the muscle obliquely, at about one centimeter below the zygoma. It is also crossed by the facial (*external maxillary*) artery and the facial (*anterior facial*) vein and by branches of the facial nerve. It is lined by the mucous membrane of the mouth, between which and the muscle are a number of racemose glands called the buccal glands; a few of these glands are found on the lateral surface of the muscle, and are called molar glands.

Nerve Supply.—From the facial nerve. The long buccal (*buccinator*) nerve, a branch of the inferior maxillary (*mandibular*), pierces the buccinator muscle on its way to supply the mucous membrane of the mouth.

Action.—The two buccinator muscles widen the aperture of the mouth transversely, pressing the lips against the teeth, and contract and compress the cheeks so that during mastication the food does not remain between the cheeks and the teeth. When only one muscle acts, the angle of the mouth is drawn to that side, and the cheek is wrinkled; during the act of whistling, the muscle contracts and prevents bulging of the cheeks.

It is hardly fair to the earnest dissector to leave this subject without the consoling reminder that the most expert dissectors cannot bring out these muscles in the cadaver as they are shown in the anatomic plates. It must be remembered that some of the facial muscles belong to the panniculus carnosus group, so extensive in animals but very limited in man. In some faces the musculature is a complex network of subcutaneous fibers running in all directions. In a muscular subject, a large number of distinct fasciculi are seen crossing one another, and are

PLATE LI.

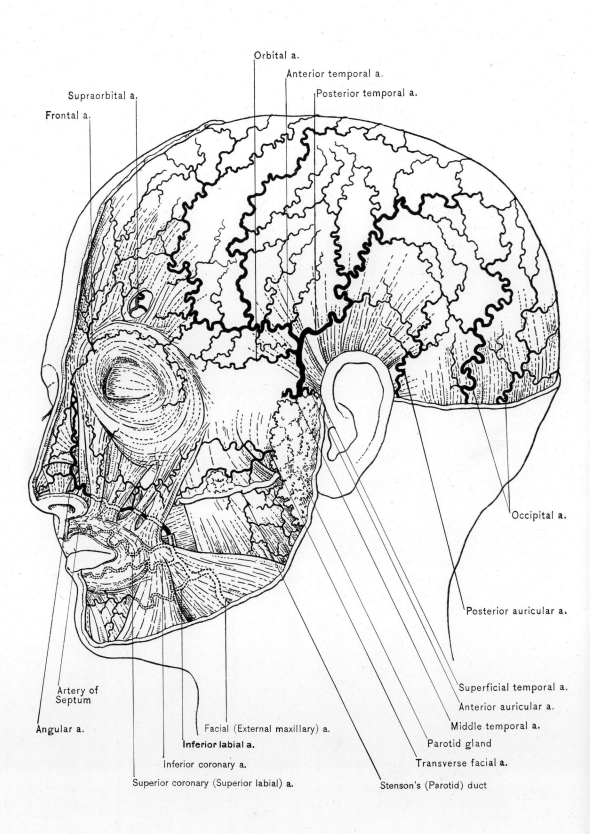

Orbital a.

Anterior temporal a.

Posterior temporal a.

Supraorbital a.

Frontal a.

Occipital a.

Posterior auricular a.

Artery of
Septum

Superficial temporal a.

Anterior auricular a.

Angular a.

Middle temporal a.

Facial (External maxillary) a.

Parotid gland

Inferior labial a.

Transverse facial a.

Inferior coronary a.

Stenson's (Parotid) duct

Superior coronary (Superior labial) a.

ARTERIES OF SCALP AND FACE.

PLATE LII.

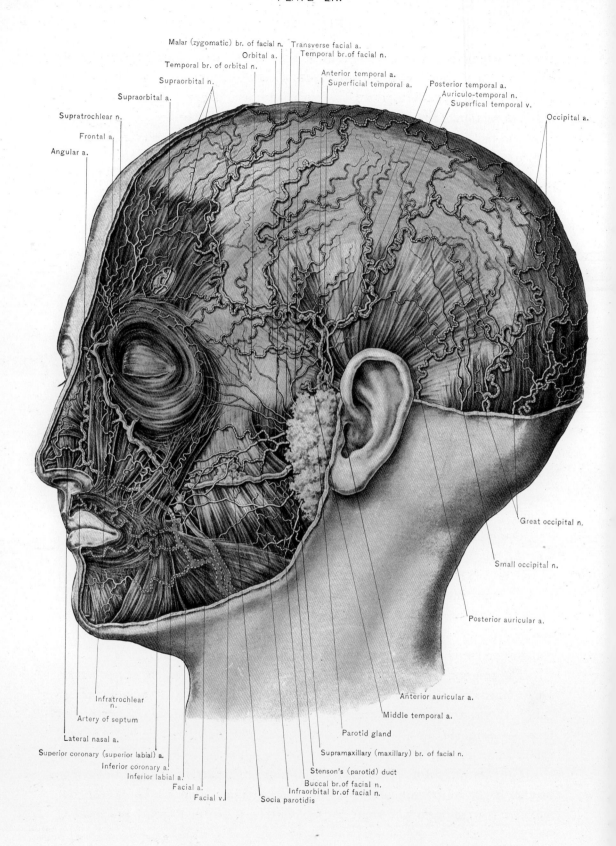

Malar (zygomatic) br. of facial n.
Orbital a.
Temporal br. of orbital n.
Supraorbital n.
Supraorbital a.
Supratrochlear n.
Frontal a.
Angular a.
Transverse facial a.
Temporal br. of facial n.
Anterior temporal a.
Superficial temporal a.
Posterior temporal a.
Auriculo-temporal n.
Superfical temporal v.
Occipital a.
Great occipital n.
Small occipital n.
Posterior auricular a.
Infratrochlear n.
Artery of septum
Lateral nasal a.
Superior coronary (superior labial) a.
Inferior coronary a.
Inferior labial a.
Facial a.
Facial v.
Socia parotidis
Anterior auricular a.
Middle temporal a.
Parotid gland
Supramaxillary (maxillary) br. of facial n.
Stenson's (parotid) duct
Buccal br.of facial n.
Infraorbital br.of facial n.

ARTERIES, NERVES, AND MUSCLES OF SCALP AND FACE.

232

more or less merged with the constant muscles of the face. This difference in the amount of facial musculature undoubtedly accounts for much of the variation in the amount of facial wrinkling observed in different persons. It is safe to say . that a dissection of the muscles of the face with their boundaries as well defined as shown in pictures does more credit to the dissector's skill in imitating a diagram than to any painstaking effort to exhibit the natural state of the parts.

The **Facial (External Maxillary) Artery** (Plates LI; LII), a branch of the external carotid, enters the face over the body of the mandible, at the antero-inferior angle of the masseter muscle, where its pulsations can readily be felt and it can be compressed against the bone; thence it ascends forward across the cheek, over the buccinator, and beneath the platysma muscle to the angle of the mouth; thence to the side of the nose, to terminate at the medial canthus of the eye as the *angular artery*. As the artery passes over the mandible it is covered by the platysma muscle and the deep fascia; near the mouth it passes beneath the zygomaticus major and the risorius muscles; along the side of the nose it is usually covered by the levator labii superioris alæque nasi (*quadrangular head of the quadratus labii superioris*) muscles. The companion vessel of the facial artery, the **facial (anterior facial) vein,** runs in an almost straight line from the medial canthus of the eye to the antero-inferior angle of the masseter muscle, being in contact with the facial (*external maxillary*) artery at these points, but elsewhere posterior to it. The artery is crossed by filaments of the facial nerve, while the levator labii superioris (*infra-orbital head of the quadratus labii superioris*) muscle separates it from the infra-orbital nerve posteriorly. The artery is usually divided into two portions, the facial and the cervical.

The **branches of the facial portion of the facial (external maxillary) artery** are: the muscular, inferior labial, inferior coronary, superior coronary (*superior labial*), lateral nasal, and angular.

The **muscular branches** are directed lateralward to supply the buccinator, masseter, and internal pterygoid muscles. They anastomose with the masseteric and buccinator branches of the internal maxillary, and with the infra-orbital and transverse facial arteries.

The **inferior labial artery** passes medialward beneath the depressor anguli oris (*triangularis*) muscle to supply the muscles and integument of the lower lip and chin. It anastomoses with the inferior coronary, the submental branch of the facial (*external maxillary*), and the mental branch of the inferior dental (*alveolar*) artery.

The **inferior coronary (branch of inferior labial) artery** arises, either independently or in common with the inferior labial, from the facial (*external maxillary*) artery near the angle of the mouth. It passes forward and medialward in a tortuous manner beneath the depressor anguli oris (*triangularis*) muscle toward the angle of the mouth, then pierces the orbicularis oris, and continues between it and the mucous membrane along the free margin of the lower lip.   It anastomoses with the inferior coronary artery of the opposite side, the inferior labial, and the mental branch of the inferior dental (*alveolar*) artery.

The **superior coronary (superior labial) artery,** which is larger and takes a more tortuous course than the inferior coronary (*branch of inferior labial*), arises from the facial (*external maxillary*) artery beneath the zygomaticus major muscle. It pierces the orbicularis oris, and runs between it and the mucous membrane along the free margin of the upper lip, to anastomose with the artery of the opposite side.   By the anastomosis of the superior coronary (*superior labial*) and inferior coronary (*branch of inferior labial*) arteries with their fellows, an arterial circle is formed which surrounds the mouth and can be felt pulsating on the internal surface of the lips, at six to twelve millimeters (one-fourth to one-half of an inch) from the junction of the skin and the mucous membrane.   A small branch, the *artery of the ala,* to the ala nasi and numerous branches to the labial glands are given off from this circle.

The **artery of the septum of the nose** is a terminal branch of the superior coronary (*superior labial*).   Its twigs are a common source of epistaxis.   The hemorrhage is readily controlled by compression of the artery of the septum, either by direct backward pressure against the upper lip, or by pressure from within outward, as when a firm pledget of cotton, paper, or other substance is pushed well up under the lip so as to put its tissues upon the stretch and occlude the lumen of the artery.   Another simple method is that of holding the cartilaginous end of the nose between the thumb and the forefinger.

The **lateral nasal artery** arises from the facial (*external maxillary*) artery opposite the ala of the nose, and passes forward over the lower part and the ala of the nose; it supplies the lateral and dorsal part of the nose, and anastomoses with its fellow of the opposite side, the nasal branch of the ophthalmic, the infra-orbital, and the artery of the septum.

The **angular artery,** the terminal part of the facial (*external maxillary*), passes to the medial canthus of the eye, where it lies on the nasal side of the lacrimal sac and the tendo oculi (*medial palpebral ligament*); it anastomoses with the nasal branch of the ophthalmic and with the infra-orbital artery, and supplies branches to the cheek.   In opening an abscess of the lacrimal sac it is important to bear in mind the situation of this artery on the medial side of the sac.

The facial (*external maxillary*) artery may require ligation after injury or preliminary to operative procedures around the mouth or tongue.   Direct ligation of the wounded branch is preferable because of the free anastomosis

PLATE VIII

PLATE LIII.

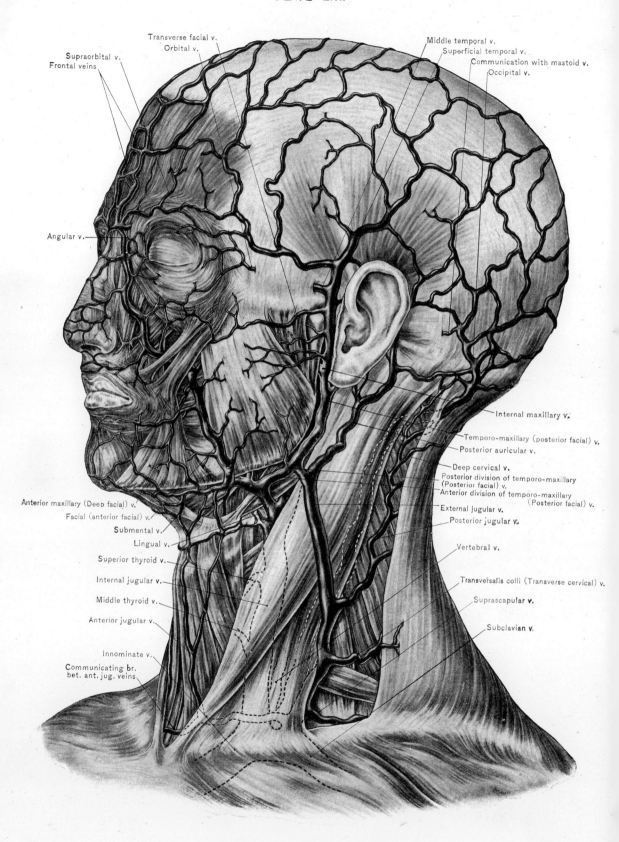

Transverse facial v.
Orbital v.
Supraorbital v.
Frontal veins
Middle temporal v.
Superficial temporal v.
Communication with mastoid v.
Occipital v.
Angular v.
Internal maxillary v.
Temporo-maxillary (posterior facial) v.
Posterior auricular v.
Deep cervical v.
Posterior division of temporo-maxillary (Posterior facial) v.
Anterior division of temporo-maxillary (Posterior facial) v.
Anterior maxillary (Deep facial) v.
Facial (anterior facial) v.
Submental v.
Lingual v.
Superior thyroid v.
Internal jugular v.
Middle thyroid v.
Anterior jugular v.
Innominate v.
Communicating br. bet. ant. jug. veins
External jugular v.
Posterior jugular v.
Vertebral v.
Transversalis colli (Transverse cervical) v.
Suprascapular v.
Subclavian v.

VEINS OF SCALP, FACE, AND NECK.

between the branches of the two sides. Preliminary to fulguration for carcinoma of the tongue, it is important to ligate the facial (external maxillary) at the same time that the lingual is ligated. The facial (*external maxillary*) artery and its branches are surrounded by a minute plexus of sympathetic fibers, *nervi molles*, not demonstrable macroscopically. These fibres are branches of the superior cervical ganglion of the sympathetic, and supply the walls of the artery and its branches; they furnish the sympathetic root to the submaxillary (*submandibular*) ganglion.

The **transverse facial artery** passes transversely across the face between the zygoma and the parotid duct, resting upon the masseter muscle. It arises from the temporal artery in the substance of the parotid gland, and sometimes from the external carotid artery. It supplies the small, often detached, part of the parotid gland (the socia parotidis) in relation with the duct, the masseter, the orbicularis palpebrarum (*orbicularis oculi*) muscles and the integument, and anastomoses with the infra-orbital, the facial (*external maxillary*), and the masseteric arteries. It is accompanied by two or three branches of the facial nerve. It is quite small except when it supplies those parts which usually receive blood from the facial (*external maxillary*) artery; it occasionally gives off the coronary and nasal arteries.

The **facial** (**anterior facial**) **vein** (Plate LIII), the continuation of the angular vein, and formed by the union of the frontal and supra-orbital veins, arises at the medial canthus of the eye and, as already stated, runs in an almost straight line to the antero-inferior angle of the masseter muscle, where it comes into relation with the lateral side of the facial (*external maxillary*) artery. In its course across the face it lies above and lateral to the artery, passing over the levator labii superioris (*infra-orbital head of the quadratus labii superioris*), beneath the zygomatic muscles, and over the parotid duct, the buccinator muscle, the antero-inferior angle of the masseter muscle and masseteric fascia, and the body of the mandible. Below the mandible it is joined by the anterior branch of the temporo-maxillary (*posterior facial*) vein, and empties into the internal jugular vein. It receives veins from the lower eyelid, the inferior palpebral, from the side of the nose, the lateral nasal, from the orbital vein, and, beneath the zygomaticus major muscle, a deep facial branch from the pterygoid plexus; it also receives muscular branches and branches corresponding to those of the facial (*external maxillary*) artery. The facial (*anterior facial*) vein arises in the angular vein, and through the latter communicates freely with the ophthalmic vein, and thus with the cavernous sinus; it also communicates with the cavernous sinus, and through the deep facial vein with the pterygoid plexus of veins, which, in turn, communicates with the sinus by means of small veins which pass through the foramen ovale, the foramen of Vesalius, and the foramen lacerum medium (*foramen lacerum*). Owing to this free communication between the vein and the cavernous sinus, the latter is endangered by an inflammatory condition of or around the facial (*anterior facial*) vein.

Disease involving the facial vein.—The facial vein, as a rule, has no valves; this explains why emboli are readily carried to the internal jugular vein and thus into the general circulation. Carbuncle of the face may prove fatal by inducing thrombosis of the cerebral sinuses through the communications previously described. Any deep inflammation of the face, such as phlegmonous erysipelas, may be complicated by thrombosis or pyemia. The injection of facial nevi in infants may result in death from thrombosis, owing to the direct communication of the facial (*anterior facial*) with the internal jugular vein. Pulmonary embolism and death have been known to follow the injection of perchlorid of iron for a nevoid growth of the face. In arteriovenous aneurysm of the cavernous sinus arterial blood flows by way of the ophthalmic and angular veins through the facial (*anterior facial*) vein, and gives rise to a pulsating varicose condition of the latter with a distinct thrill and bruit.

Vascularity of the face.—As already indicated, the tissues of the face are very vascular. In persons exposed to cold, or in those addicted to strong drink, the very small vessels of the skin, especially over the nose, appear permanently injected or varicose. Attention has been called to the fact that nevi and various forms of erectile tumors are common about the face. Wounds of the face, while they bleed freely, heal very rapidly; their edges should be carefully adjusted as soon after the accident as possible. Extensive flaps of skin which have been torn up in lacerated wounds of the face often retain their vitality in almost as marked a manner as similar flaps torn from the scalp. The anastomoses of the facial (*external maxillary*) artery are so free that when the vessel is divided, both ends bleed freely and, according to the general rule, they should both be tied.

DISSECTION.—Upon the side of the face on which the muscles have been exposed the appendages of the eye, including the eyelids, eyebrows, eyelashes, tarsal cartilages (*tarsal plates*), conjunctiva, and lacrimal caruncle, the parotid gland and the external ear should be carefully dissected before turning the head to make the dissection of the nerves.

The **eyebrows** are prominent arches of integument overlying the superciliary ridges and connected with the orbicularis palpebrarum (*orbicularis oculi*), the corrugator supercilii, and occipito-frontalis (*epicranius*) muscles. They are covered by numerous short, thick hairs which surmount the upper circumference of the orbit; although the general direction of the hairs is lateralward, they interlace, the upper ones curving downward and the lower ones upward. They serve the two-fold purpose of shielding the eye from the admission of foreign bodies, and of a multiple spring buffer reducing somewhat the impact of blows against the brow, thus often preventing serious wounds of the skin from traumatism applied against the sharp supra-orbital margin.

The **eyelids, or palpebræ,** are two movable semilunar curtains placed in front of each eyeball to protect that exceedingly delicate and important organ. The free edges, which are transverse and are studded with hairs, the eyelashes, are strengthened by the fibrous tarsal plate. The *upper lid* is the longer, so that when the lids are closed, their margin of contact lies below the center of the eye. It is also more freely movable, having a special muscle to raise it, the levator palpebræ superioris. The interval between the open eyelids is called the *fissura* or *rima palpebrarum,* or palpebral slit. At the points of union of the eyelids are the *lateral and medial canthi,* or palpebral commissures. The *medial canthus* is the larger; it contains a depressed triangular space, the *lacus lacrimalis,* and an elevation, the *caruncula lacrimalis.* At the medial extremities of the lids and upon their free surfaces are two small elevations, the *lacrimal papillæ,* in the center of which are small openings called the *puncta lacrimalia,* the orifices of the *lacrimal canaliculi.* The free margins are provided in front with eyelashes and with the orifices of sebaceous and modified sweat glands; and underneath, with small openings, the orifices of the ducts of the Meibomian (*tarsal*) glands. Medial to the orifices of the lacrimal canaliculi the eyelids are devoid of eyelashes and Meibomian (*tarsal*) glands. When the eyelids are closed, an interval exists between them and the eyeball for the passage of the tears medialward.

The **eyelashes,** or **cilia,** are two or more rows of short, thick, curved hairs fixed in the anterior margin of the free border of the eyelids. Those of the upper lid are longer and more numerous (one hundred to one hundred and fifty), and have their convexities directed downward, while those of the lower lid have their convexities directed upward. They protect the eye against the admission of dust and other foreign substances.

The conjunctiva is the mucous membrane which covers the inner surface of the eyelids and the anterior part of the eyeball. At the free margin of the lids it is continuous with the integument. Before dissecting the eyelid, the conjunctiva and the lacrimal caruncle should be examined. The conjunctiva consists of three portions: the *palpebral conjunctiva,* covering the posterior surface of the lids and closely adherent to the tarsus; the *bulbar conjunctiva,* overlying the sclera and the cornea; the *superior* and *inferior conjunctual fornices,* forming the line of transition of the conjunctiva from the eyelids to the eyeball. The palpebral portion is more vascular than the remaining parts, and is studded with a number of small papillæ. The conjunctiva covering the sclera is loosely attached by submucous tissue, while that over the cornea is very thin, consisting merely of an epithelial layer which is very adherent. In congestion of the conjunctiva with effusion into the loose subconjunctival tissue (chemosis) the membrane is at times swollen to the very edge of the cornea, where it forms a sharp elevated margin. In fractures of the frontal fossa, involving the roof of the orbit, hemorrhage first shows beneath the bulbar conjunctiva. The lacrimal ducts (excretory ducts of the lacrimal gland) empty upon the free surface of the reflected portion of the conjunctiva.

The **caruncula lacrimalis** (Plate LIV) is a small, reddish elevation situated at the medial canthus in the lacus lacrimalis. It consists of a small island of modified skin, which presents minute hairs upon its surface. It contains modified sweat glands, as well as sebaceous glands, imbedded in a small pad of fat. Lateral to the caruncle, and resting upon the eyeball, is a semilunar fold of conjunctiva, the *plica semilunaris*, with its free concave margin directed toward the cornea. It is a rudimentary membrana nictitans (the third eyelid in birds). Smooth muscle fibers have been found in this fold, and in some of the domestic animals it is known to contain a thin plate of cartilage.

Besides being continuous with the skin at the free borders of the lids, the conjunctiva is also continuous, through the lacrimal canaliculi, with the mucous membrane of the lacrimal sac, the nasal duct, and the inferior meatus of the nose. The loose subconjunctival tissue, especially in elderly persons, frequently contains small yellowish masses of fat, called pingueculæ. A triangular elevated layer of conjunctiva and subconjunctival tissue with its apex toward the cornea, called a *pterygium*, is occasionally seen.

Postconjunctival operations, such as section of the ocular muscles, require an incision into the conjunctiva; its lax attachment to the sclera is of advantage, since a loose fold is readily raised with the forceps and incised to the required extent, after which it is easily peeled back as far as necessary.

The **eyelids** are composed of skin, subcutaneous tissue, the orbicularis palpebrarum (*orbicularis oculi*) muscle, palpebral ligaments, orbito-tarsal ligaments, the tarsal plates, the Meibomian (*tarsal*) glands, and of vessels, nerves, and conjunctiva. The upper lid contains, in addition to the structures just mentioned, the aponeurotic insertion of the levator palpebræ superioris muscle. The skin of the lids and the orbicularis palpebrarum (*orbicularis oculi*) muscle have already been described.

The **subcutaneous areolar tissue** of the eyelids is notable for the entire absence of fat. Its laxity and elasticity account for the extensive ecchymosis after comparatively slight trauma, and for the marked edema sometimes present in nephritis.

PLATE LIV.

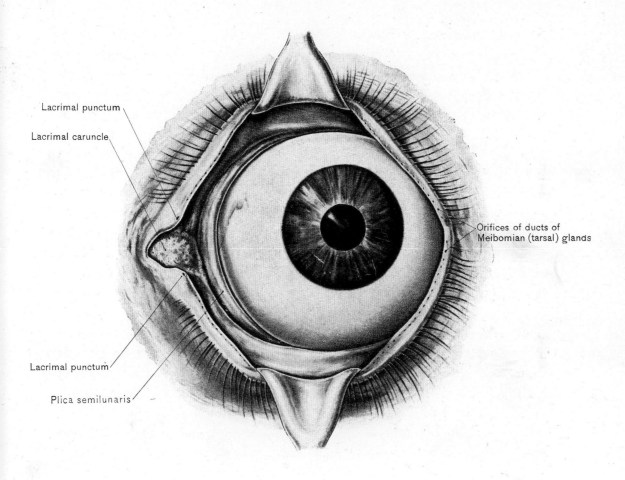

Lacrimal punctum

Lacrimal caruncle

Orifices of ducts of
Meibomian (tarsal) glands

Lacrimal punctum

Plica semilunaris

PALPEBRAL FISSURE AND EYEBALL,—EYELIDS EVERTED.

PLATE LV.

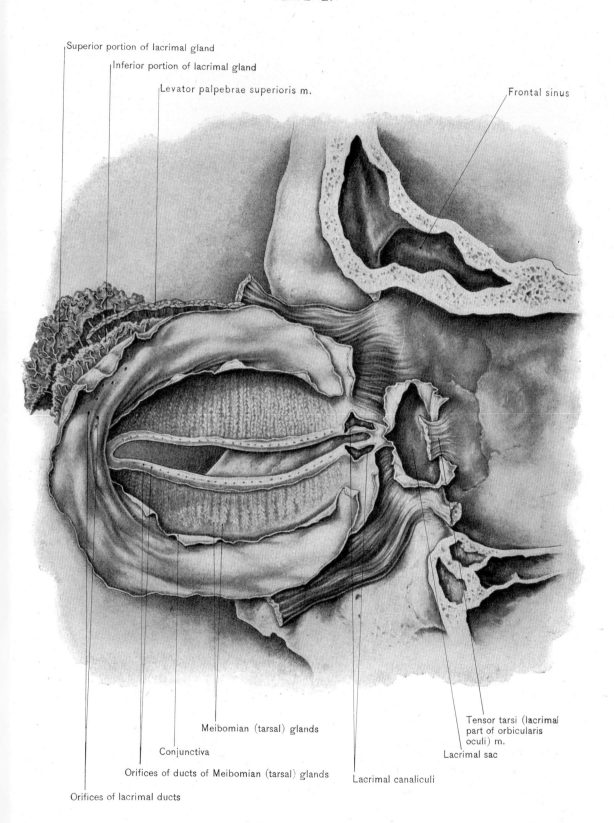

Superior portion of lacrimal gland

Inferior portion of lacrimal gland

Levator palpebrae superioris m.

Frontal sinus

Meibomian (tarsal) glands

Conjunctiva

Orifices of ducts of Meibomian (tarsal) glands

Orifices of lacrimal ducts

Tensor tarsi (lacrimal part of orbicularis oculi) m.

Lacrimal sac

Lacrimal canaliculi

LACRYMAL APPARATUS AND MEIBOMIAN (TARSAL) GLANDS.

The **palpebral ligaments,** previously described at page 220, are fibrous bands attaching the tarsal plates to the lateral and medial margins of the orbit. The *lateral* ligament is undivided, and extends from the malar (*zygomatic*) bone to the lateral extremities of the tarsal plates. The *medial* ligament, or tendo oculi, extends from the nasal process of the superior maxilla (*maxilla*) and the crest of the lacrimal bone to the medial extremities of the tarsal plates. The division of the tendo oculi (*medial palpebral ligament*) which is attached to the nasal process of the superior maxilla (*maxilla*) passes in front of the lacrimal sac, while the limb attached to the crest of the lacrimal bone passes over its lateral wall.

The **orbito-tarsal ligaments** (palpebral fasciæ) are fibrous membranes continuous with the periosteum, and extend from the superior and inferior orbital margins to the tarsal plates. In the upper lid the orbito-tarsal ligament fuses with the tendon of the levator palpebræ superioris muscle. These ligaments prevent the passage of pus from the subcutaneous areolar tissue into the orbit, and hence are called the *septa orbitale.*

The **tarsal plates,** situated in the free margins of the eyelids, are two plates of dense connective tissue. They are thickest at their free, or ciliary, margins, and give support and shape to the eyelids. The plate of the upper lid is much larger than that of the lower, and gives attachment to the aponeurosis of the levator palpebræ superioris muscle. In both lids the attached margins of the tarsal plates are continuous with the orbito-tarsal ligaments.

The **Meibomian (tarsal) glands** (Plate LV) are sebaceous glands lodged in the substance of the tarsal plates, and number between twenty-five and thirty in the upper, and somewhat less in the lower lid. The orifices of the glands open on the free borders of the lids behind the lashes. Each gland consists of a straight tube with many short, blind diverticula. The Meibomian (*tarsal*) glands secrete a sebaceous material which prevents the lids from adhering, and are readily distinguished as closely adjacent, vertical, yellow streaks across the inner surface of the lids. When the duct of one of these glands becomes occluded, a retention cyst (chalazion) similar to a wen, is formed.

Non-striated muscle fibers, *tarsal muscles,* known as the superior and inferior palpebral muscles of Müller, are also found in both lids inserted close to the attached borders of the tarsal plates. In the upper lid these fibers *arise* from the lower surface of the levator palpebræ superioris; in the lower lid they *arise* from the vicinity of the inferior oblique muscle.

BLOOD SUPPLY.—The eyelids receive their blood supply from palpebral and lacrimal branches of the ophthalmic artery, and from small branches of the temporal and transverse facial arteries. The *palpebral branches* of the ophthalmic, two in number, arise from that artery near the pulley of the superior oblique muscle; one is found in each lid running through the fibrous tissue layer of the lids between the orbicularis palpebrarum (*orbicularis oculi*) muscle and the tarsal plates near their margins. The *lacrimal branch* is the first branch and one of the largest branches of the ophthalmic artery. It accompanies the lacrimal nerve and gives off palpebral twigs which anastomose with the other palpebral arteries to form the tarsal arches.

The *veins of the eyelids* are larger and more numerous than the arteries. Those from the deeper portions, the *retrotarsal veins*, empty into the branches of the ophthalmic, while those draining the more superficial parts of the eyelid, *pretarsal veins*, empty into the frontal and facial (*anterior facial*) veins medially, and into the supra-orbital and superficial temporal laterally.

The *lymphatics of the eyelids*, consisting of a pre- and a post-tarsal set, pass to the parotid and submaxillary (*submandibular*) lymph glands.

NERVE SUPPLY.—The nerve supply is free. The nerves to the palpebral portion of the orbicularis palpebrarum (*orbicularis oculi*) muscle arise from the facial nerve and enter the lids near the lateral canthus. The cutaneous filaments of the upper lid are obtained from the lacrimal, supra-orbital, supratrochlear, and infratrochlear nerves; the lower lid derives its supply from the infra-orbital. The non-striated muscle tissue of the lids is supplied by fibers from the sympathetic system.

The **conjunctiva** has been described at p. 239.

The **levator palpebræ superioris muscle** *arises* from the inferior surface of the lesser wing of the sphenoidal bone above the optic foramen; its fibers terminate in a broad, thin aponeurosis which is *inserted* into the superior border of the superior tarsal plate. This muscle runs above the superior rectus, and its superior surface is in relation with the frontal nerve and the supra-orbital artery.

The **parotid gland** (Plate XLIX), the largest of the salivary glands, weighs from fifteen to thirty grams (one-half to one ounce). It is situated on the side of the face, and extends from the zygoma to below the level of the angle of the mandible, covering about one-third of the masseter muscle, and reaching backward to the external auditory meatus, the mastoid process, and the sterno-mastoid muscle. It is lodged in the variable space between the ramus of the mandible and the mastoid process. The main mass of the gland is triangular in shape. The superficial surface is roughly triangular, the apex extending forward over the masseter muscle and called, when detached, the socia parotidis (*accessory parotid gland*). Several processes are found passing into the intervals bounding the deep surface of the gland. The glenoid process, or lobe, occupies the non-articular part of the glenoid fossa. The extension behind the posterior margin of the mandible and between the pterygoid muscle is known as the pterygoid lobe. Where the deeper portion of the gland, the carotid lobe, comes in contact with the styloid process, the stylo-hyoid and stylo-glossus muscles, the internal carotid artery, and the internal jugular vein, are found. Owing to the position which the parotid gland holds with reference to the temporo-maxillary (*temporo-mandibular*) articulation, inflammation of the gland is attended by pain during movement of the articulation. The extent to which the mandible can be depressed under these circumstances depends upon the degree of swelling.

Parotid (parotideo-masseteric) fascia.—The parotid gland is covered by a dense and strong layer of fascia, a prolongation of the superficial layer of the deep cervical fascia, called the parotid fascia. It is attached above to the zygoma, and is continuous behind and in front with the fascia covering respectively, the sterno-mastoid and the masseter muscle. From the parotid fascia numerous processes are sent into the substance of the gland to support its lobules. The deep fascia of the neck also sends beneath the gland a thin layer continuous with the stylo-maxillary (*stylo-mandibular*) ligament, which separates the parotid from the submaxillary (*submandibular*) gland. The fibrous envelop of the parotid gland is incomplete superiorly and anteriorly, where its cavity is in communication with the pterygo-maxillary region. On account of this gap in the fascial envelop, the pus of a parotid abscess may extend into the pterygo-maxillary region, and by way of the latter, into the temporal fossa, or to the retropharyngeal space, since it meets with less resistance in taking either of these directions than in attempting to reach the surface. The abscess may also extend into the neck by ulcerating through the layer of fascia beneath the gland. Retropharyngeal abscess is often attended by swelling in the parotid region. Retropharyngeal growths of considerable size, such as sarcomata, cause bulging of the parotid region; and conversely, tumors of the parotid may bulge into the pharynx. The severe pain in a rapidly growing tumor or abscess of the gland is due to the density of the fascia covering it. This, too, makes it difficult to detect fluctuation early, and also explains why the pus in a parotid abscess is so slow to find its way to the surface, and emphasizes the importance of making an early opening. The intimate relation existing between the parotid gland, the external auditory meatus, and the temporo-maxillary (*temporo-mandibular*) articulation, should be borne in mind, as a parotid abscess may open into the meatus or cause involvement of the joint.

The **nerves** supplying the parotid gland are: the auriculo-temporal branch of the inferior maxillary (*mandibular*) nerve, the great auricular branch of the cervical plexus, the facial nerve, and branches from the carotid plexus of the sympathetic. In painful affections of the gland the pain is apt to be referred to the areas of distribution of these nerves.

The parotid lymph glands.—Lying upon the surface of the parotid gland in front of the cartilage of the ear, and close to the root of the zygoma, are one or more superficial lymph glands, enlargement of which must not be mistaken for a tumor of the parotid gland itself.

Structures within the parotid gland.—The parotid gland is important, not only on account of its function and position, as well as its relation to the surrounding parts, but also because of the important structures found within it, which mentioned from without inward are: the facial nerve, passing postero-anteriorly and spreading out into an irregular series of branches, the *pes anserinus, or parotid plexus;* the temporo-maxillary *(posterior facial)*, superficial temporal, internal maxillary, and posterior auricular veins; the origin of the external jugular vein; the external carotid artery which supplies branches to the gland and divides at the neck of the mandible into its two terminal branches, the temporal and internal maxillary arteries; the terminal part of the great auricular nerve, and one or two lymph glands. The posterior auricular branch of the external carotid artery and the transverse facial branch of the temporal artery arise in the substance of the gland.

The parotid gland is separated by a thin layer of fascia from the internal carotid artery, from the internal jugular vein, and from the vagus, the glosso-pharyngeal and the hypoglossal nerves. In stab wounds of the parotid region, involving one of the two carotid arteries, it may be difficult at first to tell which vessel has been wounded.

From an anatomic point of view removal of the entire parotid gland, including its processes would appear to be almost impossible, but the operation has been done so many times by skilful surgeons that there is no question as to its feasibility, probably due to the fact that when the gland becomes the site of a neoplasm it becomes more compact, its processes being rounded off and lifted away from the surrounding structures.

Complete removal of the parotid gland results in paralysis of the muscles of expression, for it is impossible to avoid dividing the facial nerve. The author has seen a growth of the overlying lymph gland cause facial paralysis from pressure, and thus so closely simulate a parotid neoplasm as to be pronounced a tumor of the parotid gland; but upon removal of the growth the parotid gland was seen to occupy the bottom of the wound, and to be in a very much atrophied condition.

Stenson's (parotid) duct.—Running about one centimeter below the zygoma, or in a line drawn from the lower margin of the external auditory meatus to a point midway between the free margin of the upper lip and the ala of the nose, is the parotid duct, or Stensons' duct. It is about four centimeters (two inches) in length, by three millimeters (one-eight of an inch) in diameter, being narrowest at its point of communication with the mouth. It lies between the transverse facial artery above, and the buccal branch of the facial nerve below. The duct runs over the masseter muscle, turning abruptly medialward at its anterior border, passes through the buccal fat-pad and beneath the facial (*anterior facial*) vein, and pierces the buccinator muscle and the oral mucous membrane to open into the mouth opposite the crown of the second upper molar tooth. The turn of the duct around the anterior border of the masseter muscle must be borne in mind when passing a probe into the duct from the mouth. In opening a parotid abscess a horizontal incision should be made below the line of the duct and in front of the posterior border of the ramus of the mandible. Failure to observe this precaution may result in section of the duct, with resulting salivary fistula.

The partoid, or Stenson's, duct may be divided into a *masseteric portion* resting upon the masseter muscle, and a *buccal portion* extending from the anterior border of the masseter muscle to the termination of the duct in the mucous membrane of the cheek. A fistula of the masseteric part is not easily closed, but a fistula of the buccal portion can be closed by making an opening from the duct into the mouth on the proximal side of the fistula. The author has successfully treated fistulæ of the buccal portion by exposing the duct through an incision in the cheek, dividing the duct at the proximal side of the fistula, freeing the duct from the surrounding tissues, and stitching the divided end to the margins of an opening made in the mucous membrane of the mouth.

DISSECTION.—Before turning over the head to make the dissection of the opposite side of the face, the parotid gland should be removed entire; this operation will convey an approximate idea of the difficulties which would attend the removal of the gland in the living subject. The masseter muscle should then be exposed and the external ear dissected. In exposing the parotid gland, its fascial covering is seen to be continuous anteriorly with the fascia covering the masseter muscle, so that the parotid and masseteric fasciæ are practically one. These fasciæ are derived from the superficial layer of the deep cervical fascia, which is continued upward over the body of the mandible and attached above to the zygoma. By displacing the parotid gland forward and removing the fascia covering that portion of the masseter muscle in advance of the gland, the muscle itself is exposed.

The **masseter muscle,** the most superficial muscle of mastication, is quadrate in form, and *arises* as two portions: a large, tendinous, superficial layer, and a small, fleshy, deep layer. The *superficial sheet arises* from the anterior two-thirds of the inferior border of the zygomatic arch and from the inferior border of the malar (*zygomatic*) bone; its fibers pass inferiorly and posteriorly to be *inserted* into the lateral surface of the angle and the inferior portion of the ramus of the mandible.   The *deep sheet arises* from the posterior third of the inferior border and all of the medial surface of the zygoma; it passes inferiorly and anteriorly to be *inserted* into the superior half of the ramus and the lateral surface of the coronoid process of the mandible.   The lateral portion of the muscle is concealed by the parotid gland.   In relation with the superficial surface of the muscle are the orbicularis palpebrarum (*orbicularis oculi*), the zygomaticus major and zygomaticus minor muscles, and the platysma muscle, the anterior margin of the parotid gland, the parotid duct, the transverse facial vessels, branches of the facial nerve, and at its inferior angle, the facial (*anterior facial*) vein.   In relation with its deep surface are the buccal fat-pad, the buccinator muscle and a small part of the temporal muscle, the masseteric artery and nerve, and the ramus of the mandible.

BLOOD SUPPLY.—From the masseteric branch of the internal maxillary, the transverse facial, and the facial (*external maxillary*) arteries.

NERVE SUPPLY.—From the masseteric nerve, a branch of the inferior maxillary (*mandibular*) division of the trigeminal nerve.

ACTION.—It raises the mandible, as in mastication.

The **External Ear** consists of the auricle, or pinna, and of the external auditory canal, the tube leading to the tympanic membrane.   The auricle collects the vibrations of sound and the canal conveys them to the tympanum.

The **auricle, or pinna** (Plate LVI), is pyriform in shape, with its concave surface directed lateralward and slightly forward, and consists of a layer of yellow fibrocartilage with an uneven surface covered with integument except in the lobule where the cartilage is absent.   It is attached to the commencement of the external auditory meatus, and has various elevations and depressions, each elevation having a corresponding depression on its opposite surface.   The deep hollow in its center, which is wide above and narrow below, is called the *concha*. The concha leads to the commencement of the external auditory meatus, and is partly divided into two by the beginning of the helix.   The *helix* passes upward, forms the rim of the auricle, and terminates posteriorly in the *lobule*, which is the lowest portion of the auricle and consists of fatty and areolar tissue.   Internal to the helix is the depression called the *fossa of the helix*.   Internal to this fossa, bounding the concha behind and above, is a ridge, the *antihelix;* it begins above the lobule, at a small prominence, the *antitragus*, and bifurcates at the upper part of the auricle, embracing a small triangular depression, the *fossa of the antihelix* (*fossa triangularis*).   In front of the concha and projecting backward over the orifice of the external auditory meatus is the *tragus*.   Between the tragus and antitragus is a notch, the *incisura intertragica*.

PLATE LVI.

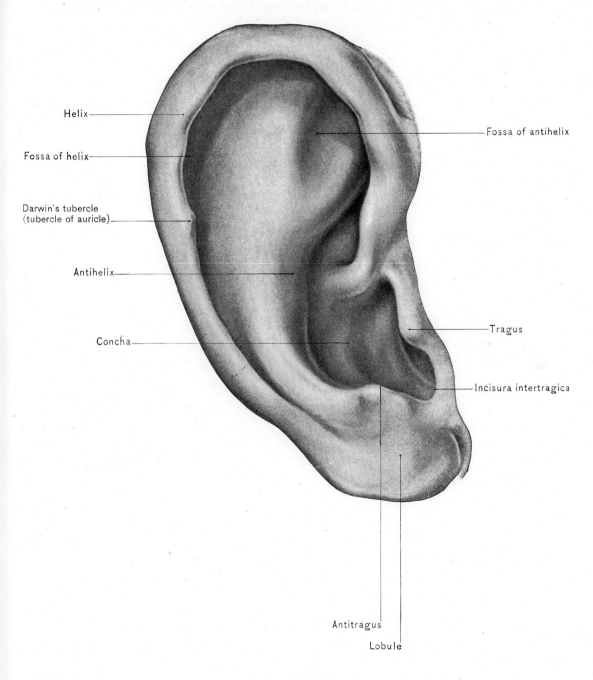

Helix

Fossa of helix

Darwin's tubercle
(tubercle of auricle)

Antihelix

Concha

Fossa of antihelix

Tragus

Incisura intertragica

Antitragus

Lobule

AURICLE.

PLATE LVII.

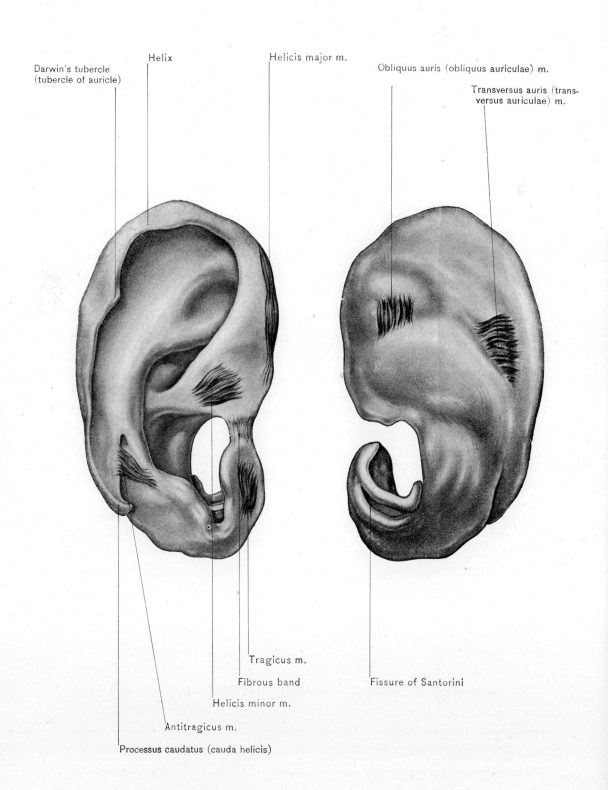

Darwin's tubercle
(tubercle of auricle)

Helix

Helicis major m.

Obliquus auris (obliquus auriculae) m.

Transversus auris (trans-
versus auriculae) m.

Tragicus m.

Fibrous band

Fissure of Santorini

Helicis minor m.

Antitragicus m.

Processus caudatus (cauda helicis)

INTRINSIC MUSCLES OF THE AURICLE.

DISSECTION.—Remove the integument from the auricle and expose the small and rudimentary muscles and the cartilage.

The integument of the auricle is thin and delicate. It contains sebaceous glands which are largest in the concha; the ducts of these glands often become filled with foreign matter, giving rise to comedones.

Upon the posterior aspect of the auricle the integument is less firmly attached to the underlying parts than elsewhere, consequently inflammatory swellings, as in erysipelas, are most marked in this situation.

Extravasations of blood beneath the skin, othematomata, or cauliflower ear, not uncommonly result from blows upon the ear, and are frequently observed in insane persons and in prize-fighters. It is said that degenerative changes in the blood-vessels and cartilage favor the occurrence of such extravasations. Cicatricial contractions may cause deformity of the auricle after the absorption or evacuation of such hematomata. Under the integument of the lobule gouty deposits (*tophi*) are sometimes found.

The three **Extrinsic Muscles,** which move the cartilage of the ear as a whole, have been described under the dissection of the scalp.

The **Intrinsic Muscles** of the auricle, which extend from one part of the cartilage to another, are six in number: the tragicus, the antitragicus, the helicis minor, the helicis major, the transversus auriculæ, and the obliquus auriculæ (Plate LVII).

The **tragicus,** the muscle of the tragus, is situated upon the lateral surface of the tragus, the vertical fibers, as a rule, being the only ones that are distinguishable.

The **antitragicus,** the muscle of the antitragus, *arises* from the lateral part of the antitragus; its fibers pass upward and are *inserted* into the posterior extremity of the helix.

The **helicis minor,** the small muscle of the helix, *arises* at the commencement of the helix and is *inserted* into the concha. This muscle is sometimes absent.

The **helicis major,** the large muscle of the helix, is situated upon the anterior margin of the helix; it *arises* above the small muscle and is *inserted* into the front of the helix, where it begins to curve backward.

The **transversus auriculæ,** the transverse muscle of the auricle, is situated on the back of the auricle in the depression between the helix and the convexity of the concha; it *arises* from the convexity of the concha and is *inserted* into the back of the helix.

The **obliquus auriculæ,** the oblique muscle of the auricle, extends from the upper back part of the concha to the convexity immediately above it.

Blood Supply.—The auricle is well supplied with freely anastomosing vessels, branches of the posterior auricular, superficial temporal, and occipital arteries. The veins accompany the corresponding arteries.

Nerve Supply.—The muscles are supplied by the temporal and the posterior auricular branches of the facial nerve. The sensory supply is from the auricular branch of the vagus (Arnold's nerve), the small occipital, the great auricular, and the auriculo-temporal nerves.

The numerous *lymphatics* empty into the pre-auricular glands and into the glands situated upon the insertion of the sterno-mastoid muscle.

The **cartilage of the auricle** is a single piece, and presents the irregularities characteristic of the external ear. It is prolonged inward in the shape of a tube which forms the outer part of the external auditory meatus; it is wanting between the tragus and the commencement of the helix, the interval between them being occupied by fibrous tissue. At the front part of the auricle, at the first bend of the helix, is a conical projection of the cartilage, the *spina helicis*, or process of the helix. At the highest part of the helix there is not infrequently another conical projection, to which Darwin first called attention, and which he regarded as the representative of the extreme tip of the auricle of some of the lower animals. At certain places the cartilage is incomplete; these gaps are known as fissures, and are located as follows: at the anterior part of the auricle, behind the process of the helix, the *fissure of the helix;* on the surface of the tragus, and at the lower part of the antihelix. In the piece of cartilage which forms the outer part of the meatus are the two *fissures of Santorini.* The auricle is attached anteriorly to the root of the zygoma and posteriorly to the mastoid process by bands of fibrous tissue; in addition, there are various intrinsic ligaments uniting the different parts.

Dissection.—Turn the head to the opposite side, fix it with hooks, and work out the facial nerve and the branches of the trigeminal nerve, both of which make their exit upon the face. Expose the facial nerve by a longitudinal incision carried into the substance of the parotid gland in front of the lobe of the ear, cutting away a little of the gland with each movement of the knife until the nerve is seen, when it can be traced backward and forward.

The **facial nerve** (the seventh cranial) is the motor nerve of the face; it consists of an intracranial, a temporal, and a facial portion (Plate LVIII). The *facial portion*, that which concerns us in this dissection, supplies all the muscles of expression, the extrinsic and intrinsic muscles of the ear, the platysma, the buccinator, the occipito-frontalis (*epicranius*), the posterior belly of the digastric, and the stylo-hyoid.

A line drawn from the anterior border of the mastoid process opposite the base of the lobule of the ear downward and forward across the face for about two

PLATE LVIII.

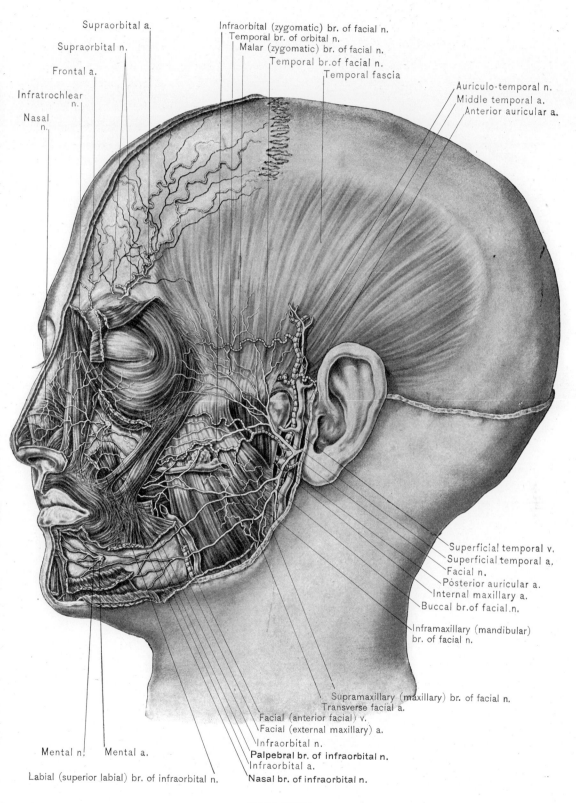

Supraorbital a.

Supraorbital n.

Frontal a.

Infratrochlear n.

Nasal n.

Infraorbital (zygomatic) br. of facial n.
Temporal br. of orbital n.
Malar (zygomatic) br. of facial n.
Temporal br. of facial n.
Temporal fascia

Auriculo-temporal n.
Middle temporal a.
Anterior auricular a.

Superficial temporal v.
Superficial temporal a.
Facial n.
Posterior auricular a.
Internal maxillary a.
Buccal br. of facial n.

Inframaxillary (mandibular) br. of facial n.

Supramaxillary (maxillary) br. of facial n.
Transverse facial a.
Facial (anterior facial) v.
Facial (external maxillary) a.
Infraorbital n.
Palpebral br. of infraorbital n.
Infraorbital a.
Nasal br. of infraorbital n.

Mental n.   Mental a.

Labial (superior labial) br. of infraorbital n.

FACIAL NERVE.

and a half centimeters (one inch) will represent the course of the *facial portion* of the trunk of the nerve.

It leaves the cranial cavity through the internal auditory meatus in company with the auditory nerve, the pars intermedia of Wrisberg (*nervus intermedius*), and the auditory artery. Reaching the bottom of the internal auditory meatus, it enters the facial canal, or aqueductus Fallopii of the temporal bone, from which it makes its exit by way of the stylo-mastoid foramen. Passing downward and forward from the foramen, it enters the parotid gland, crosses the external carotid artery, gives off a posterior auricular, a digastric, and a stylo-hyoid branch, and terminates in two divisions, the temporo-facial and the cervico-facial.

The **posterior auricular nerve,** the first extracranial branch of the facial nerve, passes upward in the groove between the ear and the mastoid process, communicates with the auricular branch of the vagus and the great auricular branch of the cervical plexus, and divides into an *auricular branch*, which supplies the attolens aurem (*superior auricular*) and retrahens aurem (*posterior auricular*) muscles, and an *occipital branch*, which passes along the superior curved line of the occipital bone, supplies the occipitalis muscle, and communicates with the small occipital branch of the cervical plexus.

The **digastric branch** supplies the posterior belly of the digastric muscle, and communicates through a twig which usually perforates that muscle, with the glossopharyngeal nerve.

The **stylo-hyoid branch** is longer than the digastric; it enters the stylo-hyoid muscle at about its middle, and communicates with filaments of the sympathetic nerve on the external carotid artery.

The **temporo-facial,** the larger of the two terminal divisions, runs obliquely upward and forward through the substance of the parotid gland, crosses the external carotid artery and the temporo-maxillary (*posterior facial*) vein. By various branchings and unions it forms an intricate looped plexus which breaks up into temporal, malar (*zygomatic*), and infra-orbital branches. It communicates with the auriculo-temporal nerve. The *temporal branches* ascend obliquely over the zygomatic arch to supply the tensor tarsi (*laminal part of the orbicularis oculi*), the orbicularis palpebrarum (*orbicularis oculi*), the corrugator supercilii, the frontalis, and the attolens aurem (*superior auricular*) and attrahens aurem (*anterior auricular*) muscles, and to communicate with the supra-orbital, the lacrimal, and the auriculo-temporal nerves and with the temporo-malar (*temporo-zygomatic*) branch of the superior maxillary (*maxillary*) nerve.

The *malar (upper zygomatic) branches* run across the malar (*zygomatic*) bone to the lateral angle of the orbit to supply the orbicularis palpebrarum (*orbicularis oculi*) muscle, and communicate with the lacrimal and the supra-orbital nerve and with the infra-orbital and temporo-malar (*temporo-zygomatic*) branches of the superior maxillary (*maxillary*) nerve. The *infra-orbital* (*lower zygomatic*), the largest branch, gives off a superficial and a deep set of branches, which pass transversely forward over the masseter and beneath the zygomatic muscles to supply the lower portion of the orbicularis palpebrarum (*orbicularis oculi*), the zygomatic muscles, the elevators of the upper lip, the muscles of the nose, and the orbicularis oris muscle. The superficial branches communicate with the nasal and the infratrochlear nerves, which are derived from the ophthalmic division of the trigeminal nerve. The deep branches form a loop with the buccal branch of the cervico-facial division, and pass beneath the levator labii superioris (*infra-orbital head of quadratus labii superioris*) muscle, where they unite with the infra-orbital branch of the superior maxillary (*maxillary*) nerve, forming the *infra-orbital plexus.*

The **cervico-facial,** the smaller of the two terminal divisions of the facial nerve, is joined by a branch of the great auricular nerve while in the substance of the parotid gland. It passes obliquely downward toward the angle of the mandible, crosses the external carotid artery and the temporo-maxillary (*posterior facial*) vein, and divides into a buccal, a supramandibular (*marginal branch of the mandible*), and inframandibular (*cervical*) branch. The *buccal branch* (*or branches*) passes forward over the masseter and buccinator muscles below the parotid duct to the angle of the mouth, to supply the buccinator and orbicularis oris muscles, and communicates with the infra-orbital nerve, the infra-orbital branches of the temporo-facial branch, and the long buccal branch of the inferior maxillary (*mandibular*) nerve. The buccal branch of the facial nerve and the long buccal branch of the inferior maxillary (*mandibular*) nerve form a plexus over the buccinator muscle and the facial vein. The *supramandibular* (*mandibular*) *branch* passes downward and forward over the masseter muscle and the facial artery, and beneath the platysma and the depressor muscles of the lower lip. It supplies the muscles of the lower lip, the risorius, and the levator menti (*mentalis*), and communicates with the buccal branch of the facial and the mental branch of the inferior dental nerve. The *inframandibular branch* (*cervical branch*) emerges from the lower border of the parotid gland in front of the external jugular vein, and passes downward and forward toward the sternum beneath the platysma muscle, which it supplies. It communicates with the great auricular and superficial cervical nerves, branches of the cervical plexus. The inframandibular (*cervical*) branch can be traced when dissecting the superficial fascia of the neck.

The **parotid plexus,** or **pes anserinus.**—The breaking up within the substance of the parotid gland of the two terminal divisions of the facial nerve, the temporo-

PLATE LIX.

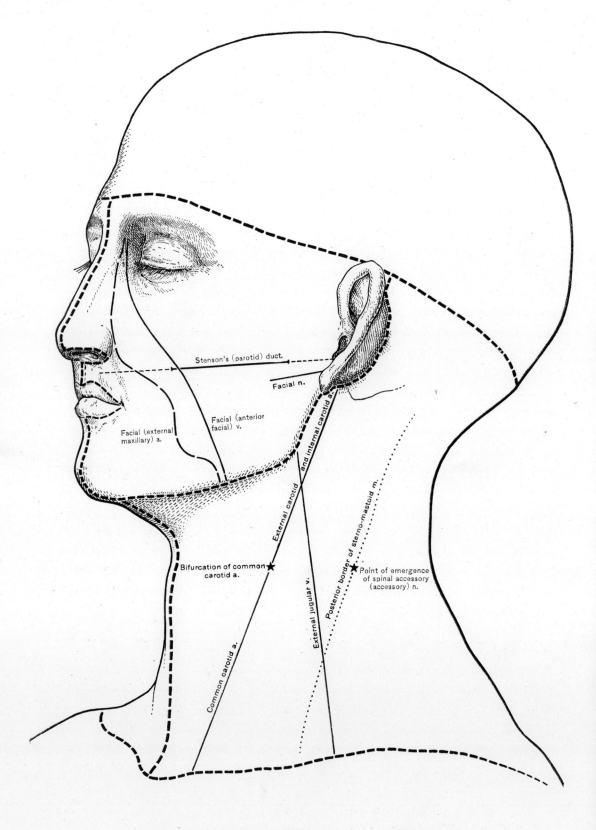

INCISIONS FOR DISSECTION AND LINES FOR VESSELS AND NERVES.

facial and the cervico-facial, gives rise to a claw-like plexus, known as the *parotid plexus,* or the pes anserinus (goose's foot).

Paralysis of the facial nerve is known as *Bell's palsy* and may be either central or peripheral. Central paralysis may be due to involvement of the nucleus of the nerve, its center in the cortex of the brain, or the fibers connecting these, as the result of pressure, by hemorrhage, abscess or tumor; it may also be brought about by degenerative processes in the brain. Peripheral paralysis is due to affection of the trunk of the nerve within the cranial cavity by tumors or by meningitis; within the facial, or Fallopian, canal, it is caused by middle ear disease or fracture of the base of the skull; if external to the stylo-mastoid foramen, it results from a growth at the stylo-mastoid foramen, rapidly growing tumors or abscess of the parotid gland, division during an operation, or exposure of the face to cold. When the lesion is situated beyond the origin of the chorda tympani nerve the muscles of expression and the buccinator muscle on the same side of the face become paralyzed, the mouth is drawn to the opposite side, and the affected side of the face becomes flattened and free from wrinkles. Through paralysis of the orbicularis palpebrarum (*orbicularis oculi*) muscle, the eye on the paralyzed side remains open, and the tears run down the cheek. Paralysis of the nasal muscles causes the anterior naris of the affected side to appear smaller than its fellow. Paralysis of the buccinator muscle causes the food to collect between the cheek and the teeth on the affected side, and when the orbicularis oris muscle is paralyzed the saliva dribbles from the mouth, and the patient is unable to whistle. When the lesion is situated in the facial, or Fallopian, canal and above the origin of the chorda tympani nerve, there is loss of the sense of taste in the anterior two-thirds of the tongue on the diseased side, and through paralysis of the stapedius muscle loud sounds are distressing. When the lesion is central, or in the brain, the brow and eyelid are not affected, that is, the frontalis, corrugator supercilii, and the orbicularis palpebrarum (*orbicularis oculi*) muscles are not involved. This is due to bilateral innervation through the upper facial fibers.

Spasm, either tonic or clonic, of the muscles supplied by the facial nerve may occur but is most commonly functional.

Operative exposure of the facial nerve (Plate LIX).—The facial nerve is exposed by carrying a vertical incision from in front of the mastoid process and behind the lobule of the ear downward toward the angle of the mandible, exposing first the posterior border of the parotid gland, which is displaced forward, and then the anterior border of the sterno-mastoid muscle at its insertion. The parotid gland should be separated from the mastoid process to the depth of about one centimeter, when the nerve may be seen. The exact location of the nerve in the wound can be ascertained by the use of the Faradic battery.

The trigeminal nerve.—The branches of the trigeminal, or fifth nerve, which make their exit upon the face are: the supra-orbital and the supratrochlear (previously described), the lacrimal, the infra-orbital, the infratrochlear, the malar (*zygomatic*), the temporal, the anterior branch of the nasal, the mental and the buccal nerve.

The **lacrimal nerve,** the smallest of the ophthalmic branches, supplies the lacrimal gland and the skin and conjunctiva around the lateral canthus of the eye. It communicates with the temporal branch of the temporo-malar (*temporo-zygomatic*) nerve in the orbit and with the temporal branch of the facial on the face.

The **infra-orbital nerve,** the terminal branch of the superior maxillary (*maxillary*) division of the trigeminal nerve, emerges from the infra-orbital foramen in company with the infra-orbital artery, under cover of the levator labii superioris (*infra-orbital head of quadratus labii superioris*) muscle. It immediately divides into palpebral, nasal, and labial branches (Plate LVIII). The *palpebral branches* (*palpebrales inferiores*), the smallest, pass upward beneath the orbicularis palpebrarum (*orbicularis oculi*) muscle, supply the conjunctiva and skin of the eyelid and communicate with the facial and the malar (*zygomatic*) branch of the orbital or temporo-malar (*temporo-zygomatic*) nerve. The *nasal branches* (*external nasal*), three or four in number, pass medialward under the levator labii superioris alæque nasi (*angular head of quadratus labii superioris*) muscle to supply the skin of the side of the nose. The *labial branches* (*superior labial*), usually four, are larger than the palpebral or nasal branches, and descend beneath the levator labii superioris (*infra-orbital head of quadratus labii superioris*) muscle to supply the skin and mucous membrane of the upper lip. Beneath the levator labii superioris (*infra-orbital head of quadratus labii superioris*) the branches assist in forming the infra-orbital plexus (see p. 260).

The **malar (zygomatico-facial) division** of the orbital, or temporo-malar (*temporo-zygomatic*), branch of the superior maxillary (*maxillary*) nerve, makes its exit through a foramen in the malar (*zygomatic*) bone, pierces the orbicularis palpebrarum (*orbicularis oculi*) muscle, and supplies the skin of the cheek covering the malar (*zygomatic*) bone. It communicates with the malar (*zygomatic*) branch of the facial nerve.

The **lateral and anterior terminal branches of the nasal (nasociliary) nerve,** emerge between the nasal bone and the lateral cartilages of the nose, supplying the tip of the nose as they descend beneath the compressor naris muscle. They communicate with the infra-orbital branches of the facial and trigeminal nerves.

PLATE LX.

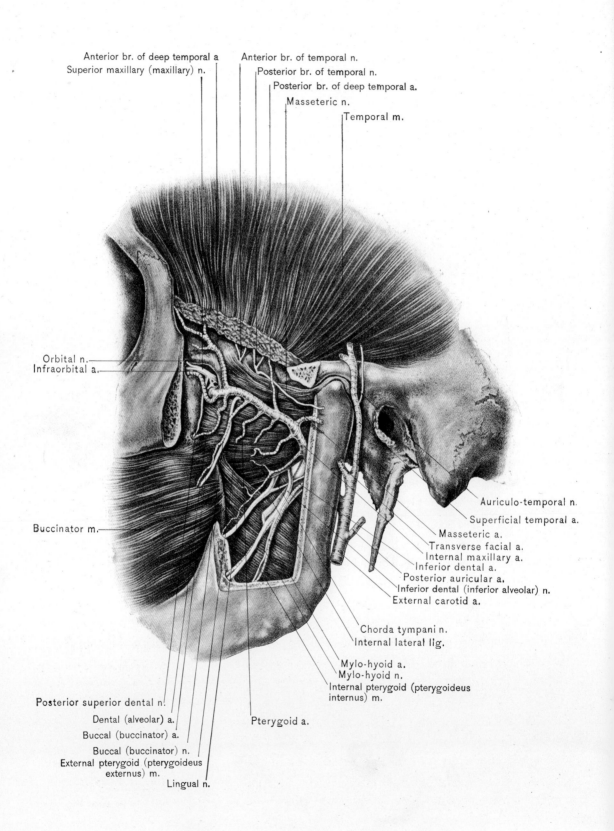

Anterior br. of deep temporal a
Superior maxillary (maxillary) n.
Anterior br. of temporal n.
Posterior br. of temporal n.
Posterior br. of deep temporal a.
Masseteric n.
Temporal m.

Orbital n.
Infraorbital a.

Auriculo-temporal n.
Superficial temporal a.
Masseteric a.
Transverse facial a.
Internal maxillary a.
Inferior dental a.
Posterior auricular a.
Inferior dental (inferior alveolar) n.
External carotid a.

Buccinator m.

Chorda tympani n.
Internal lateral lig.

Mylo-hyoid a.
Mylo-hyoid n.
Internal pterygoid (pterygoideus internus) m.

Posterior superior dental n.
Dental (alveolar) a.
Buccal (buccinator) a.
Buccal (buccinator) n.
External pterygoid (pterygoideus externus) m.
Lingual n.

Pterygoid a.

PTERYGOID MUSCLES AND INTERNAL MAXILLARY ARTERY.

The **mental nerve,** the continuation of the inferior dental (*inferior alveolar*), which is a branch of the mandibular nerve, emerges from the mental foramen in company with the mental artery. It divides beneath the depressor anguli oris (*triangularis*) muscle into a number of branches which supply the chin and lower lip. It inosculates with the supramandibular branch of the facial nerve.

The **infra-orbital artery,** a branch of the internal maxillary, accompanies the infra-orbital nerve through the infra-orbital foramen, and divides into branches which are distributed like those of the nerve. It anastomoses with the transverse facial, facial (*external maxillary*), and ophthalmic arteries.

The **infra-orbital vein** communicates with the facial (*anterior facial*) vein in front, and empties into the pterygoid plexus of veins.

The **mental artery,** the terminal portion of the inferior dental (*inferior alveolar*), supplies the chin and anastomoses with the submental, inferior labial, and inferior coronary arteries.

THE PTERYGO-MAXILLARY REGION (INFRATEMPORAL FOSSA) (Plate LX)

The pterygo-maxillary region (*infratemporal fossa*) is the space included between the ramus of the mandible, laterally; the lateral wall of the pharynx and the pterygoid process of the sphenoidal bone, medially; the zygomatic surface of the superior maxilla (*maxilla*), anteriorly, and the lower surface of the greater wing of the sphenoidal and the adjacent temporal bone, superiorly. The posterior limit of the space is represented by a plane passing directly medialward from the posterior border of the ramus of the mandible to the pharynx.

DISSECTION.—Remove the zygomatic arch by sawing through the zygomatic processes of the malar (*zygomatic*) and the temporal bones. In the latter, the point selected should be just in front of the tubercle of the zygoma. Reflect the masseter muscle from the ramus of the mandible, carrying the zygoma with it; locate the masseteric artery and nerve which pass through the mandibular notch; trace them into the masseter muscle as far as possible, and then sever them. Remove a portion of the ramus of the mandible in the following manner: saw downward behind the last molar tooth, half way through the body of the mandible, then backward to the angle; when the saw reaches the cancellous tissue, discard it and use a chisel in order to avoid dividing the inferior dental (*inferior alveolar*) vessels and nerve. Then again using the saw, direct it downward from the mandibular notch, just in front of the neck of the mandible, through the ramus to the end of the incision in the body of the bone. The removal of this portion of the mandible is tedious, as the internal pterygoid muscle, internal lateral (*spheno-mandibular*) ligament, and the inferior dental (*inferior alveolar*) vessels and nerve oppose elevation of the section of bone thus separated. Remove the posterior inferior corner of the section of the ramus with bone forceps as far as the inferior dental (*mandibular*) canal, which contains the inferior dental (*inferior alveolar*) vessels and nerve; then reflect the bone with the lower portion of the temporal muscle, taking care to avoid destroying the mylo-hyoid artery and nerve which arise from the inferior dental (*inferior alveolar*) artery and nerve, near the mandibular foramen, and pass downward and forward in a groove on the medial surface of the ramus. In making this dissection it is advisable to use the back of the scalpel, as the vessels and nerves are small and delicate and are easily severed.

The **contents of the pterygo-maxillary region** (**infratemporal fossa**) are: the internal and external pterygoid muscles, the internal maxillary artery with some of its branches and their companion veins, the pterygoid plexus of veins, the inferior maxillary (*mandibular*) nerve, and the following branches of that nerve: the anterior and posterior deep temporal, long buccal, masseteric, internal and external pterygoid, inferior dental (*inferior alveolar*), auriculo-temporal, and lingual nerves. It also contains the chorda tympani nerve, a portion of the parotid gland, the internal lateral (*spheno-mandibular*) ligament of the mandible, and the internal maxillary lymph glands.

The **internal maxillary artery,** which is closely related to the nerves of this region, passes forward either over or behind the external pterygoid muscle.

The **internal lateral** (**spheno-mandibular**) **ligament** is a thin, fibrous band which lies beneath the inferior dental (*inferior alveolar*) vessels and nerve; it passes, with the lingual and inferior dental (*inferior alveolar*) nerves, through the triangular interval between the two pterygoid muscles and the incised edge of the mandible.

The **external pterygoid muscle,** the more superficial of the two pterygoids, *arises* by an upper head from the infratemporal surface of the greater wing of the sphenoidal bone; by a lower head from the lateral surface of the lateral pterygoid lamina of the sphenoidal bone, from the tuberosities of the palatine and the superior maxillary (*maxillary*) bones. Its fibers pass horizontally backward and converge to be *inserted* into the interarticular fibrocartilage (*articular disc*) of the temporo-mandibular joint superiorly, and inferiorly, into the anterior portion of the medial surface of the neck of the mandible.

It is related, externally, with the ramus of the mandible, the temporal and masseter muscles, the superficial portion of the internal pterygoid muscle, the internal maxillary artery, the anterior and posterior deep temporal arteries, and the buccal artery and nerve. Internally it is in relation with the deep part of the internal pterygoid muscle, the middle meningeal artery, and the inferior

PLATE LXI.

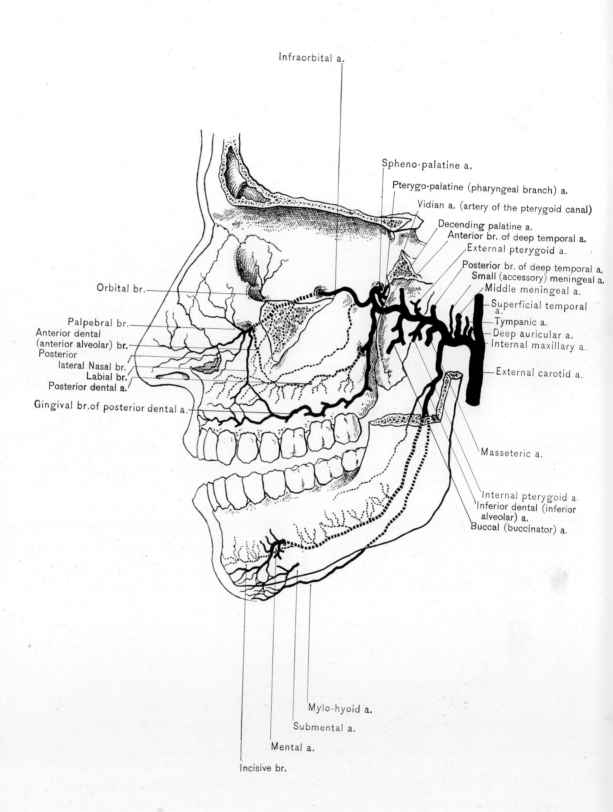

Infraorbital a.

Spheno-palatine a.

Pterygo-palatine (pharyngeal branch) a.

Vidian a. (artery of the pterygoid canal)

Decending palatine a.
Anterior br. of deep temporal a.
External pterygoid a.

Posterior br. of deep temporal a.
Small (accessory) meningeal a.
Middle meningeal a.
Superficial temporal a.
Tympanic a.
Deep auricular a.
Internal maxillary a.

External carotid a.

Orbital br.

Palpebral br.
Anterior dental
(anterior alveolar) br.
Posterior
lateral Nasal br.
Labial br.
Posterior dental a.

Gingival br. of posterior dental a.

Masseteric a.

Internal pterygoid a.
Inferior dental (inferior alveolar) a.
Buccal (buccinator) a.

Mylo-hyoid a.

Submental a.

Mental a.

Incisive br.

INTERNAL MAXILLARY ARTERY AND BRANCHES.

maxillary (*mandibular*) nerve, the internal lateral (*spheno-mandibular*) ligament of the mandible, the lingual and inferior dental (*inferior alveolar*) nerves, which emerge from beneath its lower border; the long buccal nerve, which runs between its two heads; the chorda tympani nerve, and the anterior and posterior deep temporal and masseteric nerves, which pass out from beneath the upper border of the muscle.

BLOOD SUPPLY.—From the external pterygoid branches of the internal maxillary artery.

NERVE SUPPLY.—From the mandibular division of the trigeminal nerve.

ACTION.—The external pterygoid muscles when acting together pull the mandible forward; acting alternately, they move it forward and laterally; when only one muscle acts it moves the mandible forward and to the opposite side. They are muscles of mastication.

The **internal pterygoid muscle** arises by a superficial and a deep head. The superficial, the smaller of the two, *arises* from the lower and back part of the tuberosity of the maxilla, and the lateral side of the tuberosity of the palatine bone. The deep head lies behind the lower head of the external pterygoid and *arises* from the medial surface of the lateral pterygoid lamina and from the grooved portion of the tuberosity of the palatine bone situated in the pterygoid fossa. The two heads unite at the lower margin of the external pterygoid muscle, and thence extend downward, backward, and lateralward to be *inserted* into the rough medial surface of the posterior portion of the ramus of the mandible included between the angle and the inferior dental (*mandibular*) foramen.

It is related, externally, with the ramus of the mandible, the temporal and the external pterygoid muscles, the internal lateral (*spheno-mandibular*) ligament of the mandible, the lingual or gustatory nerve, and the inferior dental (*inferior alveolar*) and mylo-hyoid vessels and nerves; internally, with the tensor palati (*tensor veli palatini*), stylo-glossus, stylo-hyoid, posterior belly of the digastric, and the superior constrictor muscle of the pharynx.

BLOOD SUPPLY.—From the mylo-hyoid and the internal pterygoid branches of the internal maxillary artery.

NERVE SUPPLY.—From the internal pterygoid branch of the inferior maxillary (*mandibular*) nerve.

ACTION.—The internal pterygoid muscles when acting together draw the mandible upward and forward; singly, they draw it upward and to the opposite side.

The **internal maxillary artery** (Plate LXI), the larger of the two terminal branches of the external carotid, arises in the parotid gland, opposite, or slightly inferior to the neck of the mandible. The artery is divided into three portions: the *first, or mandibular, portion* passes forward between the internal lateral (*spheno-mandibular*) ligament and the neck of the mandible, and reaches the lower margin of the external pterygoid muscle. The *second, or pterygoid, portion* extends obliquely upward and forward upon the lateral surface of the external pterygoid muscle, and is hidden by the insertion of the temporal muscle. The *third, or spheno-maxillary, portion* lies in the spheno-maxillary (*pterygo-palatine*) fossa. In some instances the second, or pterygoid, portion runs entirely beneath the external pterygoid muscle, but, by passing between the two heads of that muscle, appears upon the lateral surface of the muscle just before entering the spheno-maxillary (*pterygo-palatine*) fossa.

The *branches of the first, or mandibular, portion of the internal maxillary artery* are: the deep auricular, tympanic (*anterior tympanic*), middle meningeal, small (*accessory*) meningeal and inferior dental (*inferior alveolar*) arteries.

The *deep auricular artery* pierces the wall of the external auditory meatus to supply the mandibular joint, the parotid gland, the external auditory meatus, and the tympanic membrane.

The *tympanic (anterior tympanic) artery* passes behind the temporo-mandibular joint through the petro-tympanic, or Glaserian, fissure to supply the tympanum, and anastomoses with the tympanic branch (*posterior tympanic*) of the stylo-mastoid artery and with the stylo-mastoid branch of the posterior auricular artery.

The *middle meningeal artery* runs upward between the two roots of the auriculo-temporal nerve to the foramen spinosum, through which it enters the middle fossa of the cranial cavity to supply the cranium and the dura mater. After passing lateralward and upward for a short distance on the greater wing of the sphenoidal bone it divides into anterior and posterior terminal branches; within the cranium it also gives origin to four branches: *superficial petrosal; Gasserian (ganglionic) branches; tympanic (superior tympanic)*, and *orbital* branches.

The *small (accessory) meningeal artery* ascends to the foramen ovale, through which, after supplying a twig to the nasal fossa and the soft palate, it enters the cranial cavity.

The *inferior dental (inferior alveolar) artery*, with its venæ comites, accompanies the inferior dentol (*inferior alveolar*) nerve and passes downward upon the internal pterygoid muscle and the internal lateral (*spheno-mandibular*) ligament, entering the mandibular foramen together with the inferior dental (*inferior alveolar*) nerve. The artery then occupies the mandibular canal, distributing branches to the teeth; it supplies an incisive branch, and emerges, on the face, from the mental foramen as the *mental artery*, which, accompanied by the mental nerve, is distributed to the structures of the chin and the lower lip. Before entering the mandibular canal the inferior dental (*inferior alveolar*) artery gives off the lingual artery to the tongue and the *mylo-hyoid artery*, which accompanies the mylo-hyoid nerve.

The *branches of the second, or pterygoid, portion* are: the anterior and posterior deep temporal, internal and external pterygoid, and the masseteric and buccal arteries.

The *anterior and posterior deep temporal arteries* pass upward through the corresponding parts of the temporal fossa, between the temporal muscle and the pericranium, which they supply.

The *pterygoid arteries*, variable in number, supply the external and internal *pterygoid muscles.*

The *masseteric artery*, with the masseteric nerve, passes lateralward behind the temporal muscle through the mandibular notch to the masseter muscle.

The *buccal artery* accompanies the long buccal nerve in its forward course between the ramus of the mandible and the external pterygoid to supply the buccinator muscle and the mucous membrane of the mouth.

The *branches of the third, or spheno-maxillary, portion* are: the alveolar, infra-orbital, posterior, or descending, palatine, artery of the pterygoid canal, or Vidian artery, pterygo-palatine, or pharyngeal, branch, and the spheno-palatine artery.

The *alveolar (posterior superior alveolar) artery* gives off branches to the gums and the buccinator muscle, and supplies the molar and bicuspid teeth and the mucous lining of the maxillary sinus, or antrum of Highmore.

The *infra-orbital artery* immediately enters the infra-orbital groove and canal, accompanied by the superior maxillary (*maxillary*) division of the trigeminal nerve, and eventually emerges upon the face, in company with the infra-orbital nerve at the infra-orbital foramen. It gives off *orbital branches* to supply the adipose tissue of the orbit and the neighboring muscles of the eye, and *anterior superior dental branches*, which run downward in the anterior wall of the maxillary sinus and supply the incisor and bicuspid teeth and the mucous membrane of the maxillary sinus. In the face, emerging from the infra-orbital foramen, it divides into *palpebral, nasal,* and *labial* branches to these respective regions; these branches anastomose with branches of the ophthalmic, the superior labial, the transverse facial, and the buccinator arteries.

The *posterior, or descending, palatine artery* accompanies the posterior palatine branches of the spheno-palatine, or Meckel's, ganglion of the trigeminal nerve, through the posterior palatine (*pterygo-palatine*) canal, then emerges from the posterior, or greater palatine, foramen and passes forward in a groove situated near the alveolar process along the inferior surface of the hard palate; it next enters the foramen of Stenson, a subdivision of the anterior palatine (*incisive*) foramen, and anas-

18

tomoses with the naso-palatine (*spheno-palatine*) artery. It is distributed to the hard and to the soft palate, the palatine glands, and the gums.

The *Vidian artery*, or the *artery of the pterygoid canal*, runs through the Vidian (*pterygoid*) canal with the corresponding nerve to supply the upper part of the pharynx, the Eustachian (*auditory*) tube, and the tympanum.

The *pterygo-palatine artery*, or *pharyngeal branch*, is a very small artery which passes backward with the pharyngeal nerve through the pterygo-palatine canal to supply the upper pharynx, the sphenoidal cells, and the Eustachian (*auditory*) tube.

The *spheno-palatine*, the terminal artery, runs medialward through the spheno-palatine foramen into the superior meatus of the nose. Shortly after traversing the foramen it divides into two branches: an *internal (naso-palatine) branch*, which crosses the roof of this meatus between the mucous membrane and the bone to reach the septum of the nose, runs downward and forward in a groove on the vomer to anastomose with the posterior palatine artery; two or three *lateral branches*, which are distributed to the mucous lining of the lateral nasal walls, the maxillary sinus, or antrum of Highmore, and the ethmoidal and the sphenoidal cells.

It is of interest to note that the branches of the first and third portions of the internal maxillary pass through bony canals, or foramina, while those of the second portion are distributed directly to the muscles without traversing such canals.

The **veins** of the pterygo-maxillary region (*infratemporal fossa*) accompany the branches of the internal maxillary artery, and converge toward the external pterygoid muscle, around which they form a dense plexus, the **pterygoid plexus.** This is drained from its posterior part by a short venous trunk, called the *internal maxillary vein*, which accompanies the first (mandibular) portion of the internal maxillary artery into the substance of the parotid gland. The internal maxillary vein joins the temporal vein to form the temporo-maxillary (*posterior facial*) vein. The pterygoid plexus sends a branch, the *anterior maxillary*, or *deep facial*, *vein*, from its anterior part over the buccinator muscle to the facial vein. It also communicates with the cavernous sinus by means of a small emissary vein which passes through the foramen of Vesalius in the sphenoidal bone.

The **lymphatics** of this region accompany the blood-vessels, and are derived from the regions which those vessels supply and drain. They empty into the deep cervical glands.

The **nerves** of the pterygo-maxillary region (*infratemporal fossa*) are the inferior maxillary (*mandibular*) division of the fifth nerve and some of its branches, and the chorda tympani nerve. (Plate LXII.)

PLATE LXII.

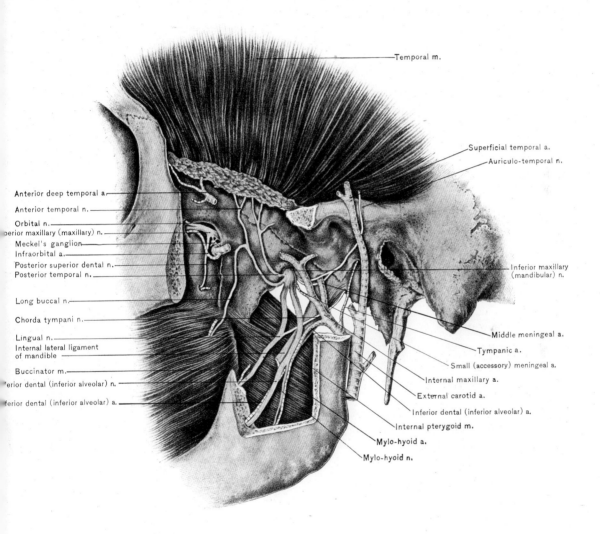

Temporal m.

Superficial temporal a.

Auriculo-temporal n.

Anterior deep temporal a.

Anterior temporal n.

Orbital n.

...erior maxillary (maxillary) n.

Meckel's ganglion

Infraorbital a.

Posterior superior dental n.

Posterior temporal n.

Long buccal n.

Chorda tympani n.

Lingual n.

Internal lateral ligament of mandible

Buccinator m.

...erior dental (inferior alveolar) n.

...ferior dental (inferior alveolar) a.

Inferior maxillary (mandibular) n.

Middle meningeal a.

Tympanic a.

Small (accessory) meningeal a.

Internal maxillary a.

External carotid a.

Inferior dental (inferior alveolar) a.

Internal pterygoid m.

Mylo-hyoid a.

Mylo-hyoid n.

INFERIOR MAXILLARY (MANDIBULAR) NERVE.

PLATE LXII.

The **inferior maxillary** (**mandibular**) **nerve** leaves the cranial cavity through the foramen ovale as a thick trunk, which lies lateral to the Eustachian tube (*auditory canal*) and beneath the external pterygoid muscle. It is the largest of the three divisions of the trigeminal nerve, and differs from the other two divisions of the fifth nerve, the ophthalmic and the superior maxillary (*maxillary*), in being composed of both motor and sensory fibers. After leaving the skull it divides into an anterior and a posterior division. The *anterior division* is motor, except for its buccal branch. It gives off the anterior and posterior deep temporal nerves, the masseteric nerve, branches to the pterygoid muscles, and the long buccal nerve. The *posterior division*, chiefly sensory, divides into three large branches: the auriculo-temporal and the lingual, both exclusively sensory, and the inferior dental (*inferior alveolar*) nerve which contains a strand of motor fibers, the mylo-hyoid nerve.

The **deep temporal nerves,** anterior and posterior, arise from the motor root of the fifth nerve, and ascend between the pericranium and the temporal muscle, which latter they supply.

The **masseteric nerve** emerges from between the external pterygoid muscle and the pterygoid ridge (*infratemporal crest*). It proceeds posteriorly along the superior border of the external pterygoid muscle; lateralward, in front of the temporo-mandibular articulation, and through the sigmoid (*mandibular*) notch of the mandible, together with the masseteric artery, entering the masseter muscle, which it supplies.

The **branch to the internal pterygoid muscle** arises from the inferior maxillary (*mandibular*) nerve before it divides; it gives off a branch to the otic ganglion, and enters the deep surface of the muscle. The **branch to the external pterygoid muscle** is usually a twig of the long buccal nerve, and divides into two branches, which enter the deep surface of the muscle.

The **long buccal,** a sensory nerve, is derived from the anterior portion of the inferior maxillary (*mandibular*) division of the fifth nerve. It runs between the two heads of the external pterygoid muscle, and passes downward and forward beneath the temporal muscle and the anterior edge of the masseter to the buccinator muscle, upon the lateral side of which it communicates with the facial nerve and forms a plexus from which filaments pass to the adjacent mucous membrane and skin of the cheek. It contains all of the sensory fibers of the anterior division of the inferior maxillary (*mandibular*) nerve. The nerve is subject to considerable variations.

The **auriculo-temporal nerve** arises by two roots, between which passes the middle meningeal artery. It runs backward and lateralward beneath the external pterygoid muscle, between the internal lateral (*spheno-mandibular*) liga-

ment and the temporo-mandibular joint, curves lateralward around the neck of
the condyle of the mandible, and pierces the upper part of the parotid gland.
It then ascends over the root of the zygoma, in front of the external auditory
meatus and beneath the temporal artery.   In its course it receives communicating twigs from the otic ganglion, and supplies branches to the external auditory
meatus, the parotid gland, and the temporo-mandibular articulation.   From the
parotid gland it sends a *communicating branch* to the temporo-facial division of
the facial nerve.   Near the level of the tragus it divides into an *anterior auricular
branch*, which supplies the upper part of the auricle; and a *superficial temporal
branch*, which lies on the lateral side of the superficial temporal vessels, divides,
and accompanies the anterior and posterior temporal arteries.

The **lingual nerve** emerges from beneath the lower edge of the external
pterygoid muscle, whence it descends medial to the inferior dental (*inferior
alveolar*) nerve between the mandible and the internal pterygoid muscle; thence it
runs beneath the mylo-hyoid nerve and over the superior constrictor of the
pharynx, the stylo-glossus, and hyoglossus muscles, Wharton's (*submandibular*)
duct and the genio-glossus muscle, to the tip of the tongue.   On the hyoglossus
muscle it is connected with the submaxillary (*submandibular*) ganglion, which will
be described with the submaxillary (*submandibular*) triangle of the neck.   It lies
above the ganglion and Wharton's (*submandibular*) duct, which it crosses at the
anterior border of the hyoglossus muscle, where it supplies a branch to the
sublingual gland and a communicating branch to the hypoglossal nerve.   Before
it emerges from behind the external pterygoid muscle it is joined by the chorda
tympani nerve.

The lingual nerve supplies branches to the hypoglossal nerve, the submaxillary (*submandibular*) ganglion, the mucous membrane of the mouth, the gums, the
sublingual gland; and lingual branches to the papillæ on the sides and tip of the tongue.   Since the lingual nerve supplies the tongue with sensory fibers, the pain due
to neuralgia or cancer of the tongue may be relieved by division of this nerve.
The incision should be made through the mucous membrane of the floor of the
mouth opposite the second molar tooth of the mandible and close to the gum,
where the nerve lies immediately beneath the mucous membrane.

The **inferior dental (inferior alveolar) nerve,** the largest branch of the
inferior maxillary (*mandibular*), emerges from beneath the lower head of the
external pterygoid muscle, and descends between the internal lateral (*spheno-
mandibular*) ligament and the ramus of the mandible to enter the inferior dental
(*mandibular*) canal.   At its origin it lies internal to the inferior dental (*inferior
alveolar*) artery, which it crosses at the inferior dental (*mandibular*) foramen;
the artery is, therefore, nearer the teeth than the nerve.   It is a sensory-motor

PLATE LXIII.

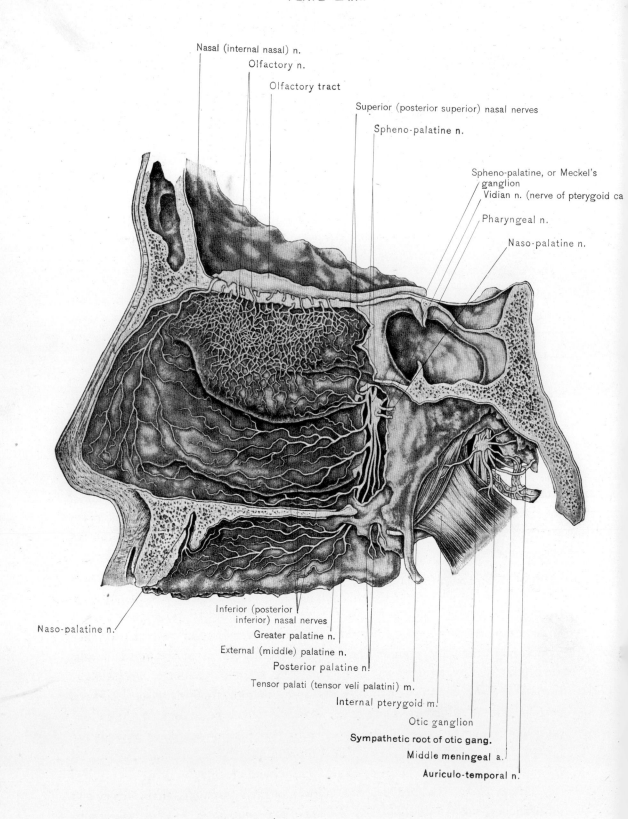

Nasal (internal nasal) n.

Olfactory n.

Olfactory tract

Superior (posterior superior) nasal nerves

Spheno-palatine n.

Spheno-palatine, or Meckel's ganglion

Vidian n. (nerve of pterygoid ca

Pharyngeal n.

Naso-palatine n.

Naso-palatine n.

Inferior (posterior inferior) nasal nerves

Greater palatine n.

External (middle) palatine n.

Posterior palatine n.

Tensor palati (tensor veli palatini) m.

Internal pterygoid m.

Otic ganglion

Sympathetic root of otic gang.

Middle meningeal a.

Auriculo-temporal n.

OLFACTORY NERVES AND INTERNAL VIEW OF MECKEL'S, OR SPHENO-PALATINE, AND OTIC GANGLIA.

nerve, lying lateral and superficial to the lingual nerve, the motor filaments being given off as the mylo-hyoid nerve just previous to its entrance into the inferior dental (*mandibular*) canal.

The **mylo-hyoid nerve** is accompanied by the mylo-hyoid artery, pierces the internal lateral (*spheno-mandibular*) ligament of the mandible, and descends to the mylo-hyoid groove upon the inner surface of the mandible. It then runs over the superficial surface of the mylo-hyoid muscle, supplying it and the anterior belly of the digastric muscle. In the inferior dental (*mandibular*) canal the inferior dental (*inferior alveolar*) nerve supplies branches to the molar and bicuspid teeth and to the gums, and divides into an incisive and a mental branch opposite the mental foramen. The *incisive branch* passes forward and inward in the inferior dental (*mandibular*) canal to supply the canine and incisor teeth and the adjacent region of the gum. The *mental branch* emerges upon the face at the mental foramen, and after communicating with the supramandibular branch of the facial nerve divides into several branches. These supply the mucous membrane of the lower lip and the fascia and skin of the lip and chin.

The **chorda tympani nerve**, containing both motor and sensory fibers, arises from the facial in the facial, or Fallopian canal, almost six millimeters (one-quarter of an inch) above the stylo-mastoid foramen. It runs in the iter chordæ posterius to the middle ear, where it passes between the handle of the malleus and the fibrous layer of the membrana tympani laterally, and the mucous membrane medially. It next enters the iter chordæ anterius, or canal of Huguier, to reach the pterygo-maxillary region, where it joins the lateral side of the lingual nerve beneath the external pterygoid muscle. Some of its fibers leave the lingual nerve to enter the submaxillary (*submandibular*) ganglion and sublingual gland.

The **otic**, or Arnold's, **ganglion** (Plate LXIII) lies upon the medial surface of the trunk of the inferior maxillary (*mandibular*) division of the fifth nerve, in front of the middle meningeal artery, and may be found by tracing any of the larger branches of the nerve until the root of the parent stem, near the foramen ovale, is reached. Its sympathetic root is derived from the plexus on the middle meningeal artery; its sensory root, from the inferior maxillary (*mandibular*) through the internal pterygoid nerve, and its motor root, from the lesser superficial petrosal nerve, which communicates with the tympanic branch of the glosso-pharyngeal nerve. It communicates with the auriculo-temporal and chorda tympani nerves. Motor fibers of the inferior maxillary (*mandibular*) nerve pass through it to the tensor veli palatini and tensor tympani muscles.

DISSECTION.—To study the first portion of the internal maxillary artery and its branches, the trunk of the inferior maxillary (*mandibular*) nerve, the origins of its branches, and the otic ganglion, it is necessary to remove the external pterygoid muscle, the condyle of the mandible, and the remainder of the ramus as far as the transverse incision in the ramus.

Fracture of the base of the skull may cause serious hemorrhage into the pterygo-maxillary region, or infratemporal fossa, because of rupture of the meningeal vessels. Lacerations of the deep temporal vessels due to cranial fracture would result in the effusion of blood into this space, its escape above the zygoma being rendered impossible because of the attachments of the temporal fascia. In these conditions pain on pressure made below the zygoma and behind the malar (*zygomatic*) bone would be a symptom of such an effusion. The effusion may also give rise to secondary irritation of the nerves in this space. Thus, irritation of the chorda tympani nerve would cause salivation; of the lingual nerve, disturbances of sensation and taste at the end of the tongue; involvement of the inferior dental (*inferior alveolar*) would cause toothache. Involvement of the motor branches would result in tonic or clonic spasms of the muscles of mastication and more or less complete fixation of the mandible by the mylo-hyoid and anterior belly of the digastric muscles.

Tumors and abscess would have similar effects, varying in degree, however, according to the exact location and rapidity of growth. Owing to the presence of important structures in this space, it is well to practise Hilton's method of opening a deep abscess in this region, as follows: through an incision in the skin push a grooved director into the abscess; then insert a pair of forceps along the director, and withdraw them with the blades sufficiently separated to make an opening large enough to insure good drainage. It is impossible to do serious damage by this procedure.

DISSECTION.—The pterygo-maxillary region should now be thoroughly cleaned, in order to study the spheno-maxillary (*inferior orbital*) and the pterygo-maxillary fissures and the spheno-maxillary (*pterygo-palatine*) fossa.

The zygomatic fossa, mentioned in connection with the contents of the pterygo-maxillary region, comprises: the lower part of the temporal muscle, the internal and external pterygoid muscles, the internal maxillary artery, the inferior maxillary (*mandibular*) nerve, branches of the artery and nerve, and the chorda tympani nerve, all of which have already been described.

The **zygomatic fossa** is the space medial to the ramus of the mandible, and corresponds closely to the upper portion of the pterygo-maxillary region *infratemporal fossa*. It is separated from the temporal fossa by a line drawn at the level of the upper border of the zygoma. It is bounded superiorly by the under surface of the greater wing of the sphenoidal and adjacent portion of the temporal bone; anteriorly, by the zygomatic surface of the maxilla; posterosuperiorly

PLATE LXIV.

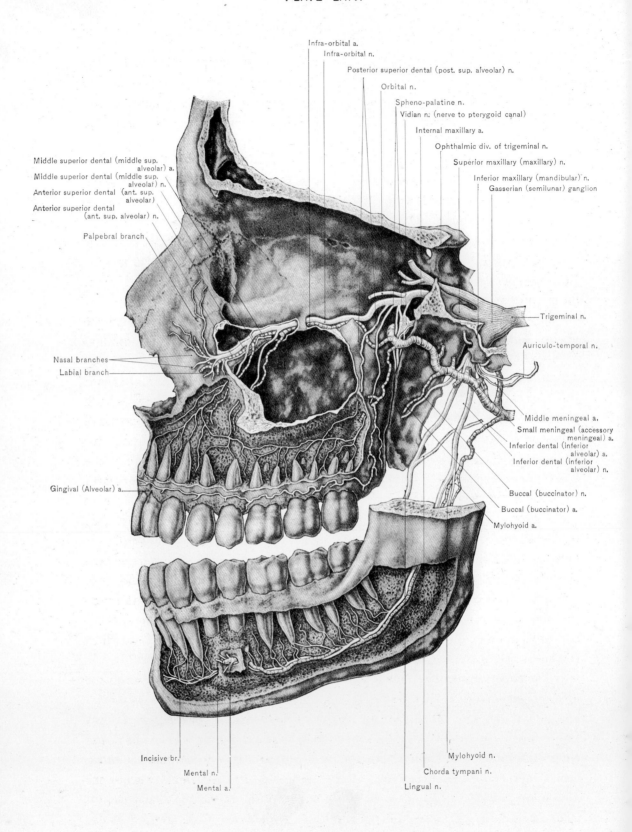

Infra-orbital a.

Infra-orbital n.

Posterior superior dental (post. sup. alveolar) n.

Orbital n.

Spheno-palatine n.

Vidian n. (nerve to pterygoid canal)

Internal maxillary a.

Ophthalmic div. of trigeminal n.

Superior maxillary (maxillary) n.

Inferior maxillary (mandibular) n.

Gasserian (semilunar) ganglion

Middle superior dental (middle sup. alveolar) a.

Middle superior dental (middle sup. alveolar) n.

Anterior superior dental (ant. sup. alveolar)

Anterior superior dental (ant. sup. alveolar) n.

Palpebral branch

Nasal branches

Labial branch

Gingival (Alveolar) a.

Trigeminal n.

Auriculo-temporal n.

Middle meningeal a.

Small meningeal (accessory meningeal) a.

Inferior dental (inferior alveolar) a.

Inferior dental (inferior alveolar) n.

Buccal (buccinator) n.

Buccal (buccinator) a.

Mylohyoid a.

Incisive br.

Mental n.

Mental a.

Mylohyoid n.

Chorda tympani n.

Lingual n.

SUPERIOR MAXILLARY (MAXILLARY) AND INFERIOR MAXILLARY (MANDIBULAR) NERVES.

284

by the posterior border of the pterygoid process of the sphenoidal bone, and the eminentia articularis; medially, by the external pterygoid plate, or lamina, and laterally, by the pterygoid ridge (*infratemporal crest*), the zygomatic arch, and the ramus of the mandible. It is open postero-inferiorly. At the upper and medial part of the zygomatic fossa there are two fissures, one horizontal, the other vertical. The horizontal one is the *spheno-maxillary (infra-orbital) fissure*, which opens into the lateroposterior part of the orbit, between the sphenoidal bone and the maxilla. It transmits the infra-orbital artery and vein, branches from the spheno-palatine, or Meckel's, ganglion, and the superior maxillary (*maxillary*) nerve and its orbital branch. It joins the pterygo-maxillary fissure at a right angle. The vertical fissure is the *pterygo-maxillary fissure*, formed by the angle between the superior maxillary (*maxillary*) bone and the front of the united pterygoid plates. It transmits the internal maxillary artery.

The **spheno-maxillary (pterygo-palatine) fossa,** which is small, lies below the greater wing of the sphenoidal bone, below and behind the apex of the orbit and at the point of junction of the pterygo-maxillary and spheno-maxillary (*infra-orbital*) fissures. It contains the terminal portion of the internal maxillary artery, the branches of this portion, the superior maxillary (*maxillary*) nerve, and Meckel's (*spheno-palatine*) ganglion. This ganglion has become of importance since the work of Sluder on a specific type of pain in a definite distribution, due to lesions of the ganglion. Three foramina are found in the posterior wall of the fossa: the *foramen rotundum*, which transmits the superior maxillary (*maxillary*) division of the fifth, or trigeminal, nerve; below this, the anterior opening of the *Vidian (pterygoid) canal*, which transmits the great superficial and deep petrosal nerves and vessels, and still lower the *pterygo-palatine foramen*, the anterior opening of the pterygo-palatine (*pharyngeal*) canal, which transmits the pterygo-palatine vessels, and the pharyngeal nerve. On the medial wall in the *spheno-palatine foramen* which opens into the nasal cavity and transmits the spheno-palatine vessels and the naso-palatine nerve. Below the spheno-palatine foramen is the orifice of the posterior (*greater*) palatine canal, which transmits the posterior, or descending, palatine vessels and nerve.

The **superior maxillary (maxillary) nerve** (Plate LXIV), second division of the fifth, or trigeminal, is purely sensory. It arises from the Gasserian (*semilunar*) ganglion at the apex of the petrous portion of the temporal bone, passes through the foramen rotundum into the spheno-maxillary (*pterygo-palatine*) fossa, and enters the infra-orbital canal with the infra-orbital artery to become the infra-orbital nerve. Its branches are: in the cranial cavity, recurrent twigs to the dura mater, which communicate with the branches of the inferior maxillary (*mandibular*) nerve; in the spheno-maxillary (*pterygo-palatine*) fossa, *temporo-malar* (*zygomatic*), or *orbital*, *spheno-palatine*, and *posterior dental (alveolar) branches; in* the infra-orbital canal, *middle superior dental (alveolar)*, and *anterior superior dental (alveolar) nerves*, and upon the face, the terminal divisions of the infra-orbital nerve, the *inferior palpebral external, nasal*, and *superior labial branches.*

DISSECTION.—Remove the lateral wall of the orbit and that portion of the greater wing of the sphenoidal bone lateral to the foramen rotundum by sawing downward from the incised edge of the skull made in removing the brain. The saw should pass through the lateral part of the sphenoidal (*superior orbital*) fissure and lateral to the foramen rotundum.

The **temporo-malar (zygomatic), or orbital, nerve** enters the orbit through the spheno-maxillary (*inferior orbital*) fissure. At the posterior part of the orbit it divides into a temporal (*zygomatico-temporal*) and a malar (*zygomatico-facial*) branch. The *temporal (zygomatico-temporal) branch* runs anteriorly in the perio-steum, lying in a groove in the bone, and passes through the spheno-malar (*spheno-zygomatic*) foramen to enter the temporal fossa. It runs upward beneath the temporal muscle, piercing it and both lamellæ of the temporal fascia to supply the skin of the temporal region; it pierces the superficial layer of the temporal fascia about two and a half centimeters (one inch) above the zygoma. It communicates in the orbit with the lacrimal nerve, and in the temporal region with the temporal branch of the facial nerve. The *malar (zygomatico-facial) branch* runs forward along the inferolateral portion of the orbit, through the malar (*zygomatic*) foramen, piercing the orbicularis palpebrarum (*orbicularis oculi*) to supply the skin of the cheek. It communicates with the malar (*zygomatic*) branch of the facial nerve and with the palpebral branches of the infra-orbital nerve.

The **spheno-palatine branches** are two or three twigs which descend directly downward to the spheno-palatine, or Meckel's, ganglion to supply its sensory root. The major portion of their fibers pass lateral to, or in front of the ganglion, only a small portion actually traversing it.

The **posterior superior dental (posterior superior alveolar) nerves** are, as a rule, two in number, and usually arise from the superior maxillary (*maxil-lary*) nerve in the spheno-maxillary (*pterygo-palatine*) fossa. They pass downward and forward through the pterygo-maxillary fissure and enter the foramina in the zygomatic surface of the superior maxilla (*maxilla*); they next run forward in canals in the lateral wall of the maxillary sinus, or antrum of Highmore, and above the roots of the molar teeth to join the middle superior dental (*alveolar*) nerve. They supply branches to the pulp of the molar teeth, to the gums, and to the mucous membrane of the maxillary sinus.

The **middle superior dental (middle superior alveolar) nerve** is given off at the posterior part of the infra-orbital canal, or it may be a branch of the anterior superior dental (*alveolar*) nerve. It passes downward in a canal in the lateral wall of the maxillary sinus. It supplies the premolar, or bicuspid, teeth and communicates with the anterior superior and posterior superior dental (*alveolar*) nerves.

The **anterior superior dental (anterior superior alveolar) nerve** is larger than the other two superior dental (*alveolar*) nerves, and arises posterior to the infra-orbital foramen; it runs downward in the anterior wall of the maxillary sinus, and supplies the incisor and canine teeth, and also gives off a branch to the nasal fossa. The anterior and middle superior dental (*alveolar*) nerves may be seen by raising the superior maxillary (*maxillary*) nerve from the floor of the infra-orbital canal.

The **infra-orbital nerve** emerges upon the face at the infra-orbital foramen, which lies beneath the levator labii superioris (*infra-orbital head of the quadratus labii superioris*) muscle. It divides here into palpebral, nasal, and labial branches, which, with the infra-orbital branch of the facial nerve, form the *infra-orbital plexus*.

The *inferior palpebral branches* pierce the origin of the levator labii superioris (*infra-orbital head of the quadratus labii superioris*) muscle and supply the integument and conjunctiva of the lower eyelid.

The *external nasal branches* pass medialward under the levator labii superioris alæque nasi (*angular head of the quadratus labii superioris*) muscle to supply the skin of the nose.

The *superior labial branches* are the largest and most numerous. They run downward beneath the levator labii superioris (*infra-orbital head of the quadratus labii superioris*) muscle to supply the skin, mucous membrane, and other tissues of the upper lip.

The **spheno-palatine, or Meckel's, ganglion** (Plate LXIII) is situoted in the spheno-maxillary (*pterygo-palatine*) fossa below the superior maxillary (*maxillary*) nerve. It is triangular in shape, of a reddish-gray color, and measures about five millimeters (one-fifth of an inch) in its longest diameter. It is regarded as a sympathetic ganglion. Its *sensory root* is derived from the superior maxillary (*maxillary*) through the spheno-palatine nerve, most of the fibers of which do not enter the ganglion but pass anterior and lateral to it. Its *motor root* is the great superficial petrosal nerve. It arises from the facial nerve in the facial canal, passes through the hiatus of the latter canal (hiatus Fallopii) and a groove in the petrous portion of the temporal bone, thence under the Gasserian (*semilunar*) ganglion to the foramen lacerum, where it joins with the *great deep petrosal* which is the *sympathetic root* of the ganglion, and is derived from the carotid plexus. The great superficial and the great deep petrosal nerves enter the spheno-maxillary (*pterygo-palatine*) fossa as the nerve of the pterygoid canal, or Vidian nerve. While in the canal the Vidian nerve receives a branch from the otic ganglion. The branches of the spheno-palatine ganglion are classified into ascending, descending, internal, and posterior branches.

The **ascending, or orbital, branches** pass through the spheno-maxillary (*inferior orbital*) fissure, and] pierce the medial wall of the orbit to supply the mucous membrane of the sphenoidal sinus and posterior ethmoidal cells.

The **descending, or palatine, branches** are derived mainly from the spheno-palatine branches of the superior maxillary (*maxillary*) nerve. They are divided into the anterior, or greater, the external, or middle, and the posterior palatine nerves.

The anterior, or *greater, palatine nerve* passes downward in the posterior (*greater*) palatine canal together with the posterior (*greater*) palatine artery, and appears on the hard palate at the posterior (*greater*) palatine foramen. It runs forward in a groove on the under surface of the hard palate, and joins the terminal portion of the naso palatine nerve. It supplies the gums and the muco-periosteum of the hard palate. In the posterior (*greater*) palatine canal it gives off two branches, inferior nasal nerves, which pierce the vertical plate of the palatine bone to supply the mucous membrane of the back part of the middle and inferior meatuses and the inferior turbinate.

The *posterior, or small, palatine nerve* descends in the accessory (*lesser*) palatine canal to supply the tonsil, the adjacent mucous membrane, and the levator veli palatini and uvular muscles. With the external (*middle*) palatine nerve it joins a branch from the glossopharyngeal nerve to form the *circulus tonsillaris*, a plexus around the tonsil.

The *external*, or *middle, palatine nerve*, when present, is small; it descends in the accessory (*lesser*) palatine canal to supply the mucous membrane of the tonsil and adjacent soft palate.

The **internal, or nasal (superior and inferior nasal), branches** are derived partly from the spheno-palatine ganglion and partly from the spheno-palatine nerve. They are divided into septal and posterior superior nasal branches.

The *septal branches* pass through the spheno-palatine foramen with the naso-palatine artery, and cross the roof of the nasal fossa beneath the mucous membrane and below the opening of the sphenoidal sinus to reach the septum, where the smaller branches terminate.

The *naso-palatine nerve* (nerve of Cotunnius), the largest of these branches runs downward and forward on the septum of the nose, between the periosteum and the mucous membrane, to the anterior palatine (*incisive*) canal, where it passes through one of the foramina of Scarpa (subdivisions of the anterior palatine (*incisive*) foramen) to supply the mucous membrane of the anterior portion of the hard palate and to join the terminal portion of the anterior palatine nerve.

The *posterior superior nasal nerves* are several twigs which pass through the spheno-palatine foramen to supply the mucous membrane of the posterior part of the middle and superior turbinated bones or conchæ, and of the posterior ethmoidal cells and the maxillary sinus, or antrum of Highmore.

The **posterior branch** is the pterygo-palatine, or pharyngeal, nerve.

The **pterygo-palatine, or pharyngeal, nerve** runs backward through the pterygo-palatine (*pharyngeal*) canal in company with the pterygo-palatine artery (*pharyngeal branch*); it supplies the upper portion of the pharynx and the Eustachian (*auditory*) tube.

The **nerve of the pyterygoid canal, or Vidian nerve,** was formerly considered a posterior branch of the spheno-palatine ganglion, but it is in reality the nerve which is formed by the junction of its motor and sympathetic roots. It passes through the Vidian (*pterygoid*) canal, from which it emerges at the root of the pterygoid process, and enters the spheno-maxillary (*pterygo-palatine*) fossa to join the spheno-palatine ganglion.

The **superior maxillary (maxillary) nerve** with its many communications is especially important, because it is so frequently affected in trigeminal neuralgia. This disease is discussed in connection with the Gasserian (*semilunar*) ganglion (page 63).

Removal of the infra-orbital nerve.—The **infra-orbital notch,** or **foramen,** is on a line drawn from the supra-orbital notch to a point between the bicuspid teeth of the maxilla. It corresponds to a point about one centimeter (one-half inch) below the junction of the medial and the intermediate third of the infra-orbital margin. The infra-orbital nerve is best exposed through a semilunar incision with its convexity directed downward, and carried a short distance below the foramen. A flap, including skin, cellular tissue, and the orbicularis palpebrarum (*orbicularis oculi*) muscle, is raised. The levator labii superioris (*infra-orbital head of the quadratus labii superioris*) muscle, which covers the foramen, is now apparent, and must be displaced laterally or divided, when both the infra-orbital plexus and nerve will readily be found, surrounded by a small quantity of fatty tissue.

The removal of the nerve before it enters the canal and the division of the maxillary division of the trigeminal are rarely practiced at the present time, and their discussion is omitted in this revision.

The **Lymph Glands of the Head** are divided into a superficial and a deep set. The lymphatics from the scalp pass into the **superficial set** which is composed of

19

the occipital, posterior auricular, parotid (*anterior auricular*), buccal, and sub-maxillary (*submandibular*) lymph glands.

The **occipital, or suboccipital, lymph glands,** one to three in number, are situated in the superficial fascia along the superior curved (*superior nuchal*) line of the occipital bone over the attachments of the trapezius muscle and the occipital belly of the occipito-frontalis (*epicranius*) muscle. These glands *receive* the lymph vessels from the posterior portion of the scalp or the area supplied by the occipital artery, and may be involved in wounds or infections of the occipital and post-auricular portion of the scalp. The *efferent* vessels from these glands empty into the superficial lymph glands of the neck.

The **posterior auricular, or mastoid, lymph glands,** usually two in number, are situated behind the auricle, over the mastoid process and the insertion of the sterno-mastoid muscle. They *receive* the lymph vessels from the posterior auricular region and the portion of the scalp above it. Their *efferent* vessels empty into the superficial lymph glands of the neck.

The **parotid, or anterior auricular, lymph glands** are numerous and variable in size. They lie both in and upon the parotid salivary gland in front of the auricle, below the zygoma; a few are also found in the substance of the gland. They *receive* the lymph vessels from the temporal region, the portion of the scalp above it, and the lateral portion of the eyelids and of the cheek. Their *efferent* vessels empty into the superficial lymph glands of the neck and into the submaxillary (*submandibular*) lymph glands. Chronic enlargement of the internal glands may simulate parotid tumor. Suppuration of the same nodes results in a parotid abscess. The pus may rupture into the temporo-mandibular joint, may burrow into the neck, or may extend inward, posterior to the pharynx, resulting in a retropharyngeal abscess.

The **buccal (buccinator) lymph glands** rest upon the buccinator muscle. They are three or four in number, and *receive* some of the lymphatics from the anterior portion of the face, the medial half of the eyelids, the brow, and the front of the scalp. Their *efferent* vessels empty into the submaxillary (*submandibular*) and the internal maxillary (*deep facial*) lymph glands.

The **submaxillary (submandibular) lymph glands,** the most numerous group, are small in size and somewhat scattered below the border of the mandible, most of them lying in the submaxillary (*submandibular*) triangle in relation with the submaxillary (*submandibular*) salivary gland; two or three supra-hyoid lymphatics lie above the body of the hyoid bone, between the anterior bellies of the two digastric muscles. The submaxillary (*submandibular*) lymph glands *receive* the lymph vessels from the front of the scalp, medial part of the eyelids, anterior portion of the face, floor of the mouth, anterior portion of the tongue, the sublingual and submaxillary (*submandibular*) salivary glands, and some of the efferent vessels from the parotid lymph glands. Their *efferent* vessels empty into the superficial and deep cervical lymph glands.

The deep lymph glands of the head are the internal maxillary (*deep facial*), the lingual, and the retropharyngeal lymph glands.

The **internal maxillary(deep facial) lymph glands** are situated in the pterygo-maxillary region (*infratemporal fossa*); some are in relation with the internal maxillary artery, others lie upon the posterior portion of the buccinator muscle, and still other deep glands lie upon the side of the pharynx. They *receive* the lymph vessels from the orbital, nasal, temporal, and zygomatic fossæ, the roof of the mouth, and the soft palate, and some of the efferent vessels from the buccal lymph glands. Their *efferent vessels* empty into the deep cervical lymph glands and partly into the deep parotid lymph glands.

The **lingual lymph glands** lie upon the hyoglossus and genio-glossus muscles. They *receive* the lymph vessels from the upper surface and posterior part of the tongue. Their *efferent* vessels unite with the upper glands of the deep cervical chain. These lymph vessel decussate in the tongue, and may empty into the glands on the opposite side of the neck.

The **retropharyngeal lymph glands** are situated below the base of the skull, between the posterior wall of the pharynx and the rectus capitis anterior major (*longus capitis*) muscle. They *receive* the lymph vessels from the upper part of the pharynx, part of the nasal fossa, and the upper part of the prevertebral muscles. Their *efferent* vessels pass to the upper deep cervical chain.

The **lymph vessels of the scalp,** which drain the portion posterior to a vertical line passing through the external auditory meatus, terminate in the occipital and posterior auricular lymph glands; the lymphatics of the temporal region of the scalp and that portion above it empty into the superficial parotid (*anterior auricular*) and deep parotid (*parotid*) lymph glands; the lymph vessels of the frontal region of the scalp follow the frontal, supra-orbital and the facial (*antesior facial*) veins downward over the face to the submaxillary (*submandibular*) lymph glands.

The **lymph vessels of the face** are also divided into a superficial and a deep set. The superficial set of the anterior portion of the face—the medial half of the eyelids, the nose, the lips, and the anterior part of the cheek—pass downward into the submaxillary (*submandibular*) lymph glands; those of the lateral half of the eyelids and outer part of the cheek terminate in the parotid lymph glands. The lymph channels follow closely the course of the facial (*anterior facial*) vein. The lymph drainage from the chin and midportion of the lower lip is largely into the submental (*suprahyoid*) nodes. The *deep lymphatics of the* *face*—those of the orbit, part of the nasal fossa, the hard and soft palates, deeper portion of the cheek, temporal fossa, and pterygo-maxillary region (*infra-temporal fossa*)—enter the internal maxillary (*deep facial*) lymph glands.

From the course of the lymph vessels it follows that in septic conditions, such as infected wounds, erysipelas, and abscess of the posterior portions of the scalp, the occipital and posterior auricular glands may become affected, and that in the same condition of the lateral part of the scalp, the parotid lymph glands may become enlarged or inflamed, and infection from the frontal region of the scalp may eventually reach the submaxillary (*submandibular*) lymph glands. The course of the lymph vessels usually corresponds to that of the veins.

Metastasis from carcinomatous growths generally follows the lymph vessels. In septic conditions or carcinomata of the anterior portion of the face, the lips, the tongue, and the sublingual and submaxillary (*submandibular*) salivary glands, the submaxillary (*submandibular*) lymph glands become enlarged and thence the deep and superficial cervical nodes along the sterno-mastoid muscle and the deep vessels of the neck. Similar affections of the outer part of the eyelids and face involve the parotid lymph glands, and in corresponding conditions of the orbital, nasal, temporal, and zygomatic fossæ, of the deeper tissues of the cheek and of the roof of the mouth, the internal maxillary (*deep facial*) lymph glands may be affected.

THE MOUTH (Plate LXV)

Examine the mouth, the pharynx, the larynx, and the nose. These are attached to the anterior portion of the skull which has been divided previous to the dissection of the prevertebral muscles. (Plate LXVI.)

The **Mouth**, or buccal cavity, is the commencement of the alimentary canal. It contains the organs of mastication and of the sense of taste, also some of the organs of speech; it acts as a resonating cavity. It is divided by the teeth and the alveolar processes into two parts, the vestibule, or pre-oral cavity, and the buccal cavity, or mouth proper.

The **vestibule** is situated between the lips and the cheeks externally, and the teeth and the gums internally. The walls of the vestibule, except when it is distended, are in contact. In front it opens upon the face at the buccal orifice, and behind the last molar teeth it communicates with the mouth proper, even when the teeth are in contact, so that in tetanus or during treatment of fractures of the mandible a patient may be fed liquids through a tube passed from the back part of the vestibule into the mouth proper. In these circumstances gavage may be practiced by a catheter introduced through the nose.

PLATE LXV.

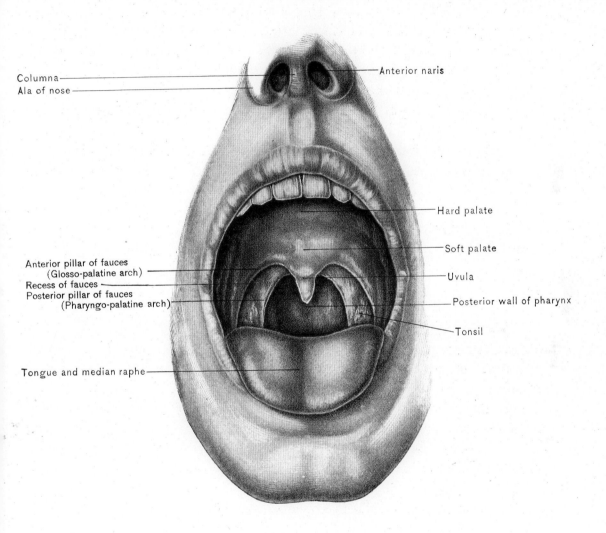

Columna

Ala of nose

Anterior naris

Hard palate

Soft palate

Anterior pillar of fauces
(Glosso-palatine arch)

Recess of fauces

Posterior pillar of fauces
(Pharyngo-palatine arch)

Uvula

Posterior wall of pharynx

Tonsil

Tongue and median raphe

ANTERIOR VIEW OF MOUTH.

PLATE LXVI.

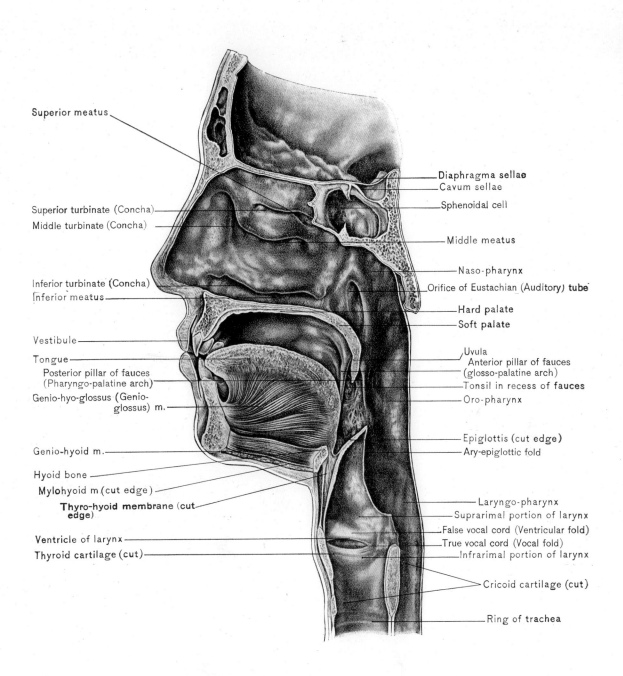

Superior meatus

Superior turbinate (Concha)
Middle turbinate (Concha)

Inferior turbinate (Concha)
Inferior meatus

Vestibule
Tongue
Posterior pillar of fauces
(Pharyngo-palatine arch)
Genio-hyo-glossus (Genio-
glossus) m.

Genio-hyoid m.

Hyoid bone
Mylohyoid m (cut edge)
Thyro-hyoid membrane (cut
edge)

Ventricle of larynx
Thyroid cartilage (cut)

Diaphragma sellae
Cavum sellae
Sphenoidal cell

Middle meatus

Naso-pharynx
Orifice of Eustachian (Auditory) tube
Hard palate
Soft palate

Uvula
Anterior pillar of fauces
(glosso-palatine arch)
Tonsil in recess of fauces
Oro-pharynx

Epiglottis (cut edge)
Ary-epiglottic fold

Laryngo-pharynx
Suprarimal portion of larynx
False vocal cord (Ventricular fold)
True vocal cord (Vocal fold)
Infrarimal portion of larynx

Cricoid cartilage (cut)

Ring of trachea

VERTICAL SECTION OF MOUTH, PHARYNX, LARYNX, AND NOSE.

The **Lips** form a transverse slit of variable length which bounds the orifice of the mouth (rima oris). They are composed of skin, superficial fascia, the orbicularis oris muscle and the muscles inserted around it, areolar tissue, and mucous membrane. The first three layers of the lips, the skin, superficial fascia, and muscular tissue, have been described with the face. The margins of the lips are covered with dry red mucous membrane, which is continuous with the skin, and contains numerous vascular papillæ and touch corpuscles. Internally, the mucous membrane is reflected from the upper and lower lips upon the gums, and in the median line forms two folds, the frenulum labii superioris and frenulum labii inferioris. The areolar tissue, or submucous layer, contains the coronary vessels, branches of the infra-orbital and mental nerves, and the labial glands. The coronary vessels completely encircle the buccal orifice near the free margin of the lips, lying immediately superficial to the mucous membrane in the submucous layer. The vascularity of the lips tends to cause extensive swelling after injuries or infections, but on the other hand, it is an important factor favoring rapid healing and avoidance of infection after surgical operations.

The **labial glands** are situated around the orifice of the mouth, in the submucous layer of the lips. They are small lobulated bodies, about the size of a small pea, and their ducts open into the mouth. They secrete a mucous fluid. When the ducts of these glands become occluded, mucous retention cysts develop.

Between the lips is the **buccal orifice,** which extends between the **angles of the mouth.**

The **lymphatics** from the median portion of the lower lip pass to lymph glands situated just above the body of the hyoid bone. These glands, however, communicate with the corresponding glands on the opposite side of the median line, allowing for metastasis to appear in the opposite side of the neck. Those from the lateral portions pass to the submaxillary (*submandibular*) lymphglands, into which the lymphatics of the upper lip also empty.

An operation frequently performed upon the upper lip is for the correction of **harelip.** This condition results from a failure of the developmental processes which normally occur in the differentiation and separation of the nasal from the buccal cavities. It occurs upon either side, opposite the interval between the canine and lateral incisor teeth and not in the median line, because the central portion of the lip, which corresponds to the four incisors, with the premaxillary bone is formed by the fronto-nasal process of the fetus, whereas each lateral portion of the upper lip develops from the maxillary process of the superior visceral arch. The deformity may be uni- or bilateral, depending upon whether the premaxillary process has united on only one or on neither side. The artery divided is the superior coronary (*superior labial*).   During the operation hemorrhage may be checked by having an assistant grasp the lip, at the angles of the mouth, between his thumbs and index fingers.   In closing the wound the artery is occluded by the pressure of the sutures.   The sutures are carried through the tissues of the lip to the mucous membrane, but not through it, and under the artery, then under the artery at the opposite side of the wound, and outward through the tissues of the lip.

The lower lip is operated upon principally for extirpation of epitheliomata. The lower lip is occasionally the site of nevus or hypertrophy.   Angio-neurotic edema of the lower lip, a rare condition, and for which operation is of no avail, must not be mistaken for hypertrophy.

The **Cheeks** are composed of five layers: skin, superficial fascia (which contains the facial vessels and some branches of the facial and trigeminal nerves), bucco-pharyngeal fascia, buccinator muscle, submucous areolar tissue, and mucous membrane.

The **bucco-pharyngeal fascia** covers the buccinator muscle, and is continued backward over the constrictor muscles of the pharynx; anteriorly the fascia thins out to become attached to the tissues of the lips.   The submucous areolar tissue contains the **buccal glands,** which resemble the labial glands.   Two or three larger glands, situated between the buccinator muscle and its fascial covering, are called **molar glands ;** their ducts open into the vestibule of the mouth opposite the last molar tooth.   Opposite the crown of the second molar tooth of the maxilla is the papilla, which marks the orifice of the duct of the parotid gland, or Stenson's duct.

The **Mouth Proper** is bounded in front and at the sides by the teeth and gums.   Its roof is formed by the hard and the soft palate, and its floor by the mucous membrane of the mouth, a large portion of the tongue, and the mylo-hyoid and genio-hyoid muscles.   Posteriorly, it opens into the pharynx at the **isthmus of the fauces.**   When the mouth is closed, the tongue lies in contact with the palate and almost fills the mouth proper.

The **Teeth** in the human subject appear as two sets: the *first, or temporary,* set is present in childhood, and comprises ten in each jaw: four incisors, two canines, and four molars.   The central incisors are the first to pierce the gums, and usually make their appearance at about the seventh month.   The lateral incisors soon follow, the last of the set to appear being the posterior molars, the eruption of which should occur in the third, or the latter half of the second year.   The *second, or permanent, set* comprises sixteen in each jaw: four incisors, two canines, four bicuspids, or premolars, and six molars.   The first molars appear at about the seventh year; the middle incisors and then the lateral incisors soon follow.

The third molars, or wisdom teeth, are the last to pierce the gums, usually at the seventeenth or eighteenth year. When a child is affected by congenital syphilis, faulty nutrition affects the development of the permanent teeth, so that they are not perfectly formed. These syphilitic teeth are uneven, and have contracted and crescentic notched cutting edges. The central incisors are the most typical, and are known as "test teeth of Hutchinson." New growths originating in the dental elements are known as odontomata.

When the mouth is wide open, a ridge produced by the pterygo-maxillary ligament (*pterygo-mandibular raphe*), which is the posterior thickened edge of the bucco-pharyngeal fascia, may be seen ascending from just behind the last molar tooth to the *pterygoid hamular process* of the medial pterygoid plate of the sphenoidal bone. This process can be felt as a resisting prominence a short distance behind, and slightly medial to the upper last molar tooth. It is the guide in division of the tensor veli palatini and levator veli palatini muscles.

The **Gums** cover the alveolar processes of the jaws and firmly surround the necks of the teeth. They are composed of dense vascular connective tissue, covered by mucous membrane. The periosteum of the alveolar processes is continued into the alveoli, forming the lining membrane of these cavities. Pus at the root of a tooth may work its way into the gum, producing a "gum boil."

In chronic lead poisoning a blue line appears upon the dental margin of the gums, and is produced by the lead sulphid formed by chemical combination of the lead in the tissues and the hydrogen sulphid derived from decomposing food.

Swelling of the gums and tenderness of the teeth during the administration of mercury indicate that the physiologic limit for that remedy has been reached, and that the dose should be decreased or the drug temporarily withdrawn.

The swollen and readily bleeding gums in scurvy assist in the diagnosis of that disease.

The **Palate** forms the roof of the mouth. It consists of the anterior, or hard, palate, and the posterior, or soft, palate.

The **hard palate** is continuous anteriorly and laterally with the alveolar processes of the maxilla, and posteriorly gives attachment to the soft palate; It separates the mouth from the nasal cavity. It is supported by the palatine process of the superior maxillary (*maxillary*) and the horizontal part of the palatine bones, clothed on their inferior surface by a dense, tough mucoperiosteum. The mucoperiosteum contains a median raphe, which marks the line of junction of the two halves of the palate. When these two halves fail to unite, cleft palate results, a malformation often associated with harelip. In the operation for cleft palate, the toughness and density of the mucoperiosteum render its manipulation more difficult, but permit the formation of firm flaps, which are essential.   The higher the arch of the palate the simpler the operation will be, since the flaps when dropped will meet with less tension.

BLOOD SUPPLY.—From the naso-palatine (*spheno-palatine*) and posterior palatine (*greater palatine*) vessels.

The posterior, or descending, palatine (*greater palatine*) arteries furnish nearly all the nutrition to the hard palate, and lie in the mucoperiosteum near the alveolar processes.   The incision into the mucoperiosteum in the operation for cleft of the hard palate should be made near and parallel with the alveolar processes, so that the descending palatine (*greater palatine*) arteries need not be divided and may be retained in the flaps to provide for their nutrition.   In dissecting up the flaps the operator should follow the bone closely, as these arteries run nearer to the bone than to the free surface of the mucoperiosteum. Bleeding from the posterior palatine (*greater palatine*) artery may be checked by plugging the posterior palatine (*greater palatine*) canal, which can be located to the medial side of the last molar tooth with a sharp probe.

NERVE SUPPLY.—From the naso-palatine and anterior, or greater, palatine nerves.

Cleft palate, as previously stated, occurs only in the median line.   The cleft may affect only the uvula and soft palate, or it may extend forward through the hard palate to the anterior palatine (*incisive*) foramen.   When the cleft extends forward beyond this foramen, it leaves the median line and follows the line of the suture at either side of the premaxillary bone (*os incisivum*), the anterior extremity of the cleft being between the lateral incisor and the canine tooth.   If the cleft follows one suture, single harelip is usually present, and if it traverses both sutures, double harelip usually exists, and the premaxillary bone (*os incisivum*) is suspended by the vomer.   In the operation for the correction of double harelip with projection of the premaxillary (*os incisivum*) bone, the attachments of this bone should be loosened and the bone pushed back in place but not removed.   Removal of the premaxillary process prevents approximation of the alveolar processes, inviting failure of the operative result, and also removes the unerupted incisor teeth.

The **soft palate** is described with the pharynx (at p. 324).

The **mucous membrane** in the floor of the mouth covers the tongue, a small area on each side of that organ, and the triangular area beneath its tip or free end. In the median line the mucous membrane is reflected upon the under surface of the tongue, forming a fold, the **frenulum linguae.** On each side of the frenulum are small papillæ, which contain the orifices of the submaxillary (*submandibular*), or Wharton's ducts.   The rounded elevation on each side of the frenulum linguae is produced by the sublingual glands, which lie immediately

PLATE LXVII.

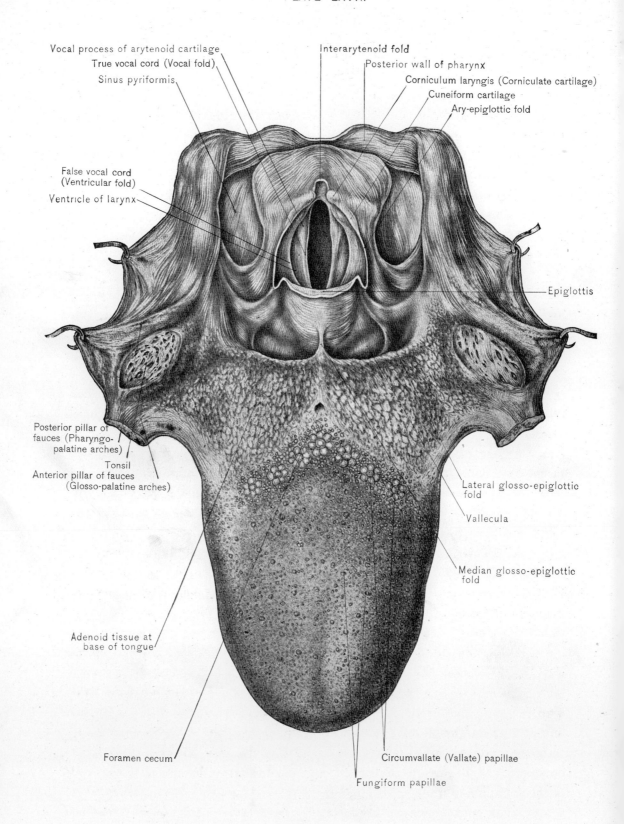

Vocal process of arytenoid cartilage
True vocal cord (Vocal fold)
Sinus pyriformis
Interarytenoid fold
Posterior wall of pharynx
Corniculum laryngis (Corniculate cartilage)
Cuneiform cartilage
Ary-epiglottic fold
False vocal cord (Ventricular fold)
Ventricle of larynx
Epiglottis
Posterior pillar of fauces (Pharyngo-palatine arches)
Tonsil
Anterior pillar of fauces (Glosso-palatine arches)
Lateral glosso-epiglottic fold
Vallecula
Median glosso-epiglottic fold
Adenoid tissue at base of tongue
Foramen cecum
Circumvallate (Vallate) papillae
Fungiform papillae

SUPERIOR APERTURE OF LARYNX AND DORSUM OF TONGUE.

beneath the mucous membrane. The orifices of the smaller sublingual ducts, or ducts of Rivinus, are situated upon these elevations. Pain in the tongue can be relieved by dividing the lingual nerve. The nerve can be felt in the floor of the mouth, opposite the second molar tooth; when the tongue is drawn out of the mouth and toward the opposite side, a ridge in the mucous membrane of the floor of the mouth, produced by this nerve, is seen extending forward from the medial side of the last molar tooth.

A *sublingual bursa*, according to Tillaux, is found immediately beneath the mucous membrane of the anterior part of the floor of the mouth, where the mucous membrane is reflected upon the posterior surface of the mandible. This bursa is affected in acute ranula.

The **Tongue** is a freely movable, muscular organ, located in the floor of the mouth. Its free surfaces—dorsum, sides and a small portion of its under surface—are covered with mucous membrane. It contains the organs of the special sense of taste, and is an important accessory in the functions of mastication, deglutition, and speech. It has a tip, a base, a dorsum, and two sides.

The **tip, or apex, of the tongue** is its most movable portion, and is covered on both its upper and lower surface by mucous membrane. Its range of motion is influenced by the length of the frenulum linguae. A short frenulum causes tongue-tie, and a long one allows the tongue to fall backward.

The **base, or root, of the tongue,** is its least movable portion. It is attached to the hyoid bone by muscular tissue and by a fibrous membrane, the *hyoglossal membrane;* to the anterior portion of the mandible, at the side of the symphysis, by the genio-glossus muscle, and to the epiglottis, by the three glosso-epiglottic folds of mucous membrane.

The **median glosso-epiglottic fold, or epiglottic frenulum,** is sharply outlined, while the **lateral glosso-epiglottic folds** are rounded and indistinct. Between the median and the lateral folds are the **glosso-epiglottic pouches, or epiglottic valleculæ,** in which small foreign bodies are apt to lodge and cause much discomfort.

The **dorsum of the tongue** (Plate LXVII) is convex and grooved in the median line, forming the *median sulcus,* a raphe from which a septum dips down between the muscles of the two sides. The raphe terminates behind at the **foramen cecum,** which is the orifice of the obliterated thyro-glossal duct. In the fetus the **thyro-glossal duct** extends from the middle lobe of the thyroid gland to the tongue. It can seldom be traced in the adult. The posterior third of the dorsum of the tongue dips downward in front of the pharynx almost to the level of the hyoid bone, and overhangs the epiglottis. It presents no papillæ, but has a somewhat uneven surface, produced by the irregular collection of lymphoid tissue, known as the **lingual tonsil.** When the lingual tonsil is much enlarged, it may depress the epiglottis and cause difficult respiration. In this region will also occasionally be found a lingual thyroid. The mucous membrane on the anterior two-thirds of the dorsum of the tongue contains numerous papillæ, which are of three varieties: filiform, fungiform, and circumvallate (*vallate*).

The **filiform papillæ,** the smallest and most numerous, are long, slender, and conical in shape, and branched at their free ends. Furred, or coated, tongue is due to increase in the thickness of the epithelium upon these papillæ.

The **fungiform papillæ,** less numerous than the filiform, resemble small knobs, and are the red spots best observed on the sides and anterior portion of the dorsum of the tongue.

The **circumvallate (vallate) papillæ,** numbering from eight to twelve, are situated at the junction of the posterior with the middle third of the dorsum of the tongue, and are arranged in the form of a **V,** with its apex directed backward toward the foramen cecum. They are surrounded by an elevated margin, or *vallum,* so that the papillæ rest in pits. They contain the special taste organs.

On the **sides of the tongue** the mucous membrane is smooth, except at the posterior part, just in front of the attachment of the anterior pillars of the fauces, where there are several parallel folds, the **papillæ foliatæ.** They are variable in size, and often rudimentary, and contain taste organs. The papillæ foliatæ are better developed in some of the lower animals than in man.

The **under surface of the tongue,** posteriorly, receives the insertion of its extrinsic muscles, but anteriorly it is free and covered by smooth, thin mucous membrane, through which the commencement of the lingual veins can be seen on each side of the median line. These veins are so superficial that they may be injured in division of the frenulum linguae for tongue-tie.

The **glands of the tongue** are found in the mucous membrane of the posterior third of the dorsum and at the sides of the organ. They are most numerous around the circumvallate (*vallate*) papillæ. Those in relation with the taste-buds secrete a *serous,* and the others a *mucous* fluid. Embedded in the substance of the lower surface of the tongue, near the tip of the organ, is a collection of mucous glands, about the size of a pea, the *glands of Nuhn or Blandin (anterior sublingual glands);* occlusion of the duct of these glands may cause the formation of a retention cyst.

DISSECTION.—Remove the mucous membrane from one side of the tongue in order to study the arrangement of its muscles. (Plate LXVIII.)

The **muscles of the tongue** compose the greater part of its mass, and are divided into an extrinsic group originating outside the tongue, and an intrinsic group contained within it. The *extrinsic muscles* are: the stylo-glossus, hyoglossus,

PLATE LXVIII.

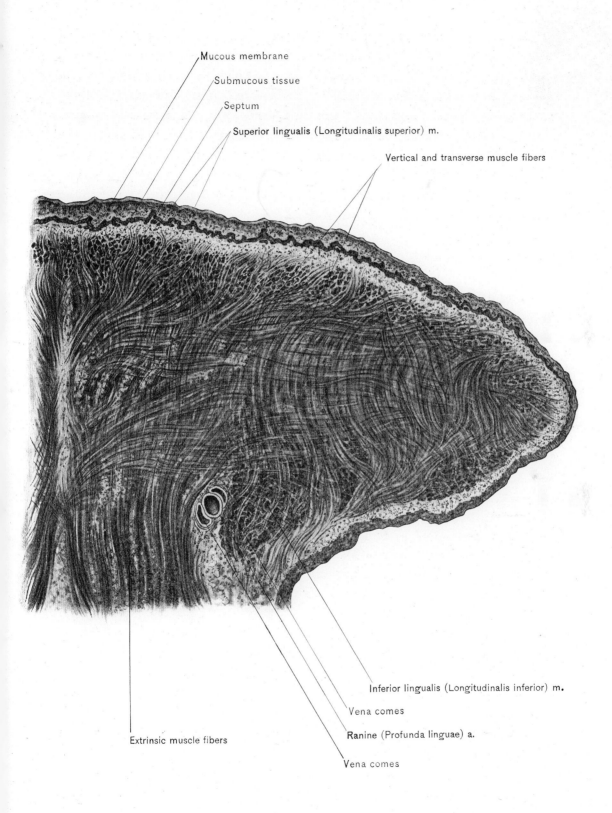

Mucous membrane

Submucous tissue

Septum

Superior lingualis (Longitudinalis superior) m.

Vertical and transverse muscle fibers

Inferior lingualis (Longitudinalis inferior) m.

Vena comes

Ranine (Profunda linguae) a.

Vena comes

Extrinsic muscle fibers

TRANSVERSE SECTION OF ONE-HALF OF TONGUE.

a small portion of the superior constrictor muscle of the pharynx, palato-glossus (*glosso-palatinus*), and genio-glossus.

The *stylo-glossus muscle* runs along the side of the tongue to its tip. The *hyoglossus* muscle is inserted medial to the stylo-glossus muscle. The superior constrictor muscle of the pharynx is seen arising from the side of the base of the tongue. The palato-glossus (*glosso-palatinus*) muscle is continuous with the transverse fibers of the intrinsic muscular tissue of the tongue. The genio-glossus muscle is next to the median line, and is separated from its fellow of the opposite side by the septum linguæ and the hyoglossal membrane. (The stylo-glossus, hyoglossus and genio-glossus are described in Vol. II; the superior constrictor and the palato-glossus at pp. 316 and 330, respectively.)

The *intrinsic muscles* contain longitudinal, transverse, and vertical fibers. The longitudinal fibers are composed of two separate bundles on each side, a superior and an inferior. The *superior lingualis (longitudinalis superior) muscle* lies beneath the mucous membrane of the dorsum, and extends from the base to the apex of the tongue. It is separated from the superior lingualis (*longitudinalis superior*) of the opposite side by the septum linguæ. The *inferior lingualis (longitudinalis inferior) muscle* is found on the under surface of the tongue, beneath the transversus linguæ. It is attached behind to the hyoid bone, and extends from the base of the tongue to its apex. Posteriorly, it lies between the hyoglossus and the genio-glossus muscles, and anteriorly, between the stylo-glossus and the genio-glossus muscles. The *transversus linguæ* forms a thick layer beneath the superior lingualis (*longitudinalis superior*) muscle, and extends from the septum linguæ to the sides of the tongue. The *verticalis linguæ* consists of thick, vertical fibers that decussate with the fibers of the transversus linguæ and pass in curved lines from the dorsum to the inferior aspect of the tongue. As the tongue is almost entirely composed of muscle tissue and contains little ✓ areolar tissue, it does not become much swollen when inflamed.

Many of the muscle fibers of the tongue are attached to the mucous membrane so that, when the mucosa is destroyed, as in ulcerative processes, the surface of the ulcer presents an uneven, ragged appearance, due, in part, to retraction of the muscle fibers.

The **septum linguæ** is a fibrous membrane which extends vertically downward from the median raphe between the halves of the tongue, and separates the linguales (*longitudinales*) and the genio-glossus muscles. Its lower portion, known as the **hyoglossal membrane,** is strong, and attaches the base of the tongue to the hyoid bone.

Paralysis and **atrophy of one-half of the tongue** may be produced by either a central or a peripheral lesion of the hypoglossal nerve, such as hemorrhage

affecting the center of that nerve in the medulla oblongata, or in disease or fracture of the occipital bone at the anterior condyloid foramen (*hypoglossal canal*),
or by pressure from an aneurysm of either the external or the internal carotid
artery, or after section of the hypoglossal nerve in operations in the neck.

Macroglossia lymphangioma cavernosum, or hypertrophy of the tongue,
is a congenital condition usually due to increased development of the lymphoid
tissue of the tongue.

The importance of chronic irritants acting on the tongue, cheeks, or lips as a
cause of malignant disease cannot be overestimated. Thickened whitish patches
(leucoplakia) are certainly precursors of epitheliomata. Carcinoma of the tongue
is a common lesion. It usually occurs in the anterior two-thirds of the tongue
which is derived from the same source as the lower lip.

Hemorrhage into the floor of the mouth may so push the tongue against
the palate as to obstruct breathing.

Blood Supply.—From the lingual, facial (*external maxillary*), and ascending pharyngeal arteries.

Nerve Supply.—From the glossopharyngeal, hypoglossal, lingual, and
chorda tympani nerves. The glossopharyngeal is the nerve of the special sense
of taste, and supplies special sensory and common sensory fibers to the mucous
membrane at the posterior third of the tongue and to the circumvallate (*vallate*)
papillæ. The hypoglossal is the motor nerve, and supplies the extrinsic muscles
and the lingual muscles, the latter being also supplied by the chorda tympani
nerve. The lingual is the common sensory nerve of the tongue, and supplies
the front and sides of that organ. Small branches of the superior laryngeal nerve
are distributed to the base of the tongue in the region of the epiglottis.

Irritation of the lingual nerve, as by an ulcer or carcinoma of the tongue,
may cause reflex disturbance in the tissues supplied by other branches of the
inferior maxillary (*mandibular*) nerve: through the auriculo-temporal nerve,
pain in the auricle, the external auditory meatus, and the temporal region;
through the inferior dental (*inferior alveolar*) nerve, pain in the lower teeth,
the lower gums, and the chin, and through the motor branches of the inferior
maxillary (*mandibular*) nerve, spasm of the muscles of mastication, excepting
the buccinator.

In **profound anesthesia** relaxation of the tissues allows the tongue to fall
backward, depressing the epiglottis, and obstructing respiration. To relieve
this condition the anesthetizer carries the mandible forward by placing his fingers
behind the angles of that bone. This procedure produces tension upon the genio-
glossus, genio-hyoid, and mylo-hyoid muscles, the hyoglossal membrane, the
glosso-epiglottic folds, and the hyo-epiglottic ligament; it draws the tongue, the

epiglottis, and the hyoid bone forward, and opens the superior aperture of the larynx.

The **lymph vessels of the lips,** together with the superficial lymph vessels of the front of the face, pass into the submaxillary (*submandibular*) and superior deep cervical lymph glands.

The **lymphatics of the roof of the mouth and deeper portion of the cheek** terminate in the internal maxillary (*deep facial*) lymph glands.

The **lymphatics of the floor of the mouth and anterior part of the tongue** pierce the mylo-hyoid muscle and join the submaxillary (*submandibular*) lymph glands.

The **lymphatics of the tongue,** excepting those of the most anterior portion, accompany the lingual vein, pass through the lingual lymph glands on the hyoglossus muscle, and terminate in the superior deep cervical glands. Any of these lymph channels may decussate with those of the opposite side.

In **excising the tongue** for carcinoma it is advisable to remove the superior deep cervical, submaxillary (*submandibular*), and lingual lymph glands, so that they may not be the source of a secondary growth. Occasionally, the submaxillary (*submandibular*) salivary gland, which contains two or more lymph glands, should also be removed.

The **isthmus of the fauces** is the large orifice of communication between the mouth and the pharynx. It is bounded above by the soft palate, below by the base of the tongue, and on each side by the pillars of the fauces.

The under surface of the **soft palate,** which is seen through the mouth, is concave, and its mucous membrane is continuous with that of the hard palate. It presents a median raphe which marks the line of union of the halves.

The **uvula** (**palatine uvula**) is the conical process which is suspended in the isthmus of the fauces from the middle of the free border of the soft palate.

The **pillars of the fauces** (**palatine arches**), or **pillars of the soft palate,** are ridges in the mucous membrane which extend lateralward and downward from the uvula. There are two on each side, an anterior pillar (*glosso-palatine arch*) and a posterior pillar (*pharyngo-palatine arch*). The *anterior pillars* (*glosso-palatine arches*) extend downward, lateralward, and forward to the sides of the base of the tongue. They contain the palato-glossus (*glosso-palatinus*) muscles. The *posterior pillars* (*pharyngo-palatine arches*) are directed downward, lateralward, and backward, and fade away upon the lateral wall of the pharynx. They are produced by the palato-pharyngeus (*pharyngo-palatinus*) muscles. A triangular depression on each side between the anterior and the posterior pillar is termed the **recess of the fauces,** or **tonsillar recess** (*sinus tonsillaris*).

The **Tonsils** are lymphoid structures situated in or around the pharynx. There are three groups: the faucial tonsils, commonly known as the tonsils, which are in the oro-pharynx, between the pillars of the fauces (*palatine arches*); the lingual tonsil, situated on the posterior surface of the tongue, and the pharyngeal tonsils, or adenoids, situated on the upper posterior wall of the naso-pharynx.

The **faucial tonsils** are two oblong, rounded bodies situated in the recesses of the fauces (*sinus tonsillaris*). They vary in size in different individuals, but should not project beyond the anterior pillars of the fauces (*glosso-palatine arches*). The medial surface of the tonsils is covered by the oral mucous membrane, and presents from ten to fifteen puncture-like orifices, which lead into recesses, called *crypts*, lined by extensions of the oral mucous membrane. The tonsils are compound follicular glands, that is, they contain a number of aggregations of lymphoid tissue similar to that of the solitary glands of the intestines. They are enveloped by a fibrous capsule. The secretion of the tonsil is derived from the mucous glands in the mucous membrane lining the crypts, and contains numerous epithelial and lymphoid cells.

Inspissation of the mucous secretion in the crypts of hypertrophied tonsils gives rise to the formation of cheesy plugs, which contain decomposing epithelium, and emit a foul odor, producing fetid breath.

It is quite probable that bacteria in the stagnant secretion in the crypts of the tonsils enter the lymph vessels, and frequently cause inflammation and tuberculosis of the deep cervical chain of lymph glands.

BLOOD SUPPLY.—From the ascending pharyngeal branch of the external carotid, the tonsillar arteries, and ascending palatine branches of the facial (*external maxillary*) artery, the dorsalis linguæ branch of the lingual artery, and the descending palatine branch of the internal maxillary artery.

NERVE SUPPLY.—From the glossopharyngeal nerve and branches of the speno-palatine, or Meckel's, ganglion.

The **veins** of the tonsil empty into the tonsillar plexus, which lies on the lateral surface of the gland and is drained by the pharyngeal veins.

The **lymphatics** of the tonsil are numerous, and empty into the lymph glands near the angle of the mandible and into the superior deep cervical lymph glands.

RELATIONS.—Laterally, each tonsil is in relation with the superior constrictor muscle of the pharynx and the pharyngeal aponeurosis, which separate it from the internal carotid and the ascending pharyngeal artery; medially, with the mucous membrane of the mouth and the pharynx.

Tonsillitis.—The tonsils are frequently affected by inflammation. In follicular tonsillitis the crypts especially are involved, and their secretion is inspissated, forming yellowish-white plugs which resemble a diphtheritic membrane, and give the throat the appearance of "ulcerated sore throat." In phlegmonous or purulent tonsillitis (quinsy), when the affection is bilateral, the tonsils may almost meet in the median line. These tonsillar abscesses should be incised with a bistoury, guarded to avoid injuring the tongue. The knife should be directed backward and medialward, and the incision be made toward the median line to avoid injuring the internal carotid artery, which lies just lateral to the gland.

Hypertrophied tonsils are not palpable externally below the angles of the mandible because the pharnygeal aponeurosis and the superior constrictor muscles of the pharynx prevent the tonsils from projecting lateralward. The masses present in these locations are enlarged lymph glands which receive lymph vessels from the tonsils. Hypertrophied tonsils project beyond the pillars of the fauces (*palatine arches*), and cause considerable annoyance through their interference with respiration and with the resonance of the voice; they should be removed. Exaggerated prominence of the anterior pillars of the fauces (*glosso-palatine arches*) may render this operation quite difficult. The relation which the tonsils bear to the internal carotid and ascending pharyngeal arteries should be borne in mind in this operation.

The ascending pharyngeal artery runs upon the lateral surface of the superior constrictor muscle of the pharynx, opposite the tonsil, and in operations upon, or in wounds of the tonsil it is more liable to injury than the internal carotid artery, which is placed further back. When the ascending pharyngeal artery is enlarged or the internal carotid artery is close to the tonsillar fossa, their pulsation is visibly transmitted to the tonsil.

The **bucco-pharyngeal fascia** is a thin, dense layer of deep fascia which covers the buccinator muscle and the constrictor muscles of the pharynx. It is continuous below, with the delicate fibrous investment of the esophagus. Anteriorly, it is continuous with the tissues of the lip, while posteriorly, it forms the pterygo-maxillary ligament (*pterygo-mandibular raphe*).

DISSECTION.—Stuff the pharynx and the esophagus with cotton, and carefully remove the fascia covering the esophagus, the trachea, and the constrictor muscles of the pharynx. The ascending pharyngeal artery, which is in relation with the superior constrictor muscle of the pharynx, and the recurrent laryngeal nerve, which lies in the groove between the esophagus and the trachea, are the structures most likely to be destroyed.

The **esophagus** is the narrow continuation of the pharynx, connecting the latter with the stomach. It begins at the lower, contracted end of the pharynx, opposite the disk between the sixth and seventh cervical vertebræ and the lower border of the cricoid cartilage, passing downward behind the trachea to enter the posterior mediastinum. It is about twenty-five centimeters (ten inches) long. At its beginning it lies in the median line, but at the lower part of the neck it inclines to the left side. Its muscular coat is continuous with the inferior constrictor muscle of the pharynx.

RELATIONS.—In front of the esophagus, in the neck, are the trachea, the left recurrent laryngeal nerve, and the posterior surface of the left lobe of the thyroid gland. Behind it are the prevertebral fascia, the bodies of the vertebræ, and the longus colli muscles. On its right side are the right carotid sheath and its contents, the right recurrent laryngeal nerve, and the right lobe of the thyroid gland. On its left side are the left carotid sheath, the left common carotid and subclavian arteries, the left recurrent laryngeal nerve, the thoracic duct, and the left lobe of the thyroid gland.

The narrowest point in the esophagus is at its beginning behind the lower border of the cricoid cartilage and in front of the lower part of the sixth cervical vertebra. Here it is only fourteen millimeters (nine-sixteenths of an inch) in diameter. This is the point at which a large foreign body, such as a set of false teeth, would be likely to lodge. The removal of foreign bodies by esophagotomy is no longer necessary since the development of esophagoscopy. The cervical esophagus, however, can be exposed as follows: an incision is made along the anterior border of the left sterno-mastoid muscle, cutting the skin and superficial fascia, the platysma muscle, some superficial vessels and nerves, the superficial layer of the deep fascia, the omo-hyoid muscle (if necessary), and the pretracheal fascia. The carotid sheath and its contents must be displaced lateralward, and the trachea, the thyroid gland, the sterno-thyroid and sterno-hyoid muscles, displaced medialward. The superior and middle thyroid veins must be avoided or else divided between ligatures; care must be taken not to injure the recurrent laryngeal nerve and the inferior thyroid artery.

Congenital and acquired diverticula may occur in this portion of the esophagus. They are exposed through an incision similar to the foregoing, and inverted and oversewn.

The thoracic portion of the esophagus is described with the chest.

THE PHARYNX

The **pharynx**, the second portion of the alimentary tract, is a conical, musculo-membranous tube, situated behind the nasal cavities, the mouth, and the larynx; it is subdivided into the naso-pharynx, oro-pharynx, and laryngo-pharynx. The **naso-pharynx** and **oro-pharynx** bridge the gap in the respiratory tract between the larynx and the nasal cavities, and assist in giving resonance to the voice; the **oro-pharynx** and **laryngo-pharynx** connect the mouth with the

PLATE LXIX.

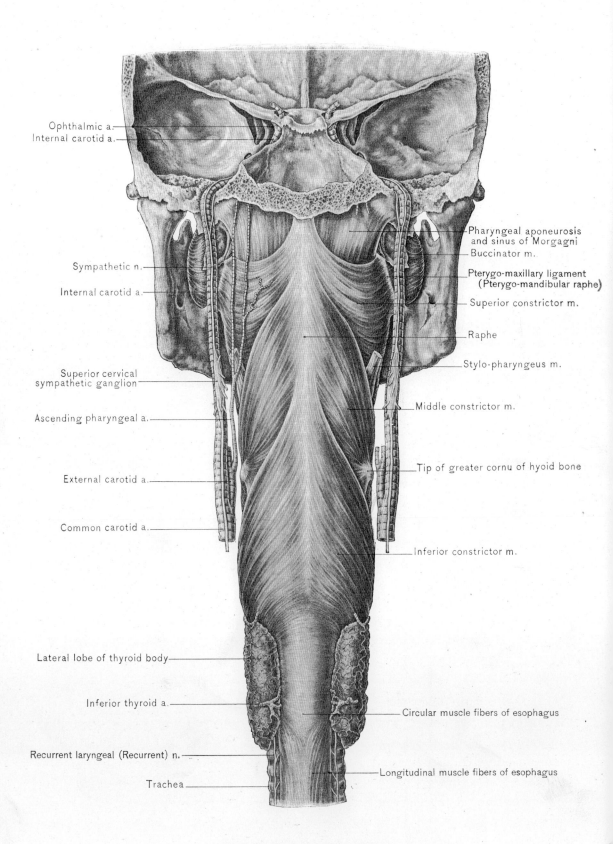

Ophthalmic a.
Internal carotid a.

Sympathetic n.

Internal carotid a.

Superior cervical
sympathetic ganglion

Ascending pharyngeal a.

External carotid a.

Common carotid a.

Lateral lobe of thyroid body

Inferior thyroid a.

Recurrent laryngeal (Recurrent) n.

Trachea

Pharyngeal aponeurosis
and sinus of Morgagni
Buccinator m.

Pterygo-maxillary ligament
(Pterygo-mandibular raphe)

Superior constrictor m.

Raphe

Stylo-pharyngeus m.

Middle constrictor m.

Tip of greater cornu of hyoid bone

Inferior constrictor m.

Circular muscle fibers of esophagus

Longitudinal muscle fibers of esophagus

CONSTRICTOR MUSCLES OF PHARYNX.

esophagus, and carry the food from the former to the latter. The pharynx is about twelve centimeters (four and a half inches) in length, and extends from the base of the skull to the lower border of the sixth cervical vertebra, opposite the lower border of the cricoid cartilage, where it becomes the esophagus. It is bounded above by the under surface of the body of the sphenoidal bone and by the basilar process of the occipital bone, which, with the spine and the prevertebral muscles and fascia covering it, form the posterior boundary. The pharynx is compressed anteroposteriorly, thus making its transverse diameter the greater. Its widest point is opposite the greater cornu of the hyoid bone, where it is about five centimeters (two inches) in width; at its narrowest point, its junction with the esophagus, opposite the lower border of the cricoid cartilage, it is about fourteen millimeters (nine-sixteenths of an inch) wide.

Although, owing to the dilatability of the pharynx, large foreign bodies may be retained in it for a long time without producing much discomfort, they more frequently give rise to alarming symptoms; they usually lodge at the lower end, which is the narrowest portion of that canal, and, remaining behind the larynx, they cause dyspnea and obstruct deglutition. In attempting to remove these bodies it is important to remember that the pharyngo-esophageal junction is about fifteen centimeters (six inches) from the teeth. Foreign bodies in the pharynx may cause suffocation by occlusion of the superior aperture of the larynx, or by producing spasm of the muscles of the larynx. In either condition sudden death may occur during eating. As the mass of food can be reached if it rests upon the superior aperture of the larynx, the proper course of procedure is to remove it with the finger used as a hook.

The basilar process of the occipital bone, the under surface of the sphenoidal bone, and the upper four cervical vertebræ may be palpated by pushing the finger up behind the soft palate along the posterior pharyngeal wall. The retropharyngeal tissue is often the site of infection leading to abscess formation. Unless promptly drained, the pus may gravitate into the mediastinum.

The pharynx has a muscular, a fibrous, and a mucous coat.

The **muscular coat of the pharynx** is composed of the inferior, middle, and superior constrictor muscles, with a few fibers from the stylo-pharyngeus (see Vol. II) and palato-pharyngeus (*pharyngo-palatinus*) muscles (see p. 330).

The **constrictor muscles of the pharynx** (Plate LXIX) are flat, and are inserted into the median raphe on the posterior aspect of the organ. This raphe is formed by the interlacing, tendinous fibers of the muscles of the opposite sides, and extends downward from the pharyngeal spine on the basilar process of the occipital bone. The constrictor muscles are so arranged that the inferior overlaps the middle, and the middle overlaps the superior.

The *inferior constrictor muscle of the pharynx*, the thickest of the three constrictors, *arises* from the posterior part of the side of the cricoid cartilage behind the crico-thyroid muscle, from the inferior cornu, the oblique line, and the superior border of the ala of the thyroid cartilage. Its fibers diverge as they pass backward around the pharynx, to be *inserted* into the median raphe. The lower fibers are almost horizontal, and are continuous with the muscular coat of the esophagus. The upper fibers ascend obliquely over the lower portion of the middle constrictor muscle, to be *inserted* into the raphe higher up. Passing beneath or through the lower border of the inferior constrictor muscle at its origin are the recurrent laryngeal nerve and the inferior laryngeal branch of the inferior thyroid artery on their way to the larynx.

The *middle constrictor muscle of the pharynx* has a narrow *origin* from the stylo-hyoid ligament, the lesser cornu of the hyoid bone, and the entire length of the upper surface of the greater cornu of the hyoid bone. Its fibers diverge as they pass to the back of the pharynx, to reach the median raphe. The lower fibers are almost horizontal, and pass beneath the upper part of the inferior constrictor muscle. The upper fibers ascend obliquely over the lower part of the superior constrictor muscle, to reach the raphe near the base of the skull. Some of its tendinous fibers continue upward to the pharyngeal spine on the basilar process of the occipital bone.

In the interval between the origins of the middle and inferior constrictor muscles, the *internal laryngeal branch of the superior laryngeal nerve* and the *superior laryngeal artery* pierce the thyro-hyoid membrane. Near the upper margin of the middle constrictor muscle runs the glossopharyngeal nerve, and passing beneath that margin is the stylo-pharyngeus muscle. Its origin is covered by the hyoglossus muscle and the lingual artery which lies between the hyoglossus and the middle constrictor muscles.

DISSECTION.—Remove the internal pterygoid muscle and expose the origin of the superior constrictor muscle. In removing the origin of the former muscle from the pterygoid fossa preserve the tensor palati (*tensor veli palatini*) muscle, which lies between the internal pterygoid muscle and the medial pterygoid plate.

The *superior constrictor muscle* is a thin, pale, quadrilateral muscle which *arises* from the lower third of the posterior border of the medial pterygoid plate, and the hamular process of that plate, from the pterygo-maxillary ligament (*pterygo-mandibular raphe*), the posterior part of the mylo-hyoid ridge of the mandible, and the side of the base of the tongue. Its fibers pass transversely to be *inserted* into the median raphe. The lower fibers are overlapped by the middle constrictor muscle. The upper fibers ascend in a curve and have a tendinous attachment to the pharyngeal spine on the basilar process of the occipital bone. The upper margin is crescentic, and is situated some distance from the base of the skull, leaving a semilunar interval, the *sinus of Morgagni*, the floor of which is formed by the pharyngeal aponeurosis. The upper border of the superior constrictor muscle of the pharynx is in relation with the levator palati (*levator veli palatini*) muscle and the Eustachian (*auditory*) tube. The superior constrictor muscle and the pharyngeal aponeurosis separate the ascending pharyngeal and internal carotid arteries from the tonsil.

NERVE SUPPLY.—The constrictor muscles of the pharynx derive their nerve supply from the pharyngeal plexus, the inferior constrictor muscle receiving additional branches from the external and recurrent laryngeal nerves.

ACTION.—In the act of deglutition, as the food enters the pharynx the elevator muscles relax and the constrictors of the pharynx contract upon the food and send it on into the esophagus.

Tetanus often presents its first symptom as spasm of the muscles of mastication which elevate the mandible—the masseter, temporal and internal pterygoid muscles—and of the constrictor muscles of the pharynx, so that the patient cannot open his mouth, and deglutition, or swallowing, is difficult or causes choking sensations. Spasm of the constrictor muscles of the pharynx and difficult deglutition are also prominent symptoms of hydrophobia.

The **pharyngeal plexus of nerves** is found chiefly upon the middle constrictor muscle. It is formed by the pharyngeal branches of the vagus, the external laryngeal, and glossopharyngeal nerves, and of the superior cervical sympathetic ganglion. It supplies the muscular coat of the pharynx. The inferior constrictor also receives fibers from the recurrent laryngeal. The mucous membrane of the pharynx is supplied by the glossopharyngeal, the vagus, the cervical sympathetic, and the pharyngeal plexus.

The **pterygo-maxillary ligament** (**pterygo-mandibular raphe**) is a fibrous raphe between the buccinator and superior constrictor muscles which would otherwise form a continuous circle around the alimentary canal, and extends from the lower extremity of the medial pterygoid plate to the posterior end of the mylohyoid, or internal oblique, line of the mandible. It is merely the posterior thickened edge of the bucco-pharyngeal fascia.

The **pharyngeal aponeurosis**, the fibrous coat of the pharynx, is situated between the mucous and the muscular coats. It is dense and strong where the muscular coat is absent, at the sinuses of Morgagni and in the triangular intervals between the origins of the constrictor muscles, and becomes delicate and fades away below. It holds the pharynx open by means of its attachment to the basilar process of the occipital bone, the cartilages in the lacerated foramina, the apices of the petrous portions of the temporal bones, the posterior borders of the medial pterygoid plates, the greater cornu of the hyoid bone, and the posterior borders of the alæ of the thyroid cartilage.

The **mucous coat,** or mucous membrane, lining the pharynx is continuous with that of the Eustachian (*auditory*) tubes, the nasal cavities, the mouth, the larynx, and the esophagus. It contains racemose mucous glands and scattered lymphoid follicles. Because of its vascularity, inflammation of this membrane, or pharyngitis, or sore throat, is common. Through the continuity of the mucous membrane of the nose and larynx the catarrhal process may extend to the mucous membrane of those cavities.

DISSECTION.—Divide the posterior wall of the pharynx in the median line, and detach it from the base of the skull as far as the lateral wall. Then turn the two flaps laterally in order to study the interior of the pharynx.

Beneath the petrous portion of the temporal bone the cavity of the pharynx extends lateralward, forming a pouch, the *pharyngeal recess.*

The **pharyngeal tonsil,** or tonsil of Luschka (Plate LXX), is a collection of lymphoid tissue in the posterior wall of the pharynx, near its junction with the roof. It usually decreases in size after childhood and often atrophies in the adult. It is commonly known as the **adenoid gland.**

The **pharyngeal bursa** is a small inconstant diverticulum in the posterior wall of the pharynx, below the occipital bone; it is most conspicuous in the fetus and in infants.

Hypertrophy of the pharyngeal tonsil is the source of the adenoid growths in the naso-pharynx, rather common among children, causing obstruction of the posterior nares, loss of nasal resonance in the voice, and resulting in mouth breathing. Extension of the hypertrophic process into the Eustachian (*auditory*) tubes causes obstruction of those tubes, tinnitus aurium, or peculiar sounds in the ears, and deafness.

Retropharyngeal abscess, usually the result of caries of the upper cervical vertebræ or suppuration of the retropharyngeal lymph glands or areolar tissue, may bulge into the pharynx and cause difficulty in deglutition or respiration. Retropharyngeal abscesses, and those arising in the pterygo-maxillary region (*infratemporal fossa*) and temporal fossa, may rupture into the pharynx.

There are **Seven Openings into the Pharynx:** the two posterior nares (*choanæ*), the two Eustachian (*auditory*) tubes, the mouth, the larynx, and the esophagus (Plate LXXI).

The **posterior nares,** or **choanæ,** are at the highest point of the anterior wall of the pharynx, and are separated from each other by the posterior margin of the septum of the nose. Through them can be seen the middle and inferior tur-

PLATE LXX.

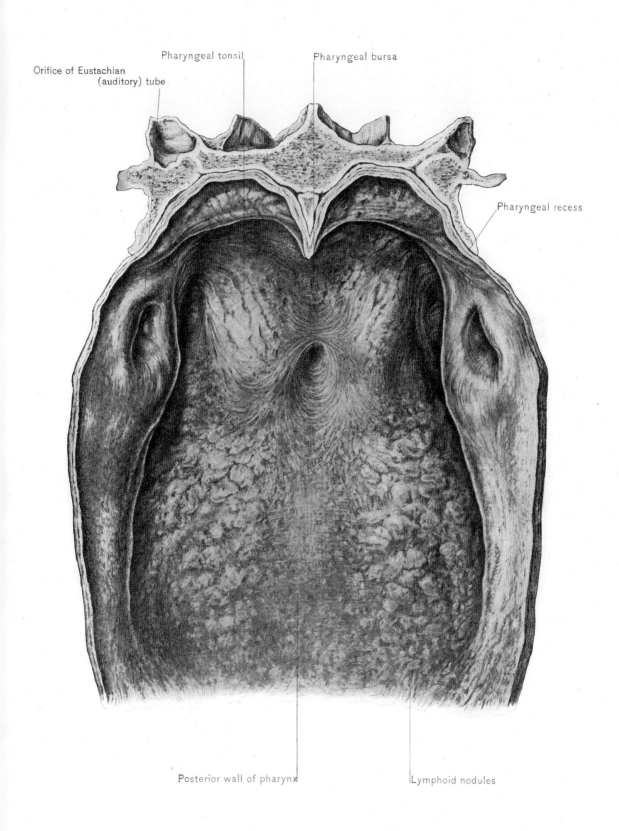

Orifice of Eustachian (auditory) tube

Pharyngeal tonsil

Pharyngeal bursa

Pharyngeal recess

Posterior wall of pharynx

Lymphoid nodules

PHARYNGEAL TONSIL AND BURSA.

PLATE LXXI.

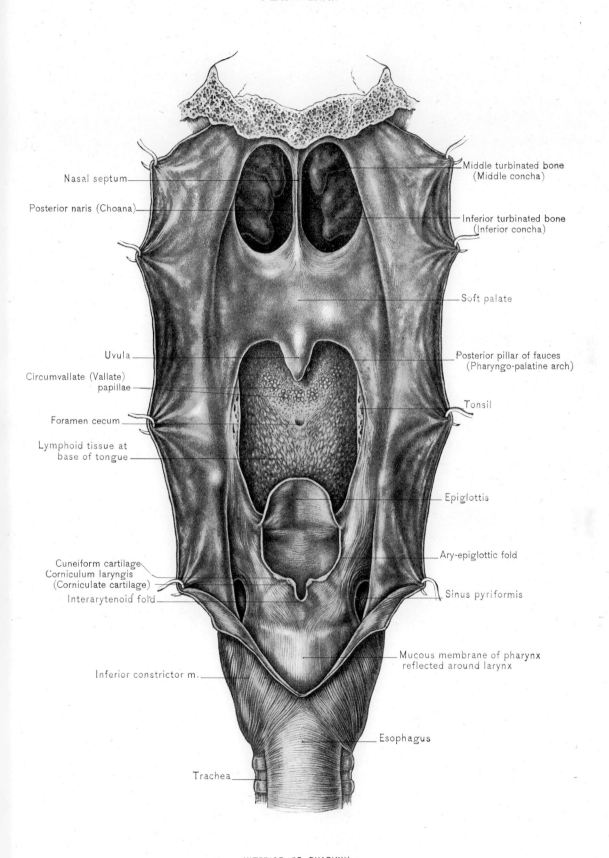

Nasal septum

Posterior naris (Choana)

Middle turbinated bone
(Middle concha)

Inferior turbinated bone
(Inferior concha)

Soft palate

Uvula

Posterior pillar of fauces
(Pharyngo-palatine arch)

Circumvallate (Vallate)
papillae

Foramen cecum

Tonsil

Lymphoid tissue at
base of tongue

Epiglottis

Ary-epiglottic fold

Cuneiform cartilage
Corniculum laryngis
(Corniculate cartilage)

Interarytenoid fold

Sinus pyriformis

Mucous membrane of pharynx
reflected around larynx

Inferior constrictor m.

Esophagus

Trachea

INTERIOR OF PHARYNX.

binated bones (*conchæ*). With a mirror placed immediately behind the soft palate, the superior turbinated bones (*conchæ*) can also be seen.

The trumpet-shaped **orifices** of the **Eustachian (auditory) tubes** are in the lateral walls of the pharynx, at about the level of the inferior turbinated bones (*conchæ*). A catheter, if carried through the inferior meatus to the posterior wall of the pharynx, and rotated lateralward and drawn forward along the lateral wall of the pharynx until it passes over the elevation at the posterior margin of the Eustachian (*auditory*) orifice, will readily slip into the Eustachian (*auditory*) tube when pushed backward again. From their orifices the Eustachian (*auditory*) tubes are directed backward, lateralward, and slightly upward, opening into the tympanic cavity at its anterior wall. The medial portion of the tube is cartilaginous on the upper and medial sides, and fibrous below; its lateral portion has bony walls, and begins in the receding angle between the squamous and petrous portions of the temporal bone.

The **isthmus of the fauces, posterior opening of the mouth,** is situated immediately below the posterior nares and soft palate. Through the isthmus some of the structures of the mouth can be examined from behind. The pillars of the fauces (*palatine arches*), the tonsils, situated in the recesses of the fauces, and the base of the tongue are more satisfactorily seen through the isthmus of the fauces than through the buccal orifice. The base of the tongue holds a vertical position, and overhangs the epiglottis. Between the tongue and the epiglottis are the three glosso-epiglottic folds and the two glosso-epiglottic pouches.

The **superior aperture of the larynx** is situated below the base of the tongue. It is a large, triangular-shaped opening, its wider portion being directed forward, and slopes obliquely downward and backward from the upper extremity of the epiglottis. It is bounded in front, by the epiglottis, behind, by the interarytenoid fold of mucous membrane, and on each side, by the ary-epiglottic fold and the tips of the arytenoid cartilages. The *recessus pyriformis* is a depression on each side of the posterior portion of the larynx, in which foreign bodies are apt to lodge. The depression is limited medially by the ary-epiglottic folds, and laterally by the greater wing of the thyroid cartilage, and the thyro-hyoid membrane. It is open posteriorly.

The **esophageal opening of the pharynx** is the narrowest portion of the pharynx, and is located behind the lower border of the cricoid cartilage.

RELATIONS OF THE PHARYNX.—In front of the pharynx are the posterior nares, the soft palate, the isthmus of the fauces, the base of the tongue, the hyoid bone, and the larynx. Behind it, are the prevertebral fascia, the retropharyngeal lymph glands, the rectus capitis anterior major (*longus capitis*) and longus colli muscles, and the bodies of the upper vertebræ. Laterally, its upper portion is in relation with the Eustachian (*auditory*) tube, the inferior maxillary (*mandibular*) nerve, the styloid process of the temporal bone, the muscles arising from that process, the internal pterygoid muscle, the parotid gland, the glossopharyngeal, vagus, spinal accessory, hypoglossal, and cervical sympathetic nerves, the ascending pharyngeal and the internal carotid arteries, and the internal jugular vein; its lower portion is in relation, laterally, with the carotid sheath and its contents, the lower part of the external carotid artery, the commencement of the superior thyroid, lingual, and facial (*external maxillary*) arteries, the lateral lobe of the thyroid gland, the sterno-thyroid muscle, and the deep cervical chain of lymph glands. Above the pharynx is that portion of the base of the skull formed by the body of the sphenoidal bone and the basilar process of the occipital bone. Below, it leads into the esophagus.

BLOOD SUPPLY.—From the ascending pharyngeal artery, the tonsillar and ascending palatine branches of the facial (*external maxillary*) artery, the superior laryngeal branch of the superior thyroid artery, and the inferior laryngeal branch of the inferior thyroid artery.

NERVE SUPPLY.—From the pharyngeal plexus of nerves.

While studying the relations of the pharynx, it is well to observe the following important facts: the body of the sphenoidal bone and the basilar process of the occipital bone and the upper three cervical vertebræ can be palpated with the finger inserted into the pharynx. The anterior arch of the atlas is in the same transverse plane as the hard palate; the body of the axis (*epistropheus*) is in the same transverse plane as the cutting edges of the upper teeth, and the body of the third cervical vertebra is just below that of the axis (*epistropheus*). In *necrosis* of the body of the sphenoidal bone, the basilar process of the occipital bone, the anterior arch of the atlas, and the bodies of the upper cervical vertebræ, pus and pieces of bone may be discharged through the pharynx and mouth. *Sharp foreign bodies* which have perforated the wall of the pharynx may wound one of the carotid arteries or the internal jugular vein.

The **veins of the pharynx** are arranged as a plexus situated between the constrictor muscles and the prevertebral fascia. This plexus communicates above with the pterygoid plexus of veins, and empties into the terminal portion of the facial (*anterior facial*) vein or into the internal jugular vein.

The **lymph vessels of the upper portion of the pharynx** terminate in the retropharyngeal glands; those of the intermediate portion, in the superior deep cervical, and those of the lower portion, in the inferior deep cervical lymph glands.

The **soft palate** (Plate LXXII) is a musculo-membranous, freely movable fold, suspended from the posterior margin of the hard palate, forming a partial

PLATE LXXII.

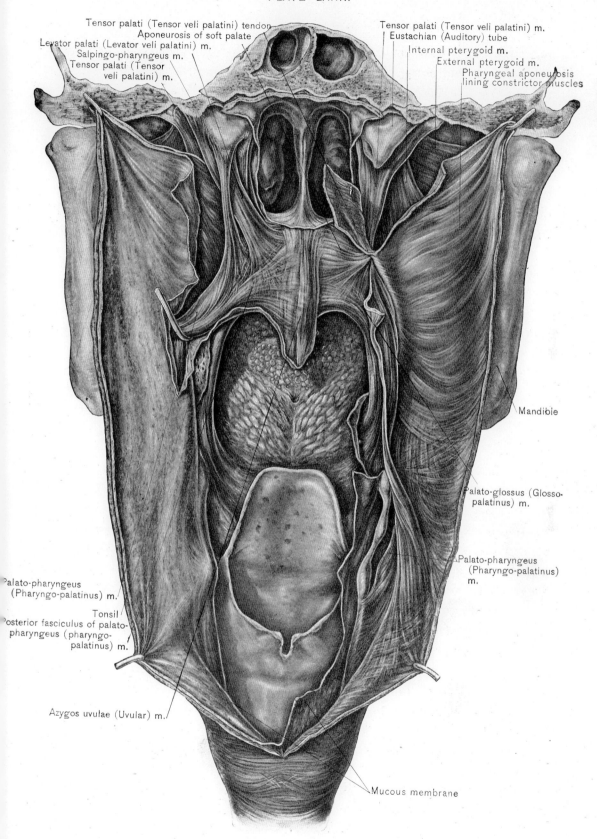

Tensor palati (Tensor veli palatini) tendon
Aponeurosis of soft palate
Levator palati (Levator veli palatini) m.
Salpingo-pharyngeus m.
Tensor palati (Tensor veli palatini) m.

Tensor palati (Tensor veli palatini) m.
Eustachian (Auditory) tube
Internal pterygoid m.
External pterygoid m.
Pharyngeal aponeurosis lining constrictor muscles

Mandible

Palato-glossus (Glosso-palatinus) m.

Palato-pharyngeus (Pharyngo-palatinus) m.

Palato-pharyngeus (Pharyngo-palatinus) m.

Tonsil

Posterior fasciculus of palato-pharyngeus (pharyngo-palatinus) m.

Azygos uvulae (Uvular) m.

Mucous membrane

MUSCLES OF SOFT PALATE.

PLATE LXXIII.

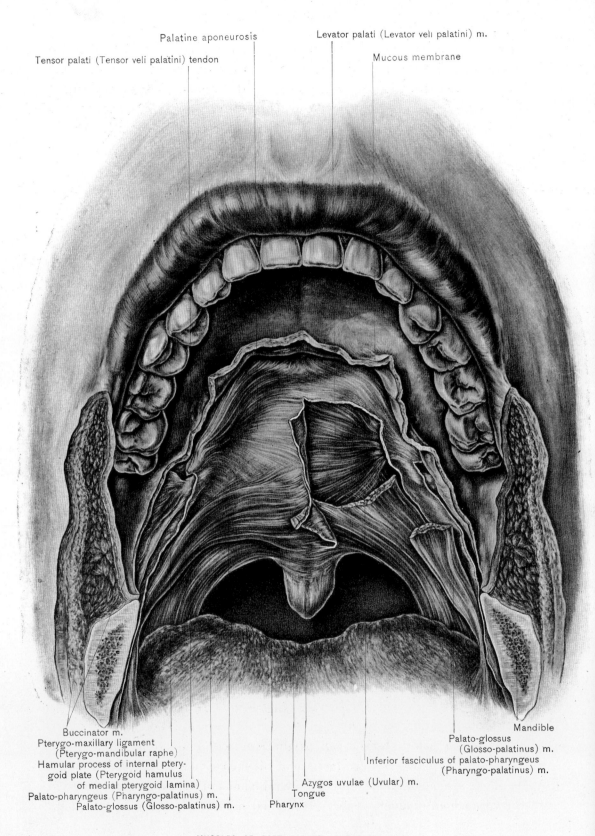

Palatine aponeurosis

Levator palati (Levator veli palatini) m.

Tensor palati (Tensor veli palatini) tendon

Mucous membrane

Buccinator m.
Pterygo-maxillary ligament
(Pterygo-mandibular raphe)
Hamular process of internal ptery-
goid plate (Pterygoid hamulus
of medial pterygoid lamina)
Palato-pharyngeus (Pharyngo-palatinus) m.
Palato-glossus (Glosso-palatinus) m.

Tongue

Pharynx

Azygos uvulae (Uvular) m.

Mandible

Palato-glossus
(Glosso-palatinus) m.
Inferior fasciculus of palato-pharyngeus
(Pharyngo-palatinus) m.

MUSCLES OF SOFT PALATE—ANTERIOR VIEW.

septum between the mouth and the naso-pharynx. Its anterior margin is attached to the posterior border of the hard palate; its lower posterior margin is free, and forms the curved upper boundary of the isthmus of the fauces. From the center of this curved margin the **uvula** (*palatine uvula*) is suspended. The lateral margins are attached to the sides of the pharynx. Its upper surface is convex; its lower, concave. The mucous membrane on the upper surface is continuous with that of the floor of the nasal cavities, and that of its lower surface with that of the roof of the mouth. Between its two layers of mucous membrane are the two levatores palati (*levatores veli palatini*), two tensores palati (*tensores veli palatini*), the palato-pharyngeus (*pharyngo-palatinus*), palato-glossus, and azygos uvulæ (*uvular*) muscles, an aponeurosis, glandular tissue, vessels, and nerves. On the under surface of the soft palate, a short distance behind the last molar tooth, there is a prominence, produced by the hamular process of the medial pterygoid plate of the sphenoidal bone, which is the guide in dividing the aponeuroses of the tensor palati (*tensor veli palatini*) and levator palati (*levator veli palatini*) muscles.

Dissection.—Render the tissues tense by means of hooks and reflect the mucous membrane from both surfaces of the soft palate and from the pillars of the fauces (*palatine arches*). Remove the mucous membrane and pharyngeal aponeurosis from the upper portion of the side of the pharynx, in order fully to expose the levatores palati (*levatores veli palatini*) and tensores palati (*tensores veli palatini*) muscles, which have been seen during the dissection of the superior constrictor muscle of the pharynx.

The **levator palati (levator veli palatini) muscle** (Plates LXXII and LXXIII) *arises* from the under surface of the petrous portion of the temporal bone in front of the carotid canal and from the lower lateral surface of the cartilaginous portion of the Eustachian (*auditory*) tube. It passes medial to the upper margin of the superior constrictor muscle of the pharynx, to reach the medial surface of that muscle, and is *inserted* into the palatine aponeurosis and into its fellow of the opposite side, in front of the azygos uvulæ (*uvular*) muscle.

Nerve Supply.—From branches of the pharyngeal plexus.

Action.—It elevates the soft palate and brings it into contact with the posterior wall of the pharynx, so as to separate the naso-pharynx from the oro-pharynx and prevent regurgitation of food from the oro-pharynx into the naso-pharynx and the nasal cavities.

The **tensor palati (tensor veli palatini) muscle** *arises* from the scaphoid fossa, which is situated behind the base of the medial pterygoid plate, from the spine of the sphenoidal bone, and the lateral lamina of the cartilaginous portion of the Eustachian (*auditory*) tube. It is a flat muscle, which lies on the lateral surface of the medial pterygoid plate and terminates in a tendon which winds around the hamular process of that plate, and forms almost a right angle with the muscle, and is *inserted* into the palatine aponeurosis, with which it is continous, and into the transverse ridge on the under surface of the horizontal plate of the palatine bone. A bursa facilitates the movement of the tendon over the pterygoid hamular process.

NERVE SUPPLY.—From twigs of the inferior maxillary (*mandibular*) nerve which pass through the otic ganglion.

ACTION.—It renders the soft palate tense and opens the Eustachian (*auditory*) tube during deglutition.

The **palato-pharyngeus (pharyngo-palatinus) muscle** is situated in the posterior pillar of the fauces. It *arises* from the soft palate by two slips, which are separated by the levator palati (*levator veli palatini*) and azygos uvulæ (*uvular*) muscles, and are continuous with the corresponding slips of the opposite muscle; it also has an *origin* from the cartilage of the Eustachian (*auditory*) tube. It passes to the side of the pharynx and joins the stylo-pharyngeus muscle, to be *inserted* into the posterior border of the thyroid cartilage below the base of the superior cornu, and by an expansion into the pharyngeal aponeurosis.

NERVE SUPPLY.—From branches of the pharyngeal plexus.

ACTION.—It elevates the pharynx and larynx and approximates the posterior pillars of the fauces (*pharyngo-palatine arches*).

The **palato-glossus (glosso-palatinus) muscle** is found in the anterior pillar of the fauces (*glosso-palatine arch*). It *arises* from the under surface of the palatine aponeurosis, and is partly continuous with the palato-glossus (*glosso-palatinus*) muscle of the opposite side in front of the azygos uvulæ (*uvular*) muscle. It is *inserted* into the side of the tongue, and is partly continuous with the transverse muscle fibers of that organ.

NERVE SUPPLY.—From the pharyngeal plexus.

ACTION.—It draws the side of the soft palate downward and elevates the sides and back part of the tongue, thus constricting the isthmus of the fauces to prevent morsels of food from being driven back into the mouth in deglutition.

The **azygos uvulæ (uvular) muscle** is a double muscle; it *arises* from the palatine aponeurosis and the posterior nasal spine on the horizontal plate of the palatine bone, and is *inserted* into the mucous membrane of the uvula.

NERVE SUPPLY.—From the pharyngeal plexus.

ACTION.—It elevates and shortens the uvula.

The **palatine aponeurosis** is a thin but dense fibrous membrane, which is attached to the posterior margin of the hard palate and gradually disappears as it approaches the posterior or free border of the soft palate. Laterally, it is continuous with the pharyngeal aponeurosis. It receives the tendinous expansion of the tensor palati (*tensor veli palatini*) muscle, and gives strength to the soft palate.

The glandular tissue of the soft palate is most abundant in its upper surface, although there is some adenoid tissue in its under surface.

Blood Supply.—From the dorsalis linguæ and the ascending pharyngeal arteries, the ascending palatine branch of the facial (*external maxillary*) artery, and the posterior palatine branch of the internal maxillary artery.

The *veins* correspond to the arteries. The *lymphatics* empty into the glands at the angle of the mandible.

Clefts of the soft palate may exist independently of those of the hard palate. They are widened by the tensor palati (*tensor veli palatini*), levator palati (*levator veli palatini*), palato-glossus (*glosso-palatinus*), and palato-pharyngeus (*pharyngo-palatinus*) muscles. These clefts give rise to difficulty in deglutition, because they allow food to pass into the naso-pharynx and nose. Before closing the cleft, the aponeuroses of these muscles are divided to prevent them from causing tension upon the sutures. The aponeuroses of the tensor palati (*tensor veli palatini*) and levator palati (*levator veli palatini*) muscles may be divided by one incision. A slender knife, with its cutting edge directed forward and upward, is inserted into the soft palate slightly in front of, and close to the medial side of the hamular process of the medial pterygoid plate of the sphenoidal bone, until it projects through the superior surface of the soft palate. As the knife is pushed upward it cuts the aponeurosis of the tensor palati (*tensor veli palatini*). The knife is then carried upward, forward, and medialward, cutting the superior surface of the soft palate for a distance sufficient to allow severance of the aponeurosis of the levator palati (*levator veli palatini*). Another simple incision is to section the soft palate near its lateral border, carrying the knife parallel with the cleft. The palato-glossus (*glosso-palatinus*) and palato-pharyngeus (*pharyngo-palatinus*) muscles can be divided by a shallow incision across each of the pillars of the fauces (*palatine arches*). The latter is seldom necessary. The attachment of the palatine aponeurosis to the posterior margin of the hard palate may also cause difficulty in approximating the freshened margins of the cleft, and should be divided in order to insure a good result. The success of the operation depends chiefly upon the relief of tension upon the sutures.

Paralysis of the muscles of the soft palate and pharynx may occur during convalescence from diphtheria. As a result, there is difficulty in swallowing and regurgitation of food through the nose.

THE LARYNX

The **larynx** is a membrano-cartilaginous, box-like organ, situated at the upper portion of the respiratory tract, above the trachea and in front of the lower portion of the pharynx. It assists in protecting the respiratory tract from the entrance of foreign bodies during deglutition and it also closes the respiratory tract, so that the chest can be rendered tense during great muscular effort. Anteriorly, it is covered by skin, superficial and deep fasciæ, two thin layers of muscle tissue, and, occasionally, by a process of the isthmus of the thyroid gland. The superficial stratum of muscle tissue is composed of the sterno-hyoid and omo-hyoid muscles, the deep stratum of the sterno-thyroid and thyro-hyoid muscles. The great vessels lie on each side of the larynx in the groove between the larynx and the sterno-mastoid muscle. It is suspended from the skull by the stylo-hyoid ligament, the muscles attached to the superior surface of the hyoid bone, and the stylo-pharyngeus and palato-pharyngeus (*pharyngo-palatinus*) muscles, which are inserted into the posterior borders of the alæ of the thyroid cartilage. It is lined internally by mucous membrane which is continuous, above, with the mucosa of the pharynx, and below, with that of the trachea. It consists of three single cartilages and three paired cartilages united by membranes, ligaments, and muscles. The single cartilages are the thyroid, cricoid, and epiglottic; the paired ones are the arytenoid, the cornicula laryngis (*corniculate cartilages*), or cartilages of Santorini, and the cuneiform cartilages, or cartilages of Wrisberg. These cartilages by change of position alter the approximation of the vocal cords, modifying their tension, producing variations in speech, and allowing air to enter and leave the trachea. The larynx is larger in all its dimensions in the male than in the female.

The **superior aperture of the larynx** (Plate LXXIV) behind the base of the tongue inclines obliquely downward and backward. It is bounded in front by the epiglottis; behind, by the interarytenoid fold of mucous membrane, and at the sides, by the ary-epiglottic folds and the tips of the arytenoid cartilages. The larynx can only be demonstrated during life by the use of a laryngeal mirror.

The **ary-epiglottic folds** extend from the sides of the epiglottis back over the summits of the arytenoid cartilages. They are composed of two layers of mucous membrane, between which are: a supporting layer of connective tissue, the cor-nicula laryngis (*corniculate cartilages*), which rest upon the summits of the ary-tenoid cartilages, the cuneiform cartilages, which lie in front of the arytenoid cartilages and the ary-epiglottic muscles. In viewing the larynx from above, the corniculum laryngis (*corniculate cartilage*) and the cuneiform cartilages appear as two small swellings in the ary-epiglottic fold. In these folds there is much loose submucous tissue, which is the chief site of the swelling in edema of

PLATE LXXIV.

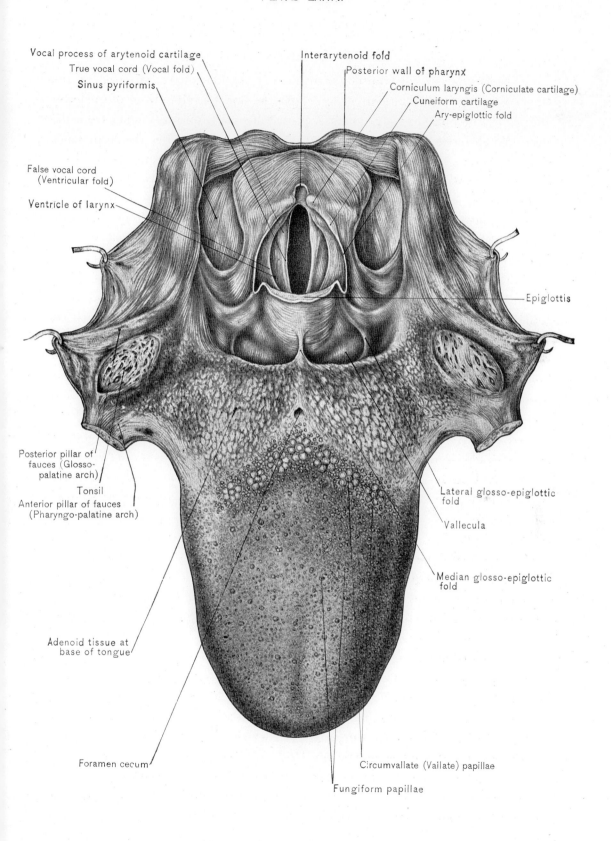

Vocal process of arytenoid cartilage

True vocal cord (Vocal fold)

Sinus pyriformis

Interarytenoid fold

Posterior wall of pharynx

Corniculum laryngis (Corniculate cartilage)

Cuneiform cartilage

Ary-epiglottic fold

False vocal cord (Ventricular fold)

Ventricle of larynx

Epiglottis

Posterior pillar of fauces (Glosso-palatine arch)

Tonsil

Anterior pillar of fauces (Pharyngo-palatine arch)

Lateral glosso-epiglottic fold

Vallecula

Median glosso-epiglottic fold

Adenoid tissue at base of tongue

Foramen cecum

Circumvallate (Vallate) papillae

Fungiform papillae

SUPERIOR APERTURE OF LARYNX.

the larynx. This swelling may be so extensive as to interfere seriously with the entrance of air into the larynx, and demand laryngotomy, tracheotomy, or ✓ intubation, for relief. Posteriorly, in the median line, is a notch where the two folds meet.

The **sinus pyriformis (recessus pyriformis)**, which is between the ary-epiglottic fold and the ala of the thyroid cartilage, the **three glosso-epiglottic** folds, and the **valleculæ**, between the epiglottis and the base of the tongue, have been described at p. 303.

Two pairs of folds may be seen stretching across the cavity of the larynx. The upper pair is formed by the **false vocal cords (ventricular folds)**, and the lower pair by the **true cords (vocal folds)**, which are more closely approximated. A depression, the **ventricle** of the **larynx,** exists between the true and false cords. The interval between the true cords (*vocal folds*) is the **rima glottidis,** or chink of the glottis. The true cords (*vocal folds*) divide the larynx into a suprarimal and an infrarimal portion so that the cavity of the larynx consists of suprarimal, or supraglottic, glottic, and infrarimal, or infraglottic, parts.

The **suprarimal portion,** or **vestibule,** of the larynx extends from the superior aperture to the true vocal cords (*vocal folds*). It is wide and triangular above, and becomes narrow below.

The **infrarimal portion** is compressed laterally above, and becomes circular below, where it is surrounded by the cricoid cartilage and leads into the trachea. In laryngotomy the knife enters this portion of the larynx and is directed downward and backward to avoid the vocal cords.

DISSECTION.—Clean the anterior portion of the lateral surface of the larynx, entirely removing the attachments of the sterno-hyoid, omo-hyoid, and thyro-hyoid muscles from the hyoid bone, those of the thyro-hyoid and sterno-thyroid muscles from the thyroid cartilage, and the attachments of the inferior constrictor muscles of the pharynx from the thyroid and cricoid cartilages. Avoid injuring: the superior laryngeal artery and the internal branch of the superior laryngeal nerve, which pierce the thyro-hyoid membrane; the external laryngeal nerve, which supplies the inferior constrictor and the crico-thyroid muscles, the crico-thyroid artery, which crosses the crico-thyroid membrane, and the recurrent laryngeal nerve and inferior laryngeal artery, which pass to the larynx behind the crico-thyroid articulation. This dissection more thoroughly exposes the thyro-hyoid membrane, thyroid cartilage, crico-thyroid muscles, crico-thyroid membrane, and cricoid cartilage.

The **thyro-hyoid membrane,** which is largely composed of elastic fibers, extends from the upper border of the thyroid cartilage to the posterior superior border of the hyoid bone. Its central portion, the *middle thyro-hyoid ligament,* is thick and strong, and its lateral portions, the *lateral thyro-hyoid ligaments*, are thin and are pierced by the superior laryngeal arteries and the internal laryngeal nerves on their way to the interior of the larynx. The *thyro-hyoid bursa* intervenes between the thyro-hyoid membrane and the posterior surface of the hyoid bone; it may become enlarged and produce a cystic tumor and swelling in the median line of the neck. Laterally, the thyro-hyoid membrane is continuous with the thyro-hyoid ligaments. Behind the thyro-hyoid membrane lies the epiglottis, from which it is separated by a small amount of loose areolar tissue.

The **thyro-hyoid ligaments** are elastic bands connecting the superior cornua of the thyroid cartilage with the tips of the greater cornua of the hyoid bone. They frequently contain a nodule of cartilage, known as the *cartilago triticea*, which sometimes is ossified.

The **thyroid and cricoid cartilages** are described at pp. 358 and 360 respectively.

The **intrinsic muscles of the larynx** are: the posterior crico-arytenoid, thyro-epiglottic, lateral crico-arytenoid, thyro-arytenoid, thyro-epiglottic and ary-epiglottic. They are all paired muscles with the exception of the arytenoid.

The **crico-thyroid muscle** (Plate LXXV) *arises* from the anterior portion of the side of the cricoid cartilage, passes upward and lateralward, and is *inserted* into the anterior border of the inferior cornu and the lateral surface of the lower border of the ala of the thyroid cartilage. Its fibers diverge and appear as two groups: its upper or anterior fibers, forming the *pars recta*, pass obliquely upward and backward, and its lower fibers, constituting the *pars obliqua*, pass horizontally backward. At its insertion the crico-thyroid blends with the origin of the inferior constrictor muscle of the pharynx. It rests upon the cricoid cartilage and the lateral portion of the crico-thyroid membrane (*conus elasticus*). In the interval between the two crico-thyroid muscles the central portion of the crico-thyroid membrane (*median crico-thyroid ligament of the conus elasticus*) is seen.

Nerve Supply.—From the external laryngeal branch of the superior laryngeal nerve.

Action.—It depresses the anterior portion of the thyroid cartilage, thus making the vocal cords tense.

Dissection.—Remove the crico-thyroid muscle on one side, in order more fully to expose the crico-thyroid membrane.

The **crico-thyroid membrane** (**conus elasticus**) (Plate LXXVI) is composed chiefly of elastic fibers. It is divided into an anterior, or central, portion and two lateral portions, which are lined by the mucous membrane of the larynx. The **anterior portion** (**median crico-thyroid ligament**) is thicker and stronger than the lateral portions, and extends from the middle of the upper border of the anterior

PLATE LXXV.

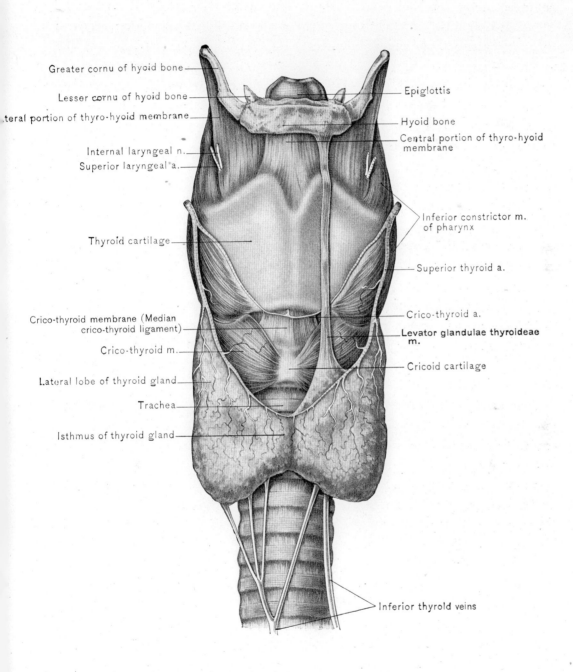

Greater cornu of hyoid bone

Lesser cornu of hyoid bone

teral portion of thyro-hyoid membrane

Internal laryngeal n.

Superior laryngeal a.

Thyroid cartilage

Crico-thyroid membrane (Median
crico-thyroid ligament)

Crico-thyroid m.

Lateral lobe of thyroid gland

Trachea

Isthmus of thyroid gland

Epiglottis

Hyoid bone

Central portion of thyro-hyoid
membrane

Inferior constrictor m.
of pharynx

Superior thyroid a.

Crico-thyroid a.

**Levator glandulae thyroideae
m.**

Cricoid cartilage

Inferior thyroid veins

LARYNX AND CRICO-THYROID MUSCLE.

PLATE LXXVI.

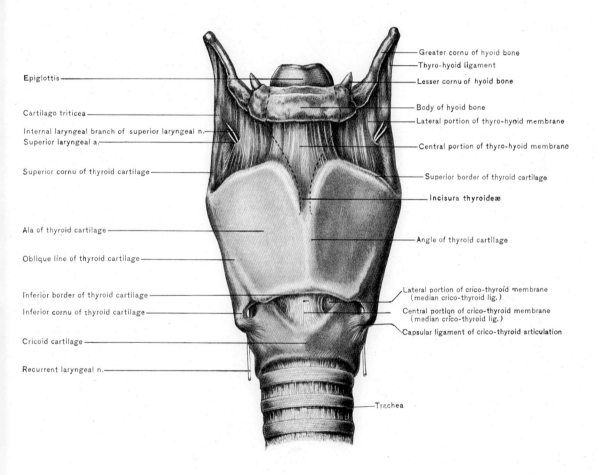

Epiglottis

Cartilago triticea

Internal laryngeal branch of superior laryngeal n.
Superior laryngeal a.

Superior cornu of thyroid cartilage

Ala of thyroid cartilage

Oblique line of thyroid cartilage

Inferior border of thyroid cartilage
Inferior cornu of thyroid cartilage

Cricoid cartilage

Recurrent laryngeal n.

Greater cornu of hyoid bone
Thyro-hyoid ligament
Lesser cornu of hyoid bone

Body of hyoid bone
Lateral portion of thyro-hyoid membrane

Central portion of thyro-hyoid membrane

Superior border of thyroid cartilage

Incisura thyroideæ

Angle of thyroid cartilage

Lateral portion of crico-thyroid membrane
(median crico-thyroid lig.)
Central portion of crico-thyroid membrane
(median crico-thyroid lig.)
Capsular ligament of crico-thyroid articulation

Trachea

ANTERIOR VIEW OF LARYNX, INCLUDING CRICO-THYROID MEMBRANES (MEDIAN CRICO-THYROID LIGAMENTS).

PLATE LXXXI.

PLATE LXXVII.

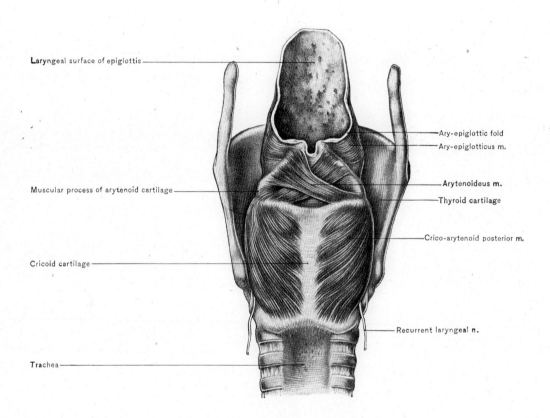

Laryngeal surface of epiglottis

Ary-epiglottic fold

Ary-epiglotticus m.

Arytenoideus m.

Thyroid cartilage

Muscular process of arytenoid cartilage

Crico-arytenoid posterior m.

Cricoid cartilage

Recurrent laryngeal n.

Trachea

MUSCLES OF LARYNX—POSTERIOR VIEW.

PLATE LXXVIII.

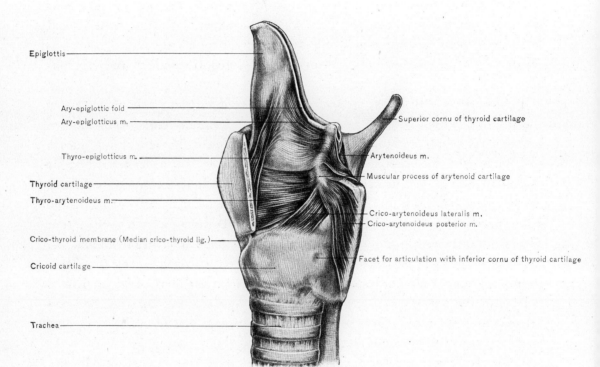

Epiglottis

Ary-epiglottic fold
Ary-epiglotticus m.

Thyro-epiglotticus m.

Thyroid cartilage
Thyro-arytenoideus m.

Crico-thyroid membrane (Median crico-thyroid lig.)

Cricoid cartilage

Trachea

Superior cornu of thyroid cartilage

Arytenoideus m.

Muscular process of arytenoid cartilage

Crico-arytenoideus lateralis m.
Crico-arytenoideus posterior m.

Facet for articulation with inferior cornu of thyroid cartilage

MUSCLES OF LARYNX—LATERAL VIEW.

portion of the cricoid cartilage to the corresponding portion of the lower border of the thyroid cartilage. Near the lower border of the thyroid cartilage it is crossed by the anastomosing crico-thyroid branches of the superior thyroid arteries, and is pierced by one or two branches of the arch formed by the crico-thyroid arteries. It lies immediately beneath the interval between the two sterno-hyoid muscles and the two sterno-thyroid muscles, and may be seen in the triangular interval between the medial margins of the crico-thyroid muscles. Laryngotomy is performed through the lower border of this portion of the membrane.

The **lateral portions** of the crico-thyroid membrane (*conus elasticus*) are thin, and pass upward from the medial margin of the superior border of the cricoid cartilage to become continuous with the true vocal cords (*vocal folds*); they are covered by the crico-thyroid, lateral crico-arytenoid, and thyro-arytenoid muscles.

DISSECTION.—Place the larynx, with the anterior aspect down, upon a board and fasten it in that position with pins or tacks. Carefully remove the pharyngeal mucous membrane from its posterior aspect, preserving the recurrent laryngeal nerve and the inferior laryngeal artery, which is a branch of the inferior thyroid artery. Then remove the mucous membrane from the lateral surface of the ary-epiglottic fold and the portion of the thyroid cartilage bounding the sinus (*recessus*) pyriformis. Next cut through the crico-thyroid articulation on one side, and divide the ala of the thyroid cartilage about eight millimeters (one-fourth inch) to the same side of the angle of that cartilage. This dissection requires care to avoid injuring the underlying muscles, the vocal cords, the lateral portion of the crico-thyroid membrane (*conus elasticus*), the superior laryngeal artery, the internal laryngeal nerve, and the terminal portion of the recurrent laryngeal nerve, and the inferior laryngeal artery.

The **posterior crico-arytenoid muscle** (Plates LXXVII; LXXVIII) is a distinct, triangular muscle *arising* from the surface at the side of the posterior median ridge of the cricoid cartilage. It is *inserted* into the posterior portion of the lateral angle, or muscular process, of the arytenoid cartilage. Its upper fibers pass transversely lateralward; its middle fibers, obliquely upward and lateralward, and its lower fibers, vertically upward.

NERVE SUPPLY.—From the recurrent laryngeal nerve.

ACTION.—It pulls the muscular processes of the arytenoid cartilage downward and medialward, and swings the vocal processes and the vocal cords laterally, thus opening the rima glottidis.

The **arytenoid muscle** is an unpaired muscle, situated between the arytenoid cartilages. It consists of superficial oblique fibers and a transverse portion.

The *oblique fibers* arise from the lateral angle of one arytenoid cartilage, and pass upward and lateralward to the summit of the opposite arytenoid cartilage, crossing the oblique fibers from the other side in the form of the letter X. Some of these fibers pass around the apex of the arytenoid cartilage, and join the ary-epiglottic muscle to form a sphincter for the superior aperture of the larynx. The *transverse portion* is thicker, and connects the posterior concave surfaces of the arytenoid cartilages.

NERVE SUPPLY.—From the recurrent and superior laryngeal nerves.

ACTION.—It draws the arytenoid cartilages together and approximates the vocal cords.

The **lateral crico-arytenoid muscle** *arises* from the upper border of the lateral part of the cricoid cartilage, in front of the crico-arytenoid articulation. It is *inserted* into the anterior and inferior aspects of the lateral angle, the muscular process, of the arytenoid cartilage. It is covered by the thyroid cartilage and the crico-thyroid muscle, and rests upon the lateral portion of the crico-thyroid membrane (*conus elasticus*). Its upper border, near its termination, blends with the thyro-arytenoid muscle, and the inferior border, occasionally, with the crico-thyroid muscle.

NERVE SUPPLY.—From the recurrent laryngeal nerve.

ACTION.—It pulls the muscular process of the arytenoid cartilage foward, relaxing the vocal cords, and rotates that cartilage medialward, approximating the cords and closing the rima glottidis.

The **thyro-arytenoid muscle** is a quadrilateral band of muscle fibers which is divided into a superior and an inferior portion. The **superior,** or **lateral, portion** is broad and thin, and is situated above the level of the vocal cords, lateral to the ventricle of the larynx and the laryngeal pouch (*ventricular appendix*). It *arises* from the lower two-thirds of the medial surface of the ala, near the angle of the thyroid cartilage, and is *inserted* into the anterior surface and lateral angle of the arytenoid cartilage. The **inferior,** or **medial, portion** is closely attached to the true vocal cord (*vocal fold*). It *arises* from the ala, near the angle of the thyroid cartilage, lateral to the attachment of the true vocal cord (*vocal fold*), and is *inserted* into the anterior angle or vocal process and the adjacent portion of the anterior surface of the arytenoid cartilage. Some of its deeps fibers, ary-vocalis of Ludwig, are said to be attached to the vocal cord at several points; although Lushka denied this, Jacobson found that some fibers were inserted into the cord.

NERVE SUPPLY.—From the recurrent laryngeal nerve.

ACTION.—It relaxes the true vocal cords (*vocal folds*) by drawing the arytenoid cartilages forward, and approximates them by drawing the vocal processes

PLATE LXXIX.

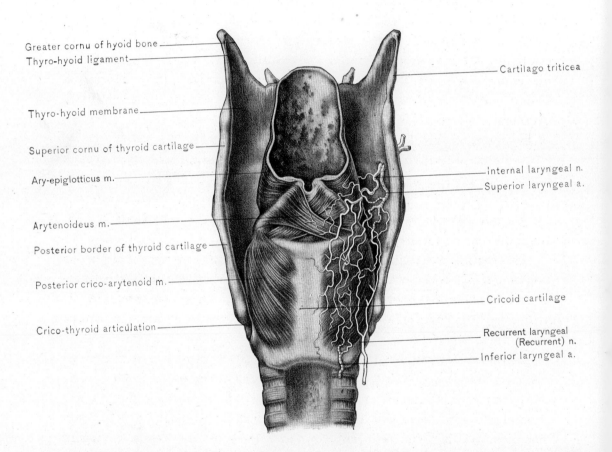

Greater cornu of hyoid bone

Thyro-hyoid ligament

Thyro-hyoid membrane

Superior cornu of thyroid cartilage

Ary-epiglotticus m.

Arytenoideus m.

Posterior border of thyroid cartilage

Posterior crico-arytenoid m.

Crico-thyroid articulation

Cartilago triticea

Internal laryngeal n.

Superior laryngeal a.

Cricoid cartilage

Recurrent laryngeal (Recurrent) n.

Inferior laryngeal a.

NERVES AND ARTERIES OF LARYNX.

downward and medialward. The ary-vocalis can make a portion of the true cord (*vocal fold*) tense while the remainder is relaxed.

The **thyro-epiglottic muscle** is composed of a few of the uppermost fibers of the thyro-arytenoid muscle, which turn upward, lateral to the laryngeal pouch (*ventricular appendix*), to be attached to the side of the epiglottis.

NERVE SUPPLY.—From the recurrent laryngeal nerve.

ACTION.—It depresses the epiglottis.

The **ary-epiglottic muscle** is situated in the ary-epiglottic fold. It *arises* from the apex and anterior border of the arytenoid cartilage, above the false vocal cord (*ventricular fold*). Its *upper fibers* are *inserted* into the mucous membrane at the margin of the ary-epiglottic fold, and its *lower fibers* are *inserted* into the side of the epiglottis. It is joined by some of the fibers of the oblique portion of the arytenoid muscle, which pass around the apex of the arytenoid cartilage.

NERVE SUPPLY.—From the recurrent laryngeal nerve.

ACTION.—It pulls the epiglottis backward and compresses the laryngeal pouch (*ventricular appendix*), and, with the assistance of the arytenoid muscle, acts as a sphincter of the superior aperture of the larynx.

The preceeding two muscles are looked upon as aberrant bundles of the lateral portion of the thyro-arytenoid muscle.

The **extrinsic muscles of the larynx** are: the sterno-thyroid, thyro-hyoid, stylo-pharyngeus described with the neck, (Vol. II) and the palato-pharyngeus (*pharyngo-palatinus*), described with the pharynx (p. 330). These muscles are assisted by all the muscles which elevate or depress the hyoid bone and larynx or hold the hyoid bone firm.

Laryngismus stridulus, or spasmodic laryngitis, a spasmodic condition of the muscles of the larynx, occurs most frequently in children, and is usually due to reflex irritation, as after eating indigestible food, or it may be caused by irritation of the nerve centers in the medulla oblongata. In adults it may result from pressure upon the recurrent laryngeal nerve by aneurysms, malignant growths of the esophagus or the posterior mediastinal glands, or enlargement of the thyroid body. It may also be produced by irritation from foreign bodies in the larynx or lower part of the pharynx. This name has also been given to a special disease in children in which the stridulus is associated with a nervous affection.

NERVE SUPPLY OF THE LARYNX.—From the superior laryngeal and recurrent laryngeal branches of the vagus nerve.

The **superior laryngeal nerve** (Plate LXXIX) divides into the external and internal laryngeal nerves. The **external laryngeal nerve** passes downward with the superior thyroid artery, supplies the crico-thyroid muscle, and sends a branch to the inferior constrictor of the pharynx. The **internal laryngeal nerve,** with the superior laryngeal artery, pierces the thyro-hyoid membrane, passes downward and backward, ramifies upon the intrinsic muscles in the lateral wall of the larynx, and supplies the mucous membrane, sending a branch to the arytenoid muscle. The internal laryngeal nerve is the *sensory nerve* of the larynx. It may be injured, as in cut-throat wounds, leading to aspiration pneumonia.

The **recurrent laryngeal (recurrent) nerve** is the *motor nerve* of the larynx which it reaches behind the crico-thyroid articulation, where it divides into an anterior and a posterior branch. The *posterior branch* supplies the arytenoid and the posterior crico-arytenoid muscles, and communicates with the internal laryngeal branch of the superior laryngeal nerve; the *anterior branch* supplies all the other intrinsic muscles except the crico-thyroid.

Paralysis of the right side of the larynx may be caused by pressure upon the right recurrent laryngeal nerve, produced by aneurysm of the first portion of the right subclavian artery or lower portion of the right common carotid artery, enlargement of the thyroid body, malignant disease of the esophagus, and cicatrices at the apex of the right pleura, as in phthisis.

Paralysis of the left side of the larynx may be caused by pressure upon the left recurrent laryngeal nerve, produced by aneurysm of the arch of the aorta and the lower portion of the left common carotid artery, malignant disease of the esophagus, and enlargement of the thyroid body. The left side of the larynx is more frequently paralyzed than the right; this is due to the longer course of the left recurrent laryngeal nerve, and its relation with the arch of the aorta, which is more commonly affected by aneurysm than the first portion of the right subclavian artery. Moderate pressure upon one of the recurrent laryngeal nerves causes spasm of the muscles of one side of the larynx, dyspnea, and change of voice; greater pressure causes paralysis and change of voice. Both nerves may be paralyzed by a lesion of the medulla oblongata, as in labio-glosso-pharyngeal paralysis or disseminated sclerosis, or by pressure from a goiter or a malignant growth of the esophagus. In bilateral paralysis the true vocal cords (*vocal folds*) are immovable, and the rima glottidis is in the position assumed in quiet breathing.

BLOOD SUPPLY OF THE LARYNX.—From the superior and inferior laryngeal arteries, and some twigs from the dorsalis linguæ artery, which supply the epiglottis.

The **superior laryngeal artery** is a branch of the superior thyroid artery, and pierces the thyro-hyoid membrane with the internal laryngeal division of the superior laryngeal nerve. It runs downward and backward with that nerve to anastomose with the inferior laryngeal artery.

PLATE LXXX.

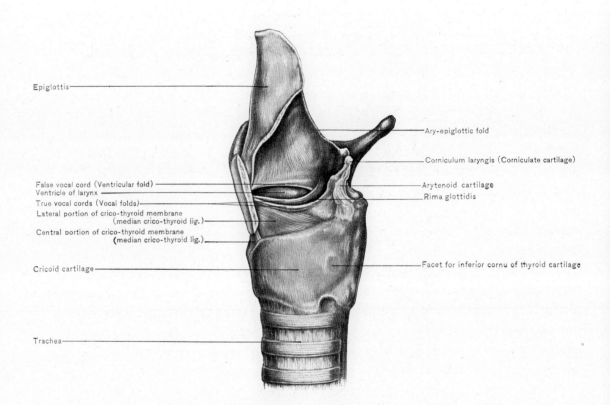

Epiglottis

Ary-epiglottic fold

Corniculum laryngis (Corniculate cartilage)

False vocal cord (Ventricular fold)
Ventricle of larynx
True vocal cords (Vocal folds)
Lateral portion of crico-thyroid membrane
(median crico-thyroid lig.)
Central portion of crico-thyroid membrane
(median crico-thyroid lig.)

Arytenoid cartilage
Rima glottidis

Cricoid cartilage

Facet for inferior cornu of thyroid cartilage

Trachea

LATERAL VIEW OF INTERIOR OF LARYNX.

The **inferior laryngeal artery** is derived from the inferior thyroid artery, and accompanies the terminal portion of the recurrent laryngeal nerve.

The veins of the larynx.—The superior laryngeal veins empty into the superior thyroid veins, and the inferior laryngeal veins, into the inferior thyroid veins.

The **lymphatics of the larynx** terminate in the deep cervical chain of lymph glands. The lymphatics from the upper, or suprarimal, portion of the larynx pass through the thyro-hyoid membrane with the superior laryngeal vessels and join the superior set of deep cervical glands near the bifurcation of the common carotid artery. The lymphatics from the lower, or infrarimal, portion of the larynx pierce the crico-thyroid membrane, join the prelaryngeal glands situated upon that membrane, and pass to some lateral laryngeal glands situated between the lower portion of the larynx and the lateral lobes of the thyroid body. The efferent vessels from the lateral, or inferior, laryngeal glands terminate in the inferior set of deep cervical glands.

DISSECTION.—Remove the lateral crico-thyroid, thyro-arytenoid, thyro-epiglottic, and ary-epiglottic muscles from one side of the larynx. Next on the same side cut away the mucous membrane and connective tissue from the upper border of the true vocal cord (*vocal fold*) to the upper margin of the ary-epiglottic fold, preserving intact the cuneiform cartilage which lies in that fold. This exposes the lateral portion of the crico-thyroid membrane (*conus elasticus*), the true vocal cords (*vocal folds*), and one side of the interior of the larynx. (Plate LXXX.)

The **true, or inferior, vocal cords** (**vocal folds**), sometimes called the inferior thyro-arytenoid ligaments, are two pearly white, fibro-elastic bands stretching between the anterior angles, vocal processes, of the arytenoid cartilages, and the retiring angle of the thyroid cartilage on each side of the median line. They are continuous with the lateral portions of the crico-thyroid membrane (*conus elasticus*), and on transverse section are prismatic in form. Their free borders are directed upward and medialward, and vibrate to produce the voice. They are covered internally by a very thin layer of mucous membrane, through which in laryngoscopic examination they appear as white bands. They are longer in men than in women and children. The region of the true vocal cords (*vocal folds*) is often the seat of warty or polypoid growths. Tuberculosis and carcinoma may also be observed here.

The **rima glottidis,** or aperture, or chink, of the glottis, is the narrowest portion of the air passages. It is bounded in its anterior portion on each side by the true vocal cords (*vocal folds*), and in its posterior portion on each side by the internal surfaces of the arytenoid cartilages. Its length is said to vary from nineteen to twenty-five millimeters in the male, and from fourteen to seventeen

23

millimeters in the female. The portion of the chink between the true cords (*vocal folds*) is named the **glottis vocalis (intermembranous part)**, for it is closely related to phonation; the portion between the bases of the arytenoid cartilages is named the **glottis respiratoria (intercartilaginous part)**, because it is closed in phonation, and affords additional space for the passage of air in respiration. In ordinary respiration the rima glottidis is triangular and somewhat lanceolate in form, as there is a slight angle at the junction of the true cord (*vocal fold*) with the arytenoid cartilage. The apex of the triangle, or point of the lance, is directed forward, and is situated at the retiring angle of the thyroid cartilage, the base lying between the arytenoid cartilages. During phonation the rima glottidis is closed, and air is forced through the narrow slit thus formed, causing vibration of the thin free borders of the true cords (*vocal folds*).

The **false, or superior, vocal cords (ventricular folds)** are not concerned in phonation. They are two rounded folds of mucous membrane which cover two elastic bands, the **superior thyro-arytenoid ligaments.** Below they present a free, arched border, which bounds the ventricle of the larynx above. They are situated above the true cords (*vocal folds*) upon each side of the larynx, but as they are more widely separated, the true cords (*vocal folds*) are seen between them in a laryngoscopic examination. The space between them is called the **false glottis.**

The **ventricles, or sinuses, of the larynx,** one on each side, are the depressions between the true cords (*vocal folds*) and false cords (*ventricular folds*). They permit free vibration of the true cords (*vocal folds*), and partially undermine the false cords (*ventricular folds*). A probe or grooved director passed into one of them will enter a diverticulum, the **laryngeal pouch, or sac (ventricular appendix),** which passes beneath the anterior portion of the false cord (*ventricular fold*) and which usually projects upward as high as the upper border of the ala of the thyroid cartilage. The ventricles of the larynx may retain small foreign bodies which have entered the larynx, and the irritation from which may cause spasm of the muscles of the larynx and eventually asphyxia.

The **fossa innominata** is a depression situated behind the margin of the epiglottis on the lateral wall of the larynx, and between the ary-epiglottic fold and the false vocal cord (*ventricular fold*). It is indistinct except during phonation.

The **mucous membrane of the larynx** is thin and closely adherent over the true cords (*vocal folds*), but is thicker, more vascular, and loosely adherent elsewhere, except over the epiglottis where it is closely adherent and forms the epiglottic folds at the entrance of the larynx. It is continuous above with the mucous membrane of the pharynx, and below with that of the trachea, so that an inflammation of the mucous membrane may spread, by continuity, from the

PLATE LXXXI.

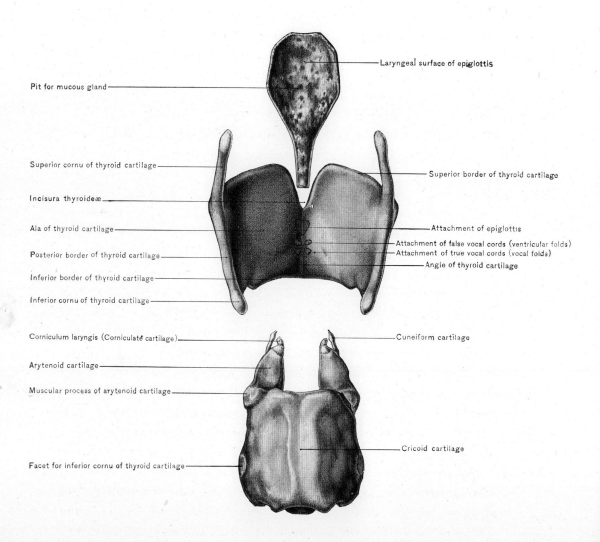

Laryngeal surface of epiglottis

Pit for mucous gland

Superior cornu of thyroid cartilage

Superior border of thyroid cartilage

Incisura thyroideæ

Ala of thyroid cartilage

Attachment of epiglottis

Attachment of false vocal cords (ventricular folds)

Attachment of true vocal cords (vocal folds)

Posterior border of thyroid cartilage

Angle of thyroid cartilage

Inferior border of thyroid cartilage

Inferior cornu of thyroid cartilage

Corniculum laryngis (Corniculate cartilage)

Cuneiform cartilage

Arytenoid cartilage

Muscular process of arytenoid cartilage

Cricoid cartilage

Facet for inferior cornu of thyroid cartilage

CARTILAGES OF LARYNX.

pharynx to the larynx, to the trachea, a course frequently observed in diphtheria. Irritation of this membrane by a foreign body or by mucus causes a cough, or a spasm of the muscles of the larynx, as in croup or laryngismus stridulus.

Edema of the mucous membrane of the larynx, or **edema of the glottis,** is frequently associated with severe attacks of acute laryngitis, as after swallowing hot or irritating liquids or after the inhalation of irritating vapors or in acute infections in contiguous structures, such as infection occurring in Ludwig's angina. Unless the submucous effusion of serum is allowed to escape by scarification, death may result from asphyxia. Intubation of the larynx, laryngotomy or tracheotomy may be required to prevent suffocation. As the submucous tissue is more plentiful at the superior aperture of the larynx, and especially upon the epiglottis, the swelling is most extensive in this location.

The **mucous glands of the larynx** are found in the mucous membrane of all portions of the larynx except over the true cords (*vocal folds*). They are especially numerous in the ary-epiglottic folds, in front of the arytenoid cartilages, in the laryngeal sacs (*ventricular appendices*), and upon the posterior surface of the epiglottis, where they are lodged in pits. These glands keep the larynx moist, those in the laryngeal sacs (*ventricular appendices*) being especially active in lubricating the true vocal cords (*vocal folds*) during phonation. After long-continued speaking, especially if in the open air, these glands are unable to preserve the moisture on the true vocal cords (*vocal folds*), and the voice becomes husky. These same conditions are likely to cause a hyperemia in the larynx and produce an acute laryngitis. When the ducts of these glands become occluded, cystic tumors appear in the mucous membrane of the larynx.

DISSECTION.—Clean the cartilages of the larynx, preserving the slender ligament connecting the corniculum laryngis (*corniculate cartilage*) with the cricoid cartilage known as the ligamentum jugale, the superior thyro-arytenoid ligaments, which are located in the false cords (*ventricular folds*), the inferior thyro-arytenoid ligaments, or true vocal cords (*vocal folds*), and the glosso-epiglottic fold and hyo-epiglottic ligaments.

The **Cartilages of the Larynx** (Plate LXXXI) are nine in number, three single and three paired. The single ones are: the epiglottis, thyroid, and cricoid. The paired ones are: the arytenoid, cornicula laryngis (*corniculate cartilages*), and the cuneiform cartilages.

The **epiglottis** is composed of yellow elastic cartilage, shaped like a leaf, with its stalk directed downward and attached to the angle of the thyroid cartilage by an elastic band, the *thyro-epiglottic ligament*. Its uppermost portion is free, and is situated behind the lowermost portion of the base of the tongue, the greater part of which holds a vertical position above it. Its *postero-inferior* *surface* is covered by mucous membrane. It is concave from side to side, looks toward the larynx, and contains numerous pits, which are occupied by mucous glands. Near its center this surface projects backward and forms a low eminence, the cushion, or *tubercle, of the epiglottis.* The *anterosuperior surface* of the epiglottis, except its uppermost portion, is not covered by mucous membrane. It is convex from side to side and looks toward the thyro-hyoid membrane, the hyoid bone, and a small portion of the base of the tongue. This surface is attached to the thyro-hyoid membrane by intervening fat and loose cellular, elastic tissue, called the *periglottis;* and to the hyoid bone by the *hyo-epiglottic ligament,* or hyoglossal membrane, also composed of elastic tissue, and to the base of the tongue by the three *glosso-epiglottic folds,* which contain three delicate elastic *glosso-epiglottic ligaments.* The *lateral margins* are curved backward, and for nearly their entire extent are attached to the ary-epiglottic folds. Into these margins the ary-epiglottic and thyro-epiglottic muscles are inserted. Its upper border is free and curls forward.

The epiglottis is the door which guards the superior aperture of the larynx. It lies in a vertical position during respiration and phonation, and, dropping backward, closes the superior aperture of the larynx during deglutition. It is drawn forward into the vertical position by muscles which are attached to the tongue and the hyoid bone: the genio-glossus, genio-hyoid, and mylo-hyoid, and is depressed by the ary-epiglottic and thyro-epiglottic muscles; they are small and weak. Occlusion of the superior aperture of the larynx is produced by elevation of that organ; by this means the larynx approaches the base of the tongue, and the epiglottis is brought against the margins of the superior aperture of the larynx.

After the epiglottis has been destroyed by ulceration, food and liquids are liable to enter the larynx during deglutition. This can be prevented by feeding the patient through a stomach tube, or a catheter passed through the nose and into the stomach, or by a duodenal bucket, or by having the patient feed himself by leaning his body far forward and sucking liquid food through a tube. After a time the muscles of the larynx may act as a sphincter, thus preventing the entrance of food into the larynx. The epiglottis is often the site of luetic or tuberculous lesions. It may also become edematous in connection with spreading inflammations in the floor of the mouth, as in Ludwig's angina.

The **thyroid cartilage** is of the hyaline variety, and forms the greater part of the anterior and lateral walls of the larynx. It is composed of two wings, or alæ (*laminæ*), which meet in the median line, almost at a right angle.

The *alæ* (*laminæ*) are irregularly quadrilateral in form. Their *upper borders,* where they meet in the median line, dip downward, leaving a *deep thyroid notch* or *incisura thyroideæ.* Behind they terminate in the anterior margins of the superior cornua. Anterior to the superior cornu each ala *(lamina)* presents a *superior tubercle,* which is placed at the upper end of the oblique line. The upper border of the ala *(lamina)* gives attachment to the thyro-hyoid membrane.

The *lower border of the cartilage* is less sinuous than the upper border; it terminates, behind, in the anterior margin of the inferior cornu, and presents the *inferior tubercle,* located at the lower end of the oblique line. It gives attachment to the central portion of the crico-thyroid membrane *(median crico-thyroid ligament)* and to the crico-thyroid muscles.

The *posterior border* is continuous with the posterior borders of the superior and inferior cornua. It gives attachment to the stylo-pharyngeus and palato-pharyngeus *(pharyngo-palatinus)* muscles and to the pharyngeal aponeurosis.

The *external surface of each ala (lamina)* presents an oblique line, which inclines downward and slightly forward, and gives attachment to the sterno-thyroid and thyro-hyoid muscles. The surface behind the oblique line is covered by the inferior constrictor muscle of the pharynx, which arises just behind the line.

The *inner surface of each ala (lamina)* is slightly concave. It is in relation with the mucous membrane of the sinus *(recessus)* pyriformis, with the thyro-hyoid and lateral crico-arytenoid muscles, and with the lateral portion of the crico-thyroid membrane *(conus elasticus).*

The *superior cornua* are longer than the inferior, and extend upward, medialward, and backward. They are attached to the greater cornua of the hyoid bone by the thyro-hyoid ligaments.

The *inferior cornua* are directed downward, forward, and medialward. On their inner surfaces they have concave facets for articulation with the cricoid cartilage. They give attachment to the inferior constrictor and crico-thyroid muscles, and to the capsular ligaments of the crico-thyroid articulations.

The *angle* is at the line of junction of the alæ *(laminæ),* is more prominent above, where it forms a subcutaneous projection, the *laryngeal prominence,* or *pomum Adami,* and lies beneath the interval between the sterno-hyoid muscles. Medially, it gives attachment, on each side of the median line, to the true vocal cords *(vocal folds)* and the false vocal cords *(ventricular folds).* In order to make the interior of the larynx accessible, the thyroid cartilage is sometimes split longitudinally, from the notch in the upper border to the lower border. In this operation it is important to divide the cartilage exactly in the median line, so as not to injure the attachments of the vocal cords. When the cartilage has been divided, the two halves are turned aside, thus exposing the interior of the larynx.

Fractures of the thyroid cartilage, although rare, are more common than of other cartilages of the larynx. They are usually produced by external direct violence, such as choking or throttling; the line of fracture is usually in the median line at the angle. The symptoms consist of pain, swelling, and tenderness in and around the larynx, with increased pain on swallowing, coughing, or talking. The moist crepitus which can be produced by forcibly moving a normal thyroid cartilage laterally must not be mistaken for that present as a result of fracture. Fracture is more apt to be seen in males because the cartilage is relatively more prominent and ossification is more complete than in the female.

Ossification of the thyroid cartilage occurs frequently, and may commence as early as the twentieth year.

The **cricoid cartilage** is the strongest of the cartilages of the larynx; it is a firm base which supports the other portions of the larynx, and rests upon the upper end of the trachea. It is hyaline in structure; it completely encircles the lower portion of the cavity of the larynx, and is shaped like a signet ring, being broader behind than in front.

Its *external surface* gives origin, in front, to the crico-thyroid muscle and, at the side, to the inferior constrictor muscle of the pharynx. At the juncture of its lateral and posterior aspects there is a facet for articulation with the inferior cornu of the thyroid cartilage. The posterior portion of the external surface presents a median ridge, which gives origin to the longitudinal muscle fibers of the esophagus, and a depression on each side of the ridge, which gives origin to the posterior crico-arytenoid muscles.

The *upper border* is horizontal for a short distance, but is soon directed obliquely downward and forward. At the beginning of the oblique portion there is a facet upon which the base of the arytenoid cartilage rests. The anterolateral portions of the upper border give attachment to the crico-thyroid membrane (*conus elasticus*) and the lateral crico-thyroid muscle.

The *lower border* is horizontal. It is attached to the first ring of the trachea by a fibrous membrane like that between the tracheal rings. The internal surface is covered by the mucous membrane of the larynx.

Ossification is not uncommon in the cricoid cartilage, but is seldom seen in the smaller cartilages of the larynx.

The **cuneiform cartilages,** or cartilages of Wrisberg, are two small, conical masses of yellow elastic cartilage situated in the ary-epiglottic folds, just anterior to the cornicula laryngis (*corniculate cartilages*). Sometimes they are long and club-shaped. Occasionally, they are absent.

The **cornicula laryngis (corniculate cartilages),** or cartilages of Santorini, are two pyramidal masses of yellow elastic cartilage situated upon the summits of the arytenoid cartilages in the ary-epiglottic folds, and are directed medial-ward. They may be separated from the arytenoid cartilages by a joint, or they may be directly continuous with those cartilages. Their summits are attached to the upper border of the posterior portion of the cricoid cartilage by the *ligamentum jugale*, a Y-shaped ligament, with its stem attached to the cricoid cartilage and the two limbs to the apices of the cornicula laryngis (*corniculate cartilages*).

In the laryngoscope, the cornicula laryngis (*corniculate cartilages*) and cunei-form cartilages appear as two whitish swellings in the posterior extremity of each ary-epiglottic fold.

The **arytenoid cartilages** are two irregularly pyramidal bodies which rest upon the upper border of the posterior portion of the cricoid cartilage. They are composed of hyaline cartilage, except at their apices, where the cartilage is of the yellow elastic type. Each has an apex, a base, three sides, three borders, and three angles. The *apex* is directed upward, backward, and medialward, and supports the corniculum laryngis (*corniculate cartilage*). The *base* is concave, and presents a smooth surface for articulation with the cricoid cartilage. The three sides are a medial, a posterior, and an anterolateral surface.

The *medial surface* is directed toward the corresponding surface of the opposite arytenoid cartilage, and is covered by mucous membrane.

The *posterior surface* is concave, and gives attachment to the arytenoid muscle.

The *anterolateral surface* is somewhat rough and irregular. It gives attach-ment to the thyro-arytenoid muscle and the superior thyro-arytenoid (*ventricular*) ligament, which supports the mucous membrane of the false voca cord (*ven-tricular fold*). Near the apex of this surface is a rounded elevation, the *colliculus*, from which a ridge, the *crista arcua*, curves backward, downward and forward to the vocal process; this ridge surrounds a circular or oval hollow, the *fovea triangularis*.

The three borders of the arytenoid cartilages are the medial, lateral, and anterior border.

The *medial border* is directed posteromedially; the *lateral border* slopes inferolaterally to the lateral angle; the *anterior border* slopes infero-anteriorly to the anterior angle.

Of the three angles of the arytenoid cartilages, the *medial angle* is situated at the posteromedial angle of the base; it gives attachment to the posterior crico-arytenoid ligament. The *lateral angle*, or *muscular process*, is located at the lateral angle of the base, and gives attachment anteriorly to the lateral crico-arytenoid muscle, and posteriorly to the posterior crico-arytenoid muscle.

The *anterior angle*, or *vocal process*, situated at the anterior angle of the base, is long and pointed, and gives attachment to the inferior thyro-arytenoid (*vocal*) ligament of the true vocal cord (*vocal fold*).

The **hyaline cartilages of the larynx**—the thyroid, cricoid, arytenoid, and cartilago triticea—frequently undergo ossification.

Fracture of any of the cartilages of the larynx should be treated by complete rest of the larynx; talking should be prohibited and feeding accomplished through the rectum. Intubation, laryngotomy, or tracheotomy may sometimes be required.

The **Joints of the Larynx** are the crico-thyroid and the crico-arytenoid.

The **crico-thyroid joints** are formed by the articulation of the inferior cornua of the thyroid with the cricoid cartilages. They are lined by synovial membrane, and have capsular ligaments which are stronger posteriorly. Their movements are gliding of the cricoid cartilage upward and backward, and rotatory around a transverse axis.

The **crico-arytenoid joints** are formed by the articulation of the cricoid cartilage with the bases of the arytenoid cartilages. They have a capsular, a posterior crico-arytenoid, and a transverse, or crico-arytenoid, ligament, and each has a synovial membrane. The *capsular ligament* is loose and allows free movement. The *posterior crico-arytenoid ligament* arrests the forward movement of the arytenoid cartilage. The *transverse*, or *crico-arytenoid*, *ligament* connects the upper border of the cricoid cartilage with the medial angles of the arytenoid cartilages. The crico-arytenoid joints permit medial or lateral gliding of the arytenoid cartilages or their rotation around a vertical axis. These movements permit the vocal processes to rotate medially and the arytenoid cartilages to be drawn together, closing the rima glottidis, as in phonation; or they allow the vocal processes to rotate laterally and the arytenoid cartilages to be separated, thus opening the rima glottidis, as in respiration.

The **Ligaments of the Larynx** not associated with the joints have been described at pp. 336; 353; 354. They are: the thyro-hyoid and crico-thyroid membranes; the thyro-hyoid ligaments; the superior thyro-arytenoid (*ventricular*) ligaments, and the inferior thyro-arytenoid (*vocal*) ligaments.

The **Hyoid Bone** is an important adjunct to the larynx. It prevents collapse of the pharynx over the superior aperture of the larynx, and from it the larynx is suspended by the thyro-hyoid membrane and thyro-hyoid ligaments. The greater cornua of this bone are important guides. The tip of the greater cornu is opposite the origin of the lingual artery, just above the level of that of the superior thyroid artery, and just below the level of the origin of the facial (*external maxillary*) artery. In the operation for ligation of the lingual artery

PLATE LXXXII.

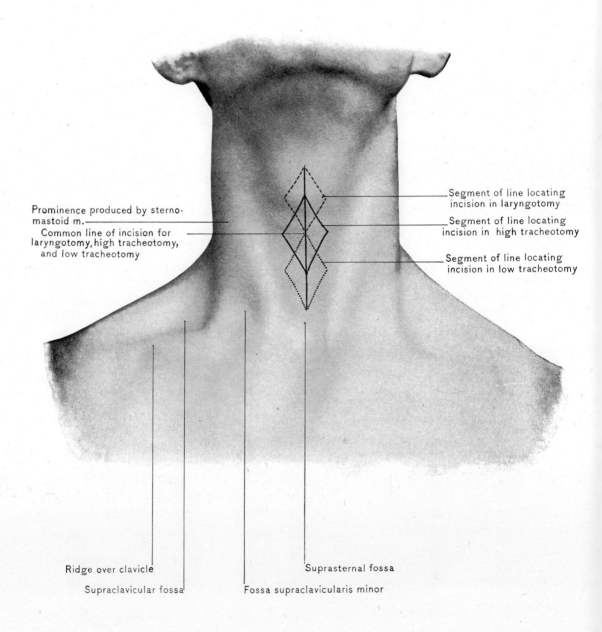

Prominence produced by sterno-
mastoid m.

Common line of incision for
laryngotomy, high tracheotomy,
and low tracheotomy

Segment of line locating
incision in laryngotomy

Segment of line locating
incision in high tracheotomy

Segment of line locating
incision in low tracheotomy

Ridge over clavicle

Supraclavicular fossa

Fossa supraclavicularis minor

Suprasternal fossa

SURFACE MARKS OF NECK AND LINES OF INCISIONS FOR LARYNGOTOMY AND TRACHEOTOMY.

PLATE LXXXIII.

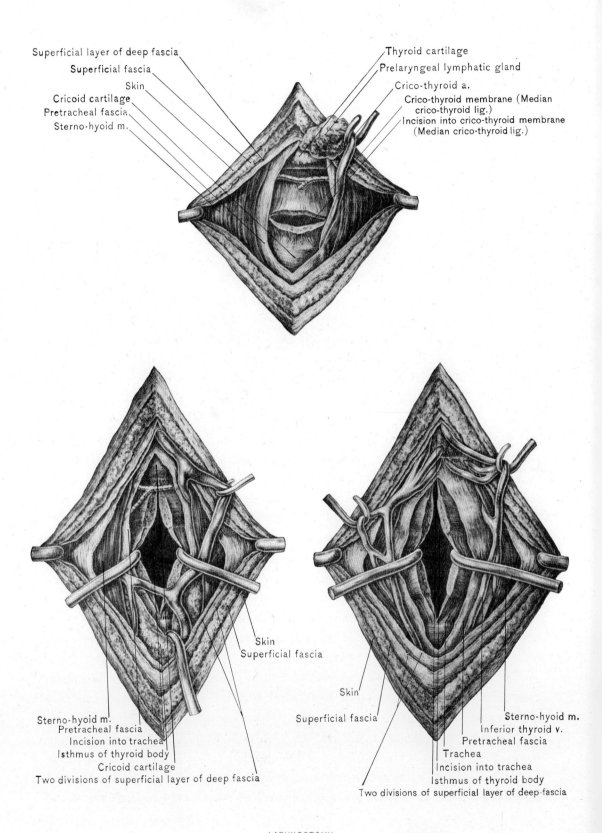

Superficial layer of deep fascia
Superficial fascia
Skin
Cricoid cartilage
Pretracheal fascia
Sterno-hyoid m.

Thyroid cartilage
Prelaryngeal lymphatic gland
Crico-thyroid a.
Crico-thyroid membrane (Median crico-thyroid lig.)
Incision into crico-thyroid membrane (Median crico-thyroid lig.)

Skin
Superficial fascia

Sterno-hyoid m.
Pretracheal fascia
Incision into trachea
Isthmus of thyroid body
Cricoid cartilage
Two divisions of superficial layer of deep fascia

Skin
Superficial fascia

Sterno-hyoid m.
Inferior thyroid v.
Pretracheal fascia
Trachea
Incision into trachea
Isthmus of thyroid body
Two divisions of superficial layer of deep fascia

LARYNGOTOMY.

HIGH TRACHEOTOMY.   366   LOW TRACHEOTOMY.

in the lingual triangle, the incision is made just above and parallel to the greater cornu of the hyoid bone.   This bone is sometimes fractured by external violence, as in choking or throttling, and also occasionally by muscular action.   The fracture usually occurs at the junction of the greater cornu with the body of the hyoid.   Swallowing and talking are painful following the fracture.   The swelling which occurs may give rise to distressing dyspnea.

The movements of the larynx *en masse* are in two directions only—upward and downward.   The most marked movements are performed during deglutition, prior to which the larynx, as well as the pharynx, is drawn upward.   By this means closure of the superior aperture of the larynx is facilitated, and elevation of the pharynx aids the constrictor muscles of the pharynx to grasp the morsel of food.   The larynx is elevated by the following muscles: the digastric, the stylo-hyoid, the mylo-hyoid, the genio-hyoid, the lower portion of the genio-glossus, the stylo-pharyngeus, and the palato-pharyngeus (*pharyngo-palatinus*).   It is depressed by the sterno-hyoid, the sterno-thyroid, and the omo-hyoid muscles.

In **laryngoscopic examination** the patient should sit at a higher level than the physician; his tongue should be drawn forward so that the base of that organ will not hang backward over the epiglottis and the superior aperture of the larynx; his head should be thrown backward so that the reflection of the interior of the larynx, instead of the image of the base of the tongue, will be seen.   When the mirror has been introduced into the oro-pharynx, its handle must usually be depressed.   The epiglottis will be seen in its upper part; the arytenoid cartilages, the cornicula laryngis (*corniculate cartilages*) and the cuneiform cartilages in its lower part; the false vocal cords (*ventricular folds*), ventricles, and true vocal cords (*vocal folds*), on their corresponding sides, and the anterior wall of the trachea.   The true vocal cords (*vocal folds*) appear as white bands more nearly approximated than the false cords (*ventricular folds*).   In acute laryngitis the true vocal cords (*vocal folds*) are of a pinkish color, and the remainder of the larynx is red and swollen.   This swelling, or edema, of the glottis is produced by a serous infiltration into the submucous areolar tissue, and if present to a marked degree, is best treated by scarification; it may, however, necessitate intubation, laryngotomy, or tracheotomy.

Thyrotomy is occasionally resorted to for the removal of intralaryngeal tumors.   The incision extends from the thyro-hyoid space to the upper portion of the cricoid cartilage.

Laryngotomy (Plates LXXXII; LXXXIII) is performed through the crico-thyroid membrane (*conus elasticus*).   The shoulders are elevated by a pillow, the head and neck are extended, a firm support is placed under the neck, and the face directed forward so that the relations of the structures in the median line of the neck may not be distorted. The thyroid and cricoid cartilages and the crico-thyroid space are outlined, the larynx is gently steadied with the thumb and fingers of one hand, and an incision about three centimeters (one and a half inches) long is made in the median line over the lower part of the thyroid carti-lage, the crico-thyroid membrane, and the cricoid cartilage. The skin, the superficial fascia, and the superficial layer of the deep fascia are divded; the sterno-hyoid and sterno-thyroid muscles are separated from the corresponding muscles of the opposite side; the pretracheal fascia is divided, and the central portion of the crico-thyroid membrane is divided transversely along the upper border of the criciod cartilage. By dividing the lowest portion of the mem-brane the crico-thyroid arteries and the true vocal cords (*vocal folds*) are avoided, and with the knife directed downward and backward, the vocal cords are also in less danger.

Excision of the larynx is sometimes performed for removal of malignant disease of that organ; but the results of the operation are so discouraging that a palliative tracheotomy is usually preferred.

The **trachea,** or **windpipe,** is directly continuous with the lower portion of the larynx, so that the larynx appears to be the upper extremity of the trachea modified for the performance of certain special functions. The trachea varies from eleven to twelve centimeters (four and a half to five inches) in length, and two to two and a half centimeters (three-fourths to one inch) in width, being always greater in the male than in the female. It extends from the cricoid cartilage to a point opposite the fourth thoracic intervertebral disc. On transverse section, it is shaped like a bar horseshoe, the indentation being posterior for the accom-modation of the esophagus. The trachea is composed of cartilaginous rings, connected by fibrous membrane. The rings are horseshoe-shaped, with the open ends posteriorly; the interval is filled by fibro-elastic membrane, which yields to pressure of bodies passing through the esophagus, thus providing additional space during deglutition. The trachea contains from sixteen to twenty of these rings, seven or eight of which are above the upper margin of the sternum. When the head and neck are in the long axis of the body, about five centimeters (two inches) of the trachea are above the sternum, and by full extension of the head and neck this distance may be increased to about six centimeters (three inches). The trachea is quite superficial at its upper extremity, but as it descends, it becomes more deeply situated owing to the forward inclination of the sternum.

RELATIONS OF THE CERVICAL PORTION OF THE TRACHEA.—In front are: the skin and superficial fascia; the superficial layer of the deep fascia, which is here composed of two layers; a communicating branch between the anterior jugular veins, situated just above the sternum; the sterno-hyoid and sterno-thyroid muscles; the isthmus of the thyroid body; the inferior thyroid veins or thyroid plexus of veins; occasionally, the thymus gland or the remains of that gland; the pretracheal fascia and the thyroidea ima artery, when present. Occasionally, a high innominate artery or the left innominate vein may be in front of the trachea at the root of the neck. Behind the cervical portion of the trachea is the esophagus. On each side of it are the lateral lobes of the thyroid body, the recurrent laryngeal nerves, the terminal portions of the inferior thyroid arteries, and the carotid sheaths enclosing the common carotid arteries, the internal jugular veins, and the vagus nerves. The trachea is more completely described under the section on the Chest (Vol. II).

Tracheotomy.—The trachea may be opened either above or below the isthmus of the thyroid gland, the former procedure being known as high, the latter, as low tracheotomy. High tracheotomy is the easier of the two operations, because the first part of the trachea, being more superficial and somewhat larger and less mobile, is more accessible than the part just above the sternum. Furthermore, the inferior thyroid veins, lying upon the trachea below the isthmus, the occasional presence of a thyroidea ima artery, and in infants the presence of the upper part of the thymus gland, add to the difficulties of the low operation; also the innominate artery or the left innominate vein may cross the trachea higher than usual and may be encountered in the low operation. However, where the operation is not of great emergency, the low operation is preferable, since intubation through the high operation, if prolonged, leads to laryngeal stenosis.

For the performance of the high operation the head is well extended and held by an assistant, so that the median line of the face will be in line with the median line of the neck. A firm cylindrical cushion is so placed under the back of the neck as to render its anterior region prominent. The parts are steadied with the fingers and thumb of one hand. The various landmarks, such as the pomum Adami (*prominentia laryngea*) and the cricoid cartilage, are located by palpation. The incision extends from about the lower border of the thyroid cartilage downward for five centimeters (two and a half inches) in the median line. It is made from below upward, and divides the skin and superficial fascia. The anterior jugular veins, which lie along the median line, may now appear, and should be avoided by cutting between them and drawing them aside. The two layers of the superficial layer of the deep cervical fascia are then divided, either upon a director or with the free hand. The interval between the flat pretracheal muscles is recognized, and the wound deepened by blunt dissection, the director or the handle of the knife being used to slit down the soft parts in the median line until the pretracheal fascia is reached. The pretracheal fascia is incised and the tracheal rings are fully exposed, the director or handle of the knife being

24

again used in order to avoid hemorrhage. The isthmus of the thyroid gland is depressed, if need be, to gain additional space.

Hemorrhage having been checked and the tracheal rings fully exposed, the trachea is held steady with a tenaculum, and a sharp narrow-bladed knife, with its cutting edge directed upward, is thrust into the windpipe, and two or three rings are divided from below upward. The edges of the tracheal wound are then held apart with a dilator, hooks, or a loop of silk passed through each side, any false membrane present is withdrawn, and the tracheal tube is inserted.

It is important during the operation that the trachea be kept exactly in the median line, otherwise it may be opened on one side, or, from being carelessly drawn to one side by the assistant, it may be missed altogether, and the operator, may expose the vertebral column before the error is recognized. It is also essential thoroughly to expose the rings of the trachea by clearing away the pretracheal fascia, in order to prevent the mistake of introducing the tracheal tube under the fascia instead of into the trachea, thereby increasing the respiratory difficulty.

In children the cricoid cartilage is sometimes divided in addition to the tracheal rings, thus converting the operation into a laryngo-tracheotomy.

In the low operation the same general rules are observed as in the high one. The incision extends from the top of the sternum to the cricoid cartilage, and after dividing the skin and fasciæ, the wound is deepened by blunt dissection, on account of the greater danger of hemorrhage in this form of the operation. The inferior thyroid veins, or thyroid plexus of veins, which lie upon the pretracheal fascia should be displaced, and the trachea thoroughly exposed, the forefinger being passed into the wound from time to time as the wound is deepened, in order to ascertain the relations of the tissues, detect abnormal vessels, and feel the tracheal rings.

THE NOSE

The **nose** is the uppermost portion of the respiratory tract. It contains the special organs of the sense of smell. It sifts particles of dust from, and warms and moistens the inhaled air. It may be divided into the **nose** proper and the **nasal cavities,** or **fossæ.**

The **nose proper** resembles a pyramid, directed toward the nasal cavities, the two lateral surfaces of which are triangular, covered by skin, and form a part of the face. The apex of the pyramid—the **root** of the nose—joins the forehead. Below the root it broadens into the **bridge,** or **dorsum,** of the nose. The two lateral borders of the nose are continuous with the face. The anterior border is free, and terminates, below, in the **lobule,** or **tip,** of the nose. The lateral surfaces, below, slope laterally into the **alæ,** or **wings,** of the nose, which form the lower borders of these surfaces.

The **base** of the nose presents two apertures, the **anterior nares,** or **nostrils,** which are separated by an anteroposterior septum, or **columna.** The anterior nares are guarded internally by short stiff hairs, or *vibrissæ*, which sift small bodies out of the inhaled air. The anterior nares open into the **vestibules** of the nose, which are the portions of the nasal cavities within the cartilaginous portion of the nose proper. As the base of the nose is in a slightly lower plane than the floor of the nasal fossæ, it should be elevated with the speculum in making an examination of the nasal cavities.

The **walls** of the nose proper are formed above, by the nasal bones, the nasal spine of the frontal bone, and the nasal processes of the superior maxillary (*maxillary*) bones, and below, by the lateral cartilages of the nose.

The **skin** is loosely adherent to the upper part of the nose, but is closely attached over the alæ and the lobule. It contains sebaceous glands, which are especially numerous at the lower part of the nose. Therefore, acne and comedones are common in this location. *Acne,* or pimples, and other inflammatory affections upon the alæ and lobule of the nose are painful on account of the density of the tissues, which prevents swelling and causes increased pressure on the nerves. The skin of the nose is also commonly affected by acne rosacea and lupus, especially lupus erythematosus, which develops on the nose, ears, and face more frequently than on other portions of the body. *Rodent ulcer,* another affection which has a predilection for the nose, frequently commences in the crease between the cheek and the ala of the nose. This also is a common site for *epithelioma.*

BLOOD SUPPLY.—The nose proper is supplied by the nasal, angular, infraorbital, lateral nasal, and superior coronary (*superior labial*) arteries. The numerous and freely anastomosing vessels of the exterior of the nose communicate with those in the mucous membrane; hence it happens that in many cases of inflammatory disease of the nasal mucosa there is congestion of the cutaneous vessels.

On account of its free blood supply, the skin of the nose offers a good field for plastic operations, or *rhinoplasty.* The flap may be derived from the forehead, as in the Indian method, or from the medial side of the arm, as in the Tagliacotian method. The flaps may also be taken from the cheeks, or flaps from the cheeks may be placed with their cutaneous surface inward and covered with a flap from the forehead. In the nose, as in the scalp, the free blood supply prevents sloughing of portions of the organ almost cut away and then replaced, and the scars formed in the repair of wounds are inconspicuous.

NERVE SUPPLY.—The nose proper is supplied by the nasal, the infratrochlear, and the infra-orbital nerves. The muscles of the nose proper, which have been considered with the description of the face (at p. 219), are supplied by the facial nerve.

The **veins** of the nose proper empty into the ophthalmic and facial (*anterior-facial*) veins. There is a network of rather large anastomosing veins in the tip of the nose.

The **lymphatics** of the nose proper, which are arranged in three sets, pass to the parotid and the submaxillary (*submandibular*) lymph glands, the latter being the more important.

Because of their exposed position and the absence of subcutaneous fat which protects the underlying vessels, the lobules and alæ of the nose, like the auricle, are easily attacked by frost, from which gangrene may result.

DISSECTION.—Remove the tissues covering the nasal bones and lateral cartilages of the nose.

The **nasal bones** are thick and narrow at their upper extremities, and thin, broad, and much exposed to injury at their lower portion. A blow at the root of the nose is far more likely to break the cribriform plate (*lamina cribrosa*) of the ethmoidal bone and the anterior walls of the frontal sinuses than the nasal bones. Fractures of the nasal bones may be reduced by manipulation of the fragments between the fingers externally and a grooved director introduced into the nasal fossæ. Owing to their vascularity, the nasal bones unite quickly. In congenital syphilis destruction of the bones, or caries, especially of those of the septum, causes the bridge of the nose to sink. Congenital protrusions of the membranes of the brain or of the brain itself may occur at the root of the nose. They are known as sincipital meningoceles and encephaloceles, and are the result of incomplete union of the frontal bone with the cribriform plate (*lamina cribrosa*) of the ethmoidal bone and with the nasal bones. The skin over these tumors may be highly vascular and present some resemblance to that over a nevus.

The **Cartilaginous Plates** (Plates LXXXIV; LXXXV) in the framework of the nose consist of a superior lateral nasal (*lateral nasal*) and an inferior lateral nasal (*greater alar*) cartilage and sesamoid (*lesser alar*) cartilages on each side, and the cartilage of the septum.

The *superior lateral nasal* (*lateral nasal*) *cartilages* are triangular. Their anterior margins are partly continuous with the anterior border of the cartilage of the septum, to which they are closely applied; their posterior margins are closely united to the superior maxillæ (*maxillæ*) and the lower borders of the nasal bones, while their inferior borders are attached to the inferior lateral nasal (*greater alar*) cartilages. Their outer surfaces are covered by the skin and the muscular and fibrous tissue of the nose, and their inner surfaces by the nasal

PLATE LXXXIV.

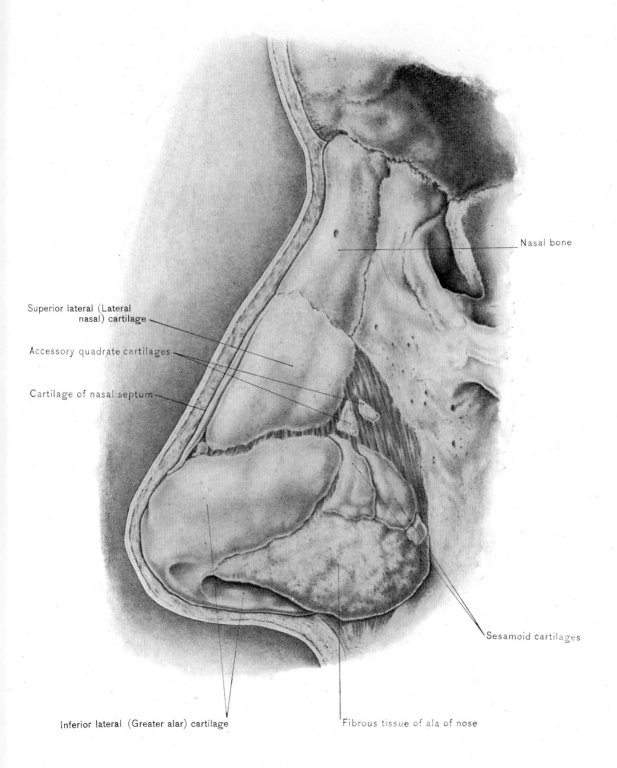

Nasal bone

Superior lateral (Lateral
nasal) cartilage

Accessory quadrate cartilages

Cartilage of nasal septum

Sesamoid cartilages

Inferior lateral (Greater alar) cartilage

Fibrous tissue of ala of nose

LATERAL CARTILAGES OF NOSE.

373

PLATE LXXXV.

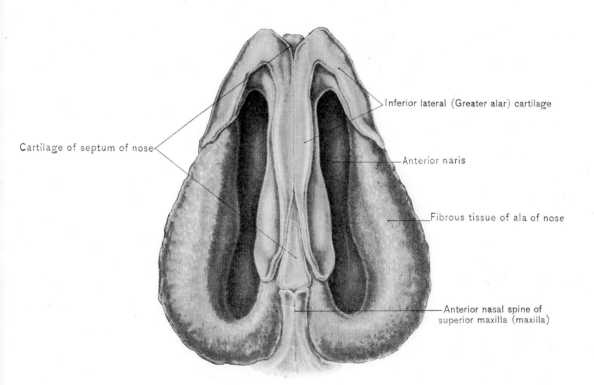

Cartilage of septum of nose

Inferior lateral (Greater alar) cartilage

Anterior naris

Fibrous tissue of ala of nose

Anterior nasal spine of
superior maxilla (maxilla)

CARTILAGES AT BASE OF NOSE.

mucous membrane.   When the superior lateral nasal (*lateral nasal*) cartilage is detached from the nasal bone by traumatism, considerable pain in the nose is produced by injury to the nasal nerve, which emerges between this cartilage and the nasal bone.

The *inferior lateral nasal (greater alar) cartilages* are sharply bent upon themselves, in front of the anterior nares, so that they compose the medial and lateral walls of the nares.   The portion which forms the medial wall, *the crus mediale*, lies in contact with the corresponding portion of the opposite inferior lateral nasal cartilage on the medial side of the anterior naris, forming part of the columna. The portion which forms the lateral wall, *the crus laterale*, is oval and curves backward in the ala of the nose.   It is attached to the superior lateral nasal (*lateral nasal*) cartilage and the superior maxilla (*maxilla*) by dense fibrous tissue, in which the sesamoid (*lesser alar*) cartilages are found.   The margin of the ala of the nose is not formed by the inferior lateral nasal (*greater alar*) cartilage, but by the dense fibrous tissue which forms the framework of the nose proper where the bones and cartilages are absent.

The *sesamoid (lesser alar), or accessory, cartilages* are usually four in number in each lateral wall of the nose proper.   Two of these are situated in the fibrous tissue which connects the inferior lateral nasal (*greater alar*) cartilage with the nasal process of the superior maxilla (*maxilla*).   Just above these are the other two, which are called the *accessory quadrate cartilages*.   Additional sesamoid (*lesser alar*) cartilages may be found in the fibrous tissue which completes the framework of the nose proper, but the four previously mentioned are the only constant ones.

The *cartilage* of the septum is placed in the antero-inferior portion of the septum, filling the angular interval between the vertical plate of the ethmoidal bone and the vomer.   It represents the anterior extremity of the primordial cartilaginous cranium.   It is quadrilateral in form.   Its posterosuperior border is in contact with the vertical plate (*perpendicular lamina*) of the ethmoidal bone, which is sometimes grooved to receive it.   Its postero-inferior border joins the anterior nasal spine of the superior maxilla (*maxilla*) and the vomer, which may be grooved for its reception.   The upper portion of its anterosuperior border is attached to the incisor crest on the under surface of the junction of the nasal bones, and below the nasal bones the sides of this border are continuous with the superior lateral nasal (*lateral nasal*) cartilages; it terminates just above the tip of the nose between the medial plates of the two inferior lateral nasal (*greater alar*) cartilages.   The antero-inferior border is short, and extends backward and downward, above the columna, to the anterior nasal spine, which it embraces.   (Plate CCXIX.)

Infections at the base of the nose or of the septum may be fatal if the infection is carried to the brain through the cribriform plate.

The cartilages and other soft tissues of the cartilaginous portion of the nose may be destroyed by *lupus vulgaris* or syphilis, without involving the bones. The nose can be repaired by one of the methods of plastic operation (rhinoplasty) previously mentioned.

Dilating specula introduced into the anterior nares should not be inserted beyond the cartilaginous portion of the nose, on account of the pain produced by pressure upon resisting bony structures.

DISSECTION.—Hold the anterior segment of the skull so that the light enters the nasal cavities through the anterior nares, or pass a probe or a grooved director into the nasal cavities to determine to which side the nasal septum is deflected. Then cut through the tissues of the upper lip and through the lateral cartilages, close to that side of the septum which does not bulge. With the hard palate facing upward, saw through the skull close to the flat or concave side of the septum. Should the superior turbinated bone on one side be accidentally broken, it can be studied on the other side after removing the septum.

The two **nasal cavities,** or **fossæ** (Plates LXXXVI; LXXXVII), are located between the base of the skull and the hard palate. They are wide below and quite narrow above where the middle and superior turbinated bones lie near the septum and, at times, in contact with it. The vertical diameter of each nasal fossa is greater than its transverse diameter; therefore, forceps inserted into the fossæ should be opened vertically. The nasal cavities open upon the face by means of the vestibules and anterior nares, and into the naso-pharynx by means of the posterior nares. They are separated by the nasal septum.

The **nasal septum** (Plate LXXXVIII) is formed by the crest at the junction of the nasal bones, the nasal spine of the frontal bone, the vertical plate of the ethmoidal bone, the cartilage of the septum, the vomer, the crest of the sphenoidal bone, and by the crest situated at the line of junction of the two palatine processes of the two superior maxillæ (*maxillæ*) and of the two horizontal plates of the palatine bones. In children, up to the seventh year, and in primitive races the septum is straight in about eighty per cent of cases; but in the adult, in about seventy-six per cent of persons, it is deflected to one side, and more frequently to the left. This deflection should not be mistaken for a bony growth of the septum.

The frequency of deviation of the nasal septum is supposed to be due to the practice of always blowing the nose with the same hand or to injuries in early life. This condition, by obstructing one nasal fossa, retards breathing and impairs the resonance of the voice.

PLATE LXXXVI.

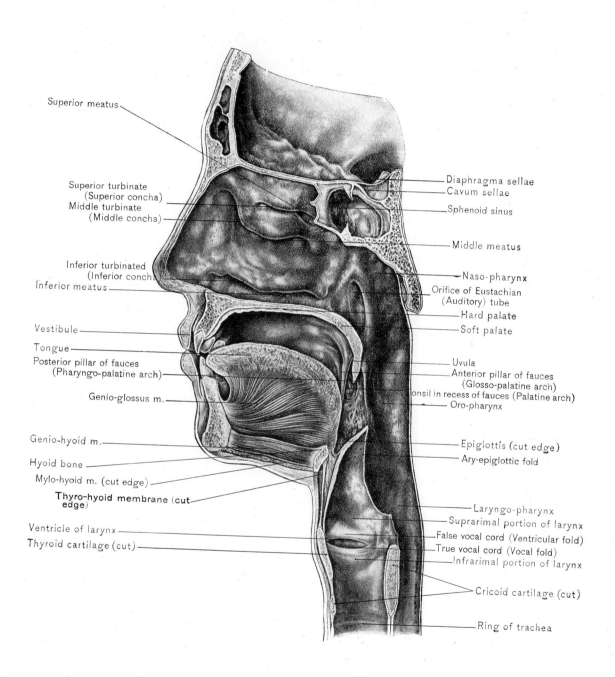

Superior meatus

Superior turbinate
(Superior concha)
Middle turbinate
(Middle concha)

Inferior turbinated
(Inferior concha)
Inferior meatus

Vestibule

Tongue
Posterior pillar of fauces
(Pharyngo-palatine arch)

Genio-glossus m.

Genio-hyoid m.

Hyoid bone

Mylo-hyoid m. (cut edge)

Thyro-hyoid membrane (cut edge)

Ventricle of larynx
Thyroid cartilage (cut)

Diaphragma sellae
Cavum sellae

Sphenoid sinus

Middle meatus

Naso-pharynx
Orifice of Eustachian
(Auditory) tube
Hard palate
Soft palate

Uvula
Anterior pillar of fauces
(Glosso-palatine arch)
onsil in recess of fauces (Palatine arch)
Oro-pharynx

Epiglottis (cut edge)
Ary-epiglottic fold

Laryngo-pharynx
Suprarimal portion of larynx
False vocal cord (Ventricular fold)
True vocal cord (Vocal fold)
Infrarimal portion of larynx

Cricoid cartilage (cut)

Ring of trachea

MEATUSES OF NOSE AND TURBINATED BONES—LATERAL VIEW.

PLATE LXXXVII.

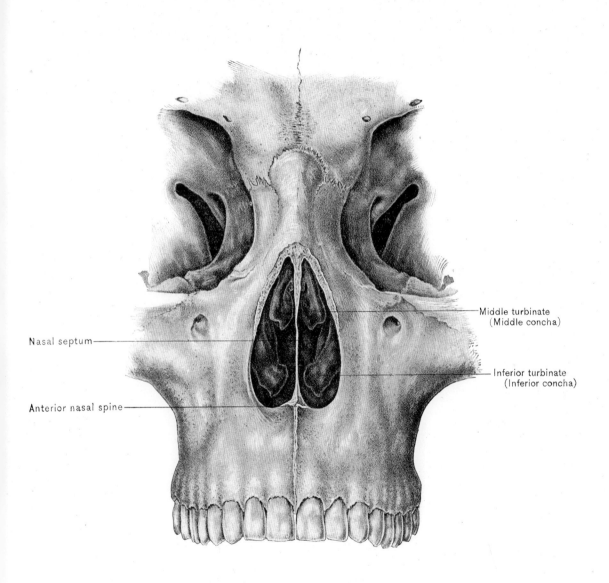

Nasal septum———

Anterior nasal spine——

Middle turbinate
(Middle concha)

Inferior turbinate
(Inferior concha)

ANTERIOR VIEW OF NASAL FOSSÆ.

PLATE LXXXVIII.

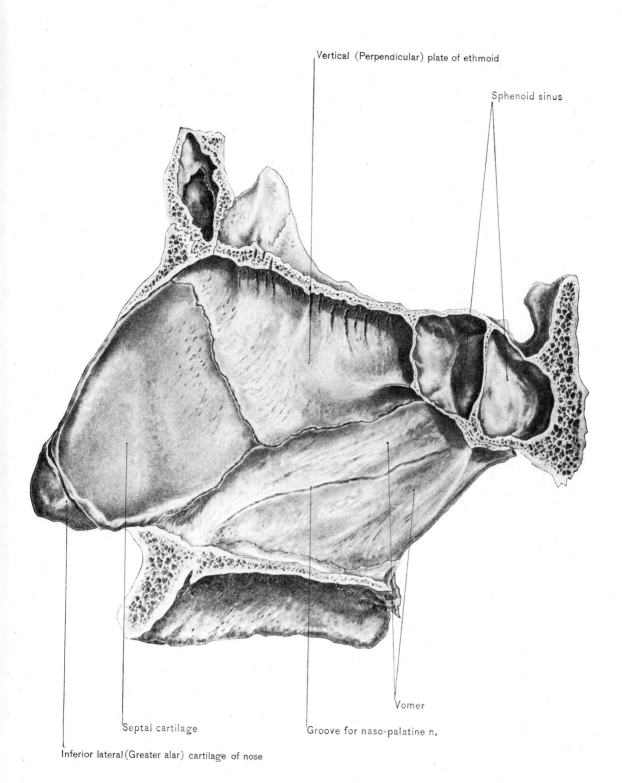

Vertical (Perpendicular) plate of ethmoid

Sphenoid sinus

Vomer

Septal cartilage

Groove for naso-palatine n.

Inferior lateral (Greater alar) cartilage of nose

NASAL SEPTUM.

Perforation of the nasal septum may be congenital, or it may result from exposure to the vapor of chromic acid in the manufacture of potassium bichromate, or from syphilis.

The **roof of the nasal fossa** is formed by the nasal bones, the nasal spine of the frontal bone, the cribriform plate of the ethmoidal bone, the sphenoidal turbinated bones, the body of the sphenoidal bone, the alæ of the vomer and the sphenoidal processes of the palatine bones. The middle portion of the roof, formed by the cribriform plate (*lamina cribrosa*) of the ethmoidal bone, is horizontal, its anterior portion slopes downward and forward, and its posterior portion downward and backward. In fracture of this portion of the base of the skull, blood or cerebro-spinal fluid may escape through the nose. A meningocele projecting through the roof of the nasal fossa into the nasal cavity may be mistaken for a polypus and removed, with a fatal result. The middle portion of the roof of the nose is so thin that it may easily be punctured and the cranial cavity entered by slender instruments or foreign bodies introduced into the nose, either intentionally or accidentally.

The **floor of the nasal fossa** is wider than the roof, being about one centimeter (one-half inch) in width. It is formed by the palatine processes of the superior maxillæ (*maxillæ*) and the horizontal plates of the palatine bones. It is somewhat concave from side to side, and slopes slightly downward and backward.

The **lateral wall** of the nasal fossa is formed by the nasal process and the medial surface of the superior maxilla (*maxilla*), the inferior turbinated bone (*inferior concha*), the lacrimal bone, the lateral mass of the ethmoidal bone, the vertical plate (*perpendicular lamina*) of the palatine bone, and the medial pterygoid plate of the sphenoidal bone. The lateral wall is made irregular by projection of the superior, middle, and inferior turbinated bones (*conchæ*) into the nasal cavity. That portion of the nasal fossa between the turbinates and the septum is called the meatus nasi communis.

The **superior turbinated bone** (**superior concha**) is situated on the upper part of the lateral wall in the posterior third of the cavity, its anterior and highest portion being about opposite the tendo oculi (*medial palpebral ligament*). The **middle turbinated bone** (**middle concha**) (Plate LXXXVI) extends along the posterior two-thirds, and the **inferior turbinated bone** (**inferior concha**) along nearly the whole length of the lateral wall of the nasal fossa. Beneath the turbinates (*conchæ*) are three recesses, or meatuses, the superior, middle, and inferior meatus, each situated beneath the corresponding turbinate (*concha*). The **superior meatus** is closed anteriorly and opens inferiorly and posteriorly. It is narrow and groove-like and about half the length of the middle meatus. It con-

25

tains the orifices of the sphenoidal cells, or sinuses, and of the posterior ethmoidal cells. The orifice of the sphenoidal cells is really in the roof of the nasal fossa at the level of the superior turbinate (*superior concha*), and when that bone is divided into two plates, the orifice is opposite the space between them, known as the **fourth meatus, or spheno-ethmoidal, recess.** The **middle meatus** is open anteriorly, posteriorly, and inferiorly. It differs from the superior meatus in being broad and arched. Anteriorly, it opens into a broad portion of the nasal cavity, called the *atrium* of the *middle meatus*. The atrium opens wide anteriorly into the vestibule, allowing most of the inhaled air to pass through the middle meatus. On the lateral wall of the middle meatus is a groove, known as the **hiatus semilunaris,** which begins at the inferior extremity of the infundibulum and curves from above posteriorly and inferiorly. The orifices leading to the maxillary sinus, or antrum of Highmore, and to the anterior ethmoidal air cells are in this groove. The **bulla ethmoidalis** is the rounded upper boundary of the hiatus semilunaris. The orifice of the maxillary sinus, or antrum of Highmore, is about two and a half centimeters (one inch) above the floor of the nose. The **inferior meatus** opens chiefly inferiorly and posteriorly, so that a greater portion of exhaled than inhaled air passes through it. It presents the inferior orifice of the lacrimo-nasal duct, which carries the tears from the lacrimal sac to the nose. The opening of the nasal duct is at the under surface of the attached margin of the inferior turbinate (*inferior concha*), about two and a half centimeters (one inch) behind the anterior nares, and two centimeters (three-fourths of an inch) above the floor of the nose. Instruments introduced into the inferior meatus must be directed toward the floor of the nose, or else the anterior end of the inferior turbinate (*inferior concha*) will guide them into the middle meatus, which is more widely open. Foreign bodies are most frequently found in the inferior meatus. If these bodies are retained for a long time, concretions of calcareous matter adhere to them, resulting in the formation of *rhinoliths*.

The turbinated bones (*conchæ*) or other portions of the walls of the nasal cavities may be the site of *necrosis*, which causes a purulent discharge, usually from one nostril. The carious bone should be removed; if the disease is situated high up, a good exposure of the nasal fossa is obtained by Rouge's operation in which the upper lip is everted, and the tissues of the lip and nose are detached from the lateral surface of the superior maxillæ (*maxillæ*). The inferior turbinate (*inferior concha*) and middle turbinate (*middle concha*) are also sometimes removed when they have hypertrophied and have caused nasal obstruction.

The nasal cavities are divided, according to function, into the **olfactory portion,** which includes the superior meatus, middle turbinate (*middle concha*), and the upper two-thirds of the septum of the nose, and the **respiratory portion,** which includes the middle meatus, inferior turbinate (*inferior concha*), inferior meatus, and lower third of the septum.

The nasal cavities are lined by a **mucous membrane** which is continuous with that of the pharynx, the sphenoidal and the ethmoidal cells, the frontal sinuses, maxillary sinuses, or antra of Highmore, the lacrimo-nasal ducts, and lacrimal sacs. This continuity with the adjacent mucous membrane and with the lining of the accessory sinuses of the nose, as the various air sinuses are called, is very important in view of the marked interrelation existing between diseases of these various parts. Empyema of the frontal and ethmoidal air sinuses, for instance, and of the *maxillary sinus,* or antrum of Highmore, is usually dependent upon disease of the nasal mucosa.

In the olfactory portion the mucosa (Schneiderian membrane) is highly specialized and of a yellowish color, which gradually fades below, making no marked line between the mucous membrane of the two portions. This specialized membrane covers only the middle of the superior turbinate (*superior concha*) and the corresponding area of the septum. It does not correspond to the entire superior turbinate (*superior concha*). Over the nasal septum it is rather firmly adherent to the underlying periosteum; sometimes submucous hematomata of the septum are seen after injury to the nose. The mucous membrane of the olfactory region contains the glands of Bowman (*olfactory glands*). They elaborate a specific, serous secretion. On the antero-inferior portion of the septum the mucous membrane presents a small diverticulum, which is the remains of the vomer nasal organ of Jacobson. This organ is more highly developed in the lower animals where it plays a part in the sense of smell, since it is supplied by twigs from the olfactory nerves, and its epithelium resembles that of the olfactory portion of the nasal fossa. At the upper two-thirds of the septum and lateral wall (in the olfactory portion) the mucous membrane is delicate and thin, and contains the branches of the olfactory nerve. In the lower, or respiratory, portion of the nasal fossa the mucous membrane is thicker, more vascular, and pale red in color. This thickness varies greatly and is especially noticeable over the lower borders and posterior extremities of the middle turbinate (*middle concha*) and inferior turbinate (*inferior concha*), where it is soft and boggy and projects beyond the bones. This condition is due to the presence of a large number of veins in the submucous layer of the mucous membrane of the middle turbinate (*middle concha*) and inferior turbinate (*inferior concha*), and to the presence of cavernous spaces of erectile tissue in that of the inferior turbinate (*inferior concha*). In chronic nasal catarrh these cavernous spaces are distended with blood, the nasal cavity is occluded, making it impossible to breathe through the nose. At times the entire mucosa atrophies. This may even affect the olfactory portion and lead to the loss of the sense of smell. The condition is characterized by an offensive nasal odor and discharge, and is known as **ozena.** The mucous membrane of the anterior extremity of the inferior turbinate (*inferior concha*), when distended, resembles a polypoid growth.

Instruments, such as specula or tubes of atomizers, introduced through the anterior nares should be directed slightly lateralward to avoid striking the septum, and to prevent injury to the mucous membrane, which often bleeds after slight traumatism.

Mucous polypi are frequently developed in the nose, and usually from the mucous membrane of the superior turbinate (*superior concha*) or middle turbinate (*middle concha*) or near the hiatus semilunaris. They occlude the nasal cavity, may broaden the nose, compressing the nasal ducts, and may project through the anterior or posterior nares. If after removal they continue to recur, a portion of the adjacent bone should also be removed, being careful to avoid fracturing the cribriform plate of the ethmoidal bone. Fibrous or sarcomatous polypi arise from the periosteum or, more frequently, from the roof of the nose.

Epistaxis, or bleeding from the nose, sometimes a prodromal symptom of typhoid fever, is more commonly due to other causes, such as engorged vessels, as in plethoric individuals with hypertension, or ulceration into an artery; it may also be a symptom of fracture of the base of the skull, purpura hemorrhagica, hemophilia, or scurvy. Hemorrhage from the nose is checked by the laity by pressure on the upper lip, which occludes the artery of the septum; by plugging the anterior nares; by raising the arm and increasing the expansion of the chest, which lessens the pressure in the veins, or by dropping a cold key down the back, or applying cold water to the back of the neck, and thus stimulating the vasomotor nerves. If the source of a serious hemorrhage cannot be found, the bleeding can be checked by plugging both the anterior and posterior nares, which is done by introducing a long silk ligature through the nose and into the pharynx, bringing it out through the mouth and attaching a plug of cotton to it; or a soft catheter, a Bellocq's cannula, may be threaded and carried through the nose into the pharynx. One end of the thread is brought out through the mouth with forceps, and the other through the nose in withdrawing the catheter. A plug of cotton or gauze is then attached to the string, the two ends of which are tied together so that the plug can be pulled against the posterior nares, or withdrawn and reapplied if necessary.

The **vestibule** of the nose is that portion of the nasal fossa within the cartilaginous portion of the nose, and is lined with skin which blends with the mucous membrane of the nose.

PLATE LXXXIX.

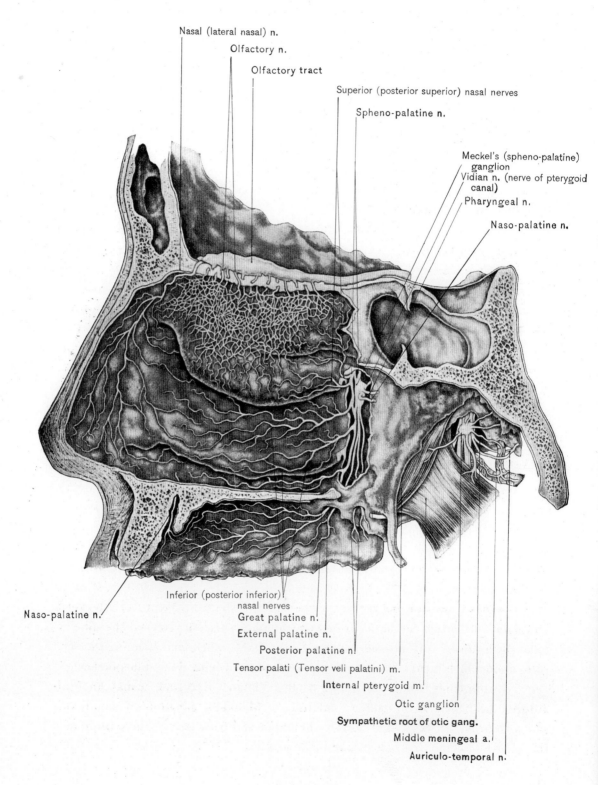

Nasal (lateral nasal) n.

Olfactory n.

Olfactory tract

Superior (posterior superior) nasal nerves

Spheno-palatine n.

Meckel's (spheno-palatine) ganglion

Vidian n. (nerve of pterygoid canal)

Pharyngeal n.

Naso-palatine n.

Naso-palatine n.

Inferior (posterior inferior) nasal nerves

Great palatine n.

External palatine n.

Posterior palatine n.

Tensor palati (Tensor veli palatini) m.

Internal pterygoid m.

Otic ganglion

Sympathetic root of otic gang.

Middle meningeal a.

Auriculo-temporal n.

OLFACTORY NERVES.

The **mucous glands** are most numerous over the posterior portion of the lateral wall and septum of the nose. The position of these glands and the postero-inferior slope of the nasal floor accounts for the gravitation of mucus to the pharynx. Occlusion of the duct of a mucous gland causes the formation of a retention cyst.

Some lymphoid tissue is also found in the nasal mucous membrane.

NERVE SUPPLY.—The nerve supply of the nasal mucous membrane is derived from the olfactory, nasal (*nasociliary*), and naso-palatine nerves, branches from the spheno-palatine or Meckel's ganglion and the nerve to the Vidian (*pterygoid*) canal, branches from the anterior superior dental (*anterior superior alveolar*) nerve, and branches from the anterior palatine nerve.

The **olfactory nerves** (Plate LXXXIX) are not so highly developed in man as in many of the lower animals. They are the central processes of the bipolar olfactory nerve cell bodies which are situated in the olfactory mucous membrane. The peripheral processess are short and extend to the surface of the mucous membrane, where each process terminates in a group of short hair-like processes, known as the olfactory hairs. The central processes pass upward from their cells and form plexuses in the mucous membrane, and from these there pass on each side through the cribriform plate about twenty filaments. These are non-medulated nerves, and comprise the olfactory nerve; passing upward, they pierce the dura mater, the arachnoid, and the pia mater, and enter the inferior surface of the olfactory bulb. *Anosmia*, or loss of the sense of smell after a severe blow upon the head, is supposed to be due to laceration of the olfactory nerves as they pass through the cribriform plate.

The **nasal** (**nasociliary**) **nerve** is a branch of the ophthalmic division of the fifth cranial, or trigeminal, nerve. It reaches the nasal fossa by passing through the nasal fissure at the side of the crista galli, runs downward in the groove on the medial surface of the nasal bone, and passes forward between the nasal bone and the superior lateral nasal (*lateral nasal*) cartilage to supply the tip of the nose. It supplies branches to the anterior portion of both the lateral wall and the septum of the nose.

The **naso-palatine nerve** is a branch of the spheno-palatine, or Meckel's, ganglion, and enters the nasal fossa with the naso-palatine artery at the spheno-palatine foramen. It crosses on the body of the sphenoidal bone to the septum, upon which it runs downward and forward, supplying its middle portion.

The **branches from the nerve to the Vidian (pterygoid) canal and the anterior branches of the spheno-palatine, or Meckel's, ganglion** are small, and can seldom be traced. They supply the upper and back part of the septum and the superior turbinated bone (*superior concha*).

The **branches of the anterior superior dental** (anterior superior alveolar) **branch of the superior maxillary** (maxillary) **nerve** supply the inferior turbinated bone (*inferior concha*) and the inferior meatus. The branches from the large palatine (*anterior palatine*) nerve, the inferior nasal nerves, run forward upon the middle and inferior turbinates (*middle and inferior conchæ*).

BLOOD SUPPLY.—The blood supply of the nasal cavities is derived from the spheno-palatine, the descending palatine (*greater palatine*), the anterior and posterior ethmoidal arteries, and the artery of the septum.

The **spheno-palatine artery,** the terminal branch of the internal maxillary, is the principal artery of the nasal fossa. It enters the cavity at the spheno-palatine foramen with the naso-palatine nerve. Its *internal branch*, the naso-palatine, accompanies the naso-palatine nerve downward and forward upon the septum toward the anterior palatine foramen (*foramen incisivum*). Its *external branch* supplies the lateral wall of the cavity, the ethmoidal cells, the frontal sinus, and the maxillary sinus, or antrum of Highmore.

The **descending palatine** (**greater palatine**) **artery** is also a branch of the internal maxillary artery. It gives off an anterior and a posterior branch. The *anterior branch* supplies the hard palate and anastomoses with the spheno-palatine artery at the anterior palatine foramen (*foramen incisivum*). The *posterior branch* supplies the soft palate and the tonsils, anastomosing with the ascending palatine branch of the facial (*external maxillary*).

The **anterior and posterior ethmoidal arteries** are branches of the ophthalmic artery. They supply the roof, upper portion of the septum, and lateral wall of the nasal fossa, the ethmoidal cells, and the frontal sinuses.

The **artery of the septum** is derived from the superior coronary branch of the facial (*external maxillary*) artery. It supplies the columna and the lower portion of the septum.

The **veins of the nasal cavities** form a plexus under the mucous membrane. The plexus is drained by: the veins which accompany the spheno-palatine artery and empty into the pterygoid plexus; those which follow the ethmoidal arteries and empty into the ophthalmic vein; some which pass through the foramina in the nasal bone and nasal process of the superior maxilla (*maxilla*) to empty into the facial (*anterior facial*) vein, and others which pass through the foramen cecum to join the superior longitudinal sinus and through the cribriform plate of the ethmoidal bone to join the intracranial veins.

The **lymph vessels** of the mucoperiosteal lining and walls of the nasal fossæ terminate in the postpharyngeal, the internal maxillary (*deep facial*), the parotid, and the superior deep cervical lymph glands. Through the cribriform plate of the ethmoidal bone these vessels communicate with the intracranial

PLATE XC.

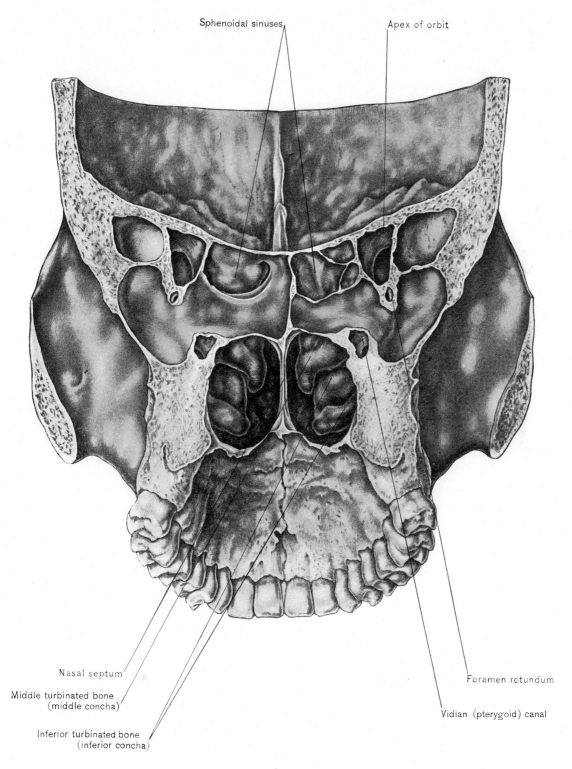

Sphenoidal sinuses

Apex of orbit

Nasal septum

Middle turbinated bone
(middle concha)

Inferior turbinated bone
(inferior concha)

Foramen rotundum

Vidian (pterygoid) canal

POSTERIOR VIEW OF NASAL FOSSÆ.

lymphatics and the subdural space, affording a channel through which meningitis may be produced by caries of the upper portion of the wall of the nose. Involvement of the postpharyngeal, the internal maxillary (*deep facial*), the parotid, and the superior deep cervical lymph glands may also result from disease of the nasal fossæ.

In **anterior rhinoscopy,** or examination of the nasal fossa through the anterior naris, the following structures can be observed: the septum, which should occupy a vertical position (if it deviates toward the fossa under examination, it is apt to be mistaken for a tumor); the floor of the nose; the inferior turbinate (*inferior concha*), which extends backward along the lateral wall of the fossa; the middle meatus; the middle turbinated bone (*middle concha*), and high up, the superior meatus and the anterior extremity of the superior turbinated bone (*superior concha*).

Posterior rhinoscopy (Plate XC), or examination of the nasal fossæ through the posterior nares is difficult, and requires considerable practice. A small mirror, similar to a laryngoscopic mirror, is inserted behind the soft palate, while the patient breathes through the nose and the tongue is depressed by the examiner. By means of light reflected through the mouth the following structures can be seen: the posterior nares, separated by the posterior margin of the nasal septum; the upper or attached portion of the inferior turbinated bone (*inferior concha*); the middle meatus; the middle turbinated bone (*middle concha*); the superior meatus; the superior turbinated bone (*superior concha*); the roof of the naso-pharynx; the upper part of the posterior wall of the naso-pharynx; the pharyngeal tonsil or adenoid; the upper part of the lateral wall of the naso-pharynx; the pharyngeal recess; the profile of the trumpet-shaped orifice of the Eustachian (*auditory*) tube.

Nasal douche.—In nasal catarrh the nasal fossæ are frequently cleansed by spraying or douching with an alkaline solution. In using the nasal douche the solution flows in one anterior naris and out through the other, elevation of the soft palate against the posterior wall of the pharynx preventing the solution from passing into the oro-pharynx. This raising of the soft palate is brought about much as in the act of swallowing it prevents regurgitation of food into the nose. The vessel containing the solution should not be placed above the level of the eyebrows, and the head should be inclined slightly forward so that the solution will not enter the Eustachian (*auditory*) tubes, the orifices of which are on a level with the posterior extremities of the inferior turbinated bones (*inferior concha*). If the solution should enter the middle ear through the Eustachian (*auditory*) tube, otitis media with resulting deafness may occur.

DISSECTION.—The student should now turn the superior turbinated bone (*superior concha*) upward, and with a probe search for the orifices of the sphenoidal sinus and the posterior ethmoidal cells.   Remove the anterior portion of the middle turbinated bone (*middle concha*), to find the orifices of the maxillary sinus, or antrum of Highmore, the anterior ethmoidal cells, and the infundibulum, and cut away the anterior portion of the inferior turbinated bone (*inferior concha*) to see the inferior opening of the lacrimo-nasal duct.   The frontal and sphenoidal sinuses, having been opened in sawing through the skull, can now be satisfactorily studied.   (Plate XCI.)

The **frontal sinuses** are situated between the inner and outer tables of the frontal bones, at the position of the superciliary eminences and the glabella. They are not recognizable until after the seventh year, when they appear as extensions of the anterior ethmoidal cells, and reach their full development at about the twentieth year.   Even in adult life they are variable as to size and shape.   The cavities are not necessarily both the same size, since one may be enlarged at the expense of the other.   The anterior, or external, bony wall of the sinuses is the thicker of the two, and upon careful examination it can usually be seen to consist of two laminæ, between which there is a thin diploic layer. The weakest and thinnest portion of this external wall is just above the medial angle of the orbit, and when a collection of pus in the frontal sinus escapes externally, it is usually at this point that the opening occurs.   Such a fistulous opening may be mistaken by the careless observer for a lacrimal fistula.

The usual shape of the frontal sinuses is pyramidal.   A thin, osseous, sometimes incomplete partition usually separates one sinus from the other. In many cases these sinuses extend backward for a considerable distance over the roof of the orbit.   Additional septa may divide the cavity into subcompartments, and furthermore, one or two of the ethmoidal cells may bulge into the sinus. In some individuals, especially in women, the sinuses are quite small, or may even be absent, this is said to be the common condition in skulls which have a mid-frontal suture.   They open into the middle meatuses of the nasal fossæ by means of the infundibula, or through a passage between the anterior attachment of the middle turbinate (*middle concha*) and the uncinate process, or occasionally through both.   Its aperture lies from two to ten millimeters from the upper end of the hiatus semilunaris.   The mucous membrane which lines them is an extension of that of the nose, and is supplied by filaments of the nasal (*naso-ciliary*) nerve.

Congestion of the mucous membrane of the frontal sinuses is likely to be associated with acute coryza, or "cold in the head," producing a dull ache over

PLATE XCI.

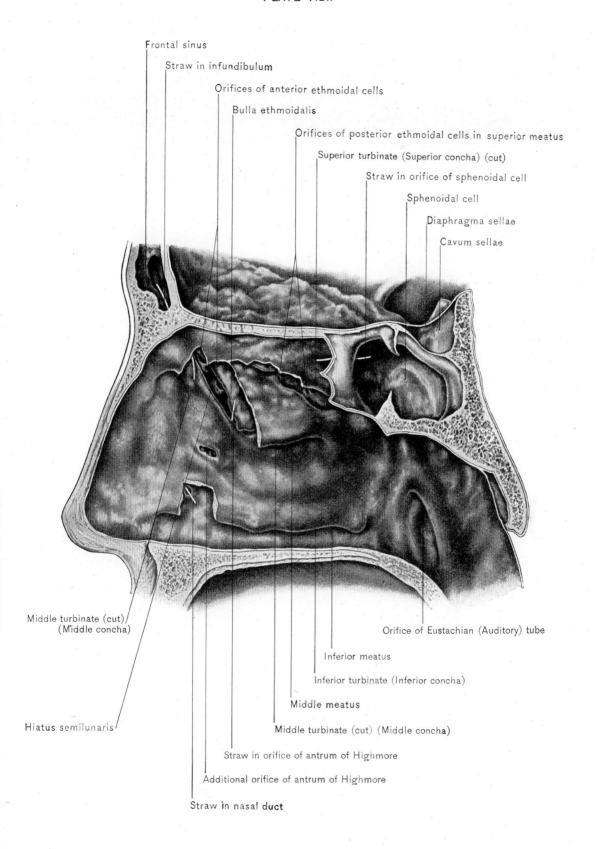

Frontal sinus

Straw in infundibulum

Orifices of anterior ethmoidal cells

Bulla ethmoidalis

Orifices of posterior ethmoidal cells in superior meatus

Superior turbinate (Superior concha) (cut)

Straw in orifice of sphenoidal cell

Sphenoidal cell

Diaphragma sellae

Cavum sellae

Middle turbinate (cut)
(Middle concha)

Orifice of Eustachian (Auditory) tube

Inferior meatus

Inferior turbinate (Inferior concha)

Middle meatus

Hiatus semilunaris

Middle turbinate (cut) (Middle concha)

Straw in orifice of antrum of Highmore

Additional orifice of antrum of Highmore

Straw in nasal duct

ORIFICES OF ACCESSORY AIR-CHAMBERS OF NOSE.

the glabella and superciliary eminences. When drainage from the sinuses is insufficient, the mucus becomes inspissated within them.

Empyema, or a purulent collection in the frontal sinus, is often associated with occlusion of the infundibulum, the resulting pain being due to the unyielding character of the walls of the sinus. If the infundibulum is patulous, the pus appears in the middle meatus of the nose. For the proper treatment of this affection it is necessary to trephine the anterior wall of the sinus, re-establish the communication with the nose, and institute drainage by means of a tube passed into the nasal fossa. The incision is made just below the supra-orbital margin, and extends from the root of the nose lateralward for about two and a half centimeters (one inch). A small trephine or a drill is applied just above the medial angle of the orbit, where the bone is thin. The trained rhinologist can occasionally pass a probe from the nasal opening in the middle meatus into the sinus and avoid the external exposure.

The *external table of the skull may be fractured* and depressed at the position of the frontal sinuses without injuring the inner table or affecting the cranial contents, and the inspissated mucus escaping from the sinus may be mistaken for brain matter. These fractures are often accompanied by emphysema, in which case the air is derived from the nose by way of the infundibulum.

Living foreign bodies, such as centipedes, maggots, and insects, may enter the frontal sinuses by passing up the infundibulum.

A *polypus* is sometimes found in one of the frontal sinuses. It may originate in the sinus or in the nose, and enter the sinus by way of the infundibulum. If it continues to enlarge, it may bulge the anterior, or orbital, wall of the sinus and displace the eyeball. It can be removed by trephining the anterior wall of the sinus.

DISSECTION.—Open the maxillary sinus, or antrum of Highmore, by sawing away part of its lateral wall.

The **maxillary sinus,** or **antrum of Highmore,** is an accessory air chamber of the nose, situated in the superior maxillary (*maxillary*) bone. It is the largest and probably the most important of the accessory sinuses. It is irregularly pyramidal in shape, the base of the pyramid being directed toward the nose, and the apex toward the malar (*zygomatic*) process of the superior maxilla (*maxilla*). The base is formed by the lateral wall of the nasal fossa, by the nasal surface of the superior maxilla (*maxilla*), the maxillary process of the inferior turbinate (*inferior concha*), the uncinate process of the ethmoidal bone, the vertical plate of the palatine bone, and the lacrimal bone. In the upper and posterior part of this surface is the orifice of the sinus, which is so situated that drainage from the antrum is defective, natural basilar drainage being impossible. This is extremely unfortunate, since this sinus is very frequently the site of pathologic processes. Consequently, mucus or pus may be retained in the cavity, forming a mucocele or empyema of the antrum. The roof of the antrum is formed by the orbital plate of the superior maxilla (*maxilla*), the floor by the alveolar process of the superior maxilla (*maxilla*), the anterior, or lateral, wall by the facial surface of the superior maxilla (*maxilla*), and the posterior wall by the malar (*zygomatic*) surface of the superior maxilla (*maxilla*).

The antrum is usually larger in the male than in the female. In young subjects it is small and its walls are quite thick, while in old age absorptive processes may cause a defect in the anterior bony wall. The two antra are frequently asymmetric in size and shape. Often the roots of the first and second molar teeth and sometimes also those of the premolars and canine teeth, form prominences in the floor of the cavity. It is evident that caries of these teeth and their roots may lead to disease of the antrum.

The *mucous membrane* of the maxillary sinus is thinner and less vascular than that of the nasal fossa.

The *orifice* of the antrum opens into the lower part of the hiatus semilunaris and the middle meatus of the nose, and is small, rounded, or elliptical. In empyema and mucocele of the antrum the orifice is usually closed by thickening of the nasal mucous membrane. There may be one or more additional orifices leading into the nasal fossa, so that infections of the latter have an easy access to the sinus.

The *tumors* which originate in the antrum may be either malignant or benign. By pressure upon the walls of the sinus they encroach upon the orbital and nasal fossæ, the lacrimal duct, the pterygo-maxillary region (*imfratemporal fossa*), and the mouth, and cause bulging of the cheek. The malignant tumors are removed by excising the superior maxilla (*maxilla*).

Empyema, or *abscess of the antrum,* may be caused by: extension of infection from the nose to the antrum, with occlusion of the antral orifice, retention of mucus, and the formation of pus; diseased roots of teeth projecting into the cavity; infectious fevers, and by injury. If the orifice of the antrum is not occluded, the pus may escape into the middle meatus by overflowing; this is favored by lying upon a horizontal surface with the opposite side of the face resting upon that surface. If the orifice is closed, it will be necessary to drain the antrum by extracting a carious bicuspid or molar tooth, which may be causing the abscess, and forcing a trocar through the alveolus into the antrum. If the teeth are not diseased, the sinus may be opened by everting the upper lip and drilling or trephining the canine fossa just above the second bicuspid tooth, or by drilling the nasal wall of the cavity in the middle or inferior meatus of the nose, which is the usual route used by the rhinologist.

In *dropsy of the antrum*, or hydrops antri, a glairy or thin serous fluid occupies the maxillary sinus. It arises from cystic degeneration of the mucous membrane.

Dentigerous cysts of the antrum develop around an unerupted tooth. *Dental cysts* are the result of infection at the root of a tooth, and *adamantine epithelio-mata* are the result of perversions of the tooth papillæ.

The **ethmoidal sinuses,** or **air cells,** are situated in the lateral masses of the ethmoidal bone, and are usually divided into an anterior, a middle, and a posterior set; sometimes, however, the cells are fused and seem to form only an anterior and a posterior cavity. In size and number they are variable. The *anterior set* forms a rounded eminence, the *bulla ethmoidalis*, situated in the lateral wall of the nasal fossa just above the hiatus semilunaris, into which many of the cells open. The middle set also opens directly into the middle meatus of the nose. The posterior ethmoidal cells open into the superior meatus of the nose. The ethmoidal cells are lined by mucoperiosteum continuous with that of the nasal fossa, and may be affected by catarrhal inflammation extending from the nose, by necrosis, mucocele, or malignant or benign growths. Infection from eth-moidal involvement may spread directly upward into the cranial cavity or it may enter the cranium by way of the ethmoidal veins or the opthalmic vein.

The **sphenoidal sinuses,** or **cells,** are located in the body of the sphenoidal bone. They are usually two in number, being separated by a delicate septum. They are lined by mucoperiosteum continuous with that of the nose and the roof of the pharynx. Their orifices are situated in the posterior part of the roof of the nose, opposite the posterior extremity of the superior turbinated bone (*superior concha*), and open into the superior meatus of the nose. They may be the site of catarrh and malignant or benign growths. They are intimately related to the cerebrum, the optic nerve, the opthalmic and internal carotid arteries and the cavernous plexus. Infection of the sphenoidal sinus is a fairly frequent source of optic neuritis.

Since the pituitary fossa forms the roof of the sinus, the transphenoidal approach for decompression or morcellation of pituitary neoplasms is frequently resorted to.

DISSECTION.—Remove the mucous membrane from the septum and the lateral wall of the nose, and trace the vessels and nerves previously described. If the otic ganglion has not been destroyed and the part is in good condition, the ganglion may be seen by carefully removing the cartilaginous portion of the Eustachian (*auditory*) tube and tracing upward the nerve to the internal ptery-goid muscle. The ganglion will be found on the medial side of the inferior maxillary (*mandibular*) nerve, below the foramen ovale. For description of the otic ganglion see page 281.

26

THE ORBIT

The **Orbits** are two irregularly conical or pyramidal cavities which contain the eyeballs and their accessory structures: muscles, fascia, vessels, nerves, and fat. The walls of the orbits are lined with a loosely attached periosteum or periorbita. Each orbit has an apex, a base, and four walls.

The **apex of the orbit** is directed posteriorly, and is situated at the optic foramen, through which the optic nerve and ophthalmic artery enter the orbit.

The **base of the orbit** is directed laterally and anteriorly, and is the only wall of the cavity which is absent since it corresponds to the opening on the face. The margins of the base are the supra-orbital and the infra-orbital margin. They project beyond the eyeball and protect it from injury by blows from large objects. The orbital margins are formed, above, by the frontal bone; laterally, by the malar (*zygomatic*) bone; medially, by the nasal process of the superior maxilla (*maxilla*); below, by the malar (*zygomatic*) bone and the body of the superior maxilla (*maxilla*). The *supra-orbital margin* contains the supra-orbital notch, a landmark in operations upon the supra-orbital and infra-orbital nerves. This notch is situated at the junction of the medial and the lateral two-thirds of that margin, and transmits the supra-orbital vessels and nerves.

The **roof of the orbit** is formed by the orbital plate of the frontal bone and the lesser wing of the sphenoidal bone. The frontal sinuses frequently project posteriorly into that part of the orbital roof formed by the frontal bone; consequently, tumors or an empyema of the frontal sinus may encroach upon the orbit and cause displacement of the eyeball with exophthalmos and double vision, or diplopia. At the lateral side, near the base of the orbit, the roof presents a large depression, the *lacrimal fossa*, for the lacrimal gland; and at the medial side, near the base of the orbit, a small depression to which the pulley of the superior oblique muscle is attached. On account of the relation between the orbit and the cranial cavity and the thinness of the intervening bony wall, a foreign body with a sharp point, such as a foil or stick, may enter the orbit, pierce its roof, and penetrate the brain without producing an apparently grave external injury.

The **floor of the orbit** is formed by the superior maxilla (*maxilla*), the malar (*zygomatic*) bone, and the orbital plate of the palatine bone. Beneath the greater portion of the floor is the maxillary sinus, or antrum of Highmore, tumors of which may encroach upon the orbit, and also displace the eyeball, and cause diplopia.

The **lateral wall of the orbit** inclines obliquely anterolaterally, and is formed by the malar (*zygomatic*) bone, the lateral angular (*zygomatic*) process of the frontal bone, and the greater wing of the sphenoidal bone. When dividing the optic nerve in excision of the eyeball, the scissors is more readily introduced on the lateral side, because of the greater space between the eyeball and ∨ the lateral wall and the lateral slope of that wall, which makes a larger angle with the optic nerve than the medial wall.

The **medial wall of the orbit** is formed by the nasal process of the superior maxilla (*maxilla*), the medial angular process of the frontal bone, the lacrimal bone, the os planum (*lamina papyracea*) of the ethmoidal bone, and a part of the body of the sphenoidal bone. Near the base of the orbit the medial wall presents a large depression, the lacrimal groove, which lodges the lacrimal sac, and below, leads into the lacrimal canal, which is lined by the mucoperiosteal wall of the lacrimo-nasal duct. In the medial wall of the orbit, and separated from it by a thin bony partition, are the ethmoidal cells and the sphenoidal cell, or sinus. Although the medial walls are slightly divergent posteriorly, they are practically parallel anteriorly.

Measurements.—The anteroposterior diameter of the adult orbit is about four centimeters (one and three-fourth inches). At the base the vertical diameter is about three and a half centimeters (one and one-fourth inches), and the transverse diameter about three centimeters (one and one-half inches).

The orbit is wide open anteriorly, while posteriorly it is in communication with the cranial cavity through the optic foramen and the sphenoidal (*superior orbital*) fissure, and with the pterygo-maxillary region (*infratemporal fossa*) and the spheno-maxillary (*pterygo-palatine*) fossa through the spheno-maxillary (*inferior orbital*) fissure. The axis of the orbit is directed upward and medialward, forming an angle of from five to twenty degrees with the horizontal plane, and one of about forty-five degrees with the orbital axis of the opposite side, the two intersecting in the region of the sella turcica. The eyeball itself fills only about one-fifth of the orbital cavity.

Blood may be extravasated into the orbit after fracture of one of the walls of that cavity, more commonly the roof, and produce subconjunctival ecchymosis. Tumors, blood, or pus may enter the orbit from the pterygo-maxillary region (*infratemporal fossa*) through the spheno-maxillary (*inferior orbital*) fissure, ∨ and from the cranial cavity through the sphenoidal (*superior orbital*) fissure, or from the frontal sinus by perforation of the medial orbital wall.

DISSECTION.—According to the level at which the calvaria has been removed, there will remain more or less of the vertical plate of the frontal bone, covered in front by the soft parts. The soft tissues should be turned down after making two incisions down to the bone, one running vertically upward from the nasion and the other running parallel to the vertical incision, and starting from the lateral angular (*zygomatic*) process of the frontal bone. If much of the vertical

plate of the frontal bone remains, it should be removed with the hammer and
chisel almost as far down as the supra-orbital arch.   The roof of the orbit should
now be removed, either entirely, or all except the supra-orbital margin.   In the
former method two cuts, converging at the optic foramen, are made with a saw,
leaving the bone around the optic foramen undisturbed, and then, by a firm tap
with a mallet, breaking away the orbital roof, and turning it forward.   In
the latter (Cunningham's) method, the thin plate of bone covering the orbit is
removed with a chisel and mallet, leaving intact the ring of bone around the optic
foramen and that constituting the supra-orbital margin.   Care should be taken
to avoid injuring two structures—the pulley of the superior oblique muscle and
the orbital periosteum.

If at the time the dissection of this portion of the body is begun the eyeball
has collapsed, it should be inflated by one of the following methods: after
opening the periosteum, carry a ligature loosely around the optic nerve by means
of an aneurysm needle; then insert a blowpipe between the optic nerve and its
sheath, thrusting it almost, if not quite, into the eyeball.   Inflate until the ball
is tense; then, while an assistant slowly withdraws the blowpipe, draw the
ligature tight.   Or the eyeball may be inflated from the front; this procedure is
less difficult, more successful, and allows reinflation when necessary.   In this
method a sharp needle is introduced obliquely at the sclero-corneal junction.
The blowpipe is then inserted through the puncture, and withdrawn after the
eyeball is distended.   The valvular character of the incision is sufficient to
prevent rapid escape of the air.

The Orbital Periosteum, or Periorbita.—The orbital roof having been removed, the periosteum comes into view.   It encloses the structures which fill the orbit,
and is loosely attached to the bony walls.   It is continuous posteriorly with
the endosteal layer of the dura mater through the optic foramen and the sphenoidal (*superior orbital*) fissure.   Anteriorly, the periorbita divides at the orbital
margins into two lamellæ, one being continuous with the periosteum on the
facial surface of the bones which form those margins, and the other blending with
the palpebral fascia of the eyelids.   The periorbita is a thin but resistant membrane and is continuous with the orbital fascia, which sends fibrous tissue prolongations into the orbital fat which serve as a support for the latter.

DISSECTION.—Two incisions are now made through the periosteum.   A
transverse one, running parallel to the supra-orbital ridge, and a longitudinal
one, running anteroposteriorly from the optic foramen to the middle of the first
incision.   Use a very sharp knife, or else make a nick in the periosteum and do
the rest of the cutting with scissors or with a knife in the trough of a small grooved
director.   The two flaps thus formed should be carefully turned aside, gently

separating them from the underlying structures. Further dissection is much facilitated by drawing the eyeball forward and retaining it in position with a suture or with hooks, taking care not to puncture the eyeball, and thus allow the escape of its contained air.

Structures Exposed by Removal of the Periosteum.—The orbital fat, orbital fascia, and frontal nerve are exposed as soon as the flaps of periosteum are reflected. Careful removal of some of the orbital fat will demonstrate a number of structures.

In the median line, *the frontal nerve* is readily demonstrable without dissection. It lies upon the levator palpebræ superioris muscle; its anterior portion is accompanied by the supra-orbital artery.

Running along the lateral wall of the orbit, and just above the lateral rectus muscle, are the *lacrimal nerve* and *artery*.

At the anterolateral part of the orbit, the *lacrimal gland* appears resting against the lacrimal fossa in the inferior surface (*pars orbitalis*) of the horizontal plate of the frontal bone.

Along the medial wall the superior oblique muscle is seen. At its anterior portion the fibrous ring or pulley through which its tendon works can be demonstrated; and well back in its course the fourth, or trochlear, nerve is seen entering its fleshy portion.

The orbital fat.—The posterior half of the orbit contains a large mass of stringy, coherent fat, which forms a soft pad, or cushion, for the support of the eyeball, and fills the interstices between the muscles, vessels, and nerves. The sinking in of the eyeball (enophthalmos), coincident with the emaciation of disease or age, is due to partial absorption of this fat. This type of enophthalmos is only apparent, but a true enophthalmos may occur if the orbital, or Müller's, muscle is paralyzed, or after injury of Tenon's capsule (*fascia bulbi*), or the check ligaments. Although this fat forms a cushion for the eyeball, the organ does not come into direct contact with it, since between the two is the capsule of Tenon (*fascia bulbi*).

Orbital abscesses are situated in the orbital fat; they may develop in the fat or they may arise from ocular inflammation, periostitis, injuries, or by extension from adjacent cavities, such as the ethmoidal or sphenoidal cells, the maxillary sinus, or antrum of Highmore, the frontal sinus, the pterygo-maxillary region (*infratemporal fossa*), or the cranial cavity. If the abscess attains a large size, it displaces the eyeball forward, retards its movements, and through pressure upon the ophthalmic vein and its tributaries causes congestion of the conjunctiva and swelling of the eyelids.

Foreign bodies may lodge in the orbital fat for a long time without causing much disturbance.

Emphysema of the orbit, or air in the orbital fat, results from rupture of the orbital periosteum and fracture of the wall intervening between the orbit and one of the accessory air-chambers of the nose—the frontal sinuses, ethmoidal cells, sphenoidal cells, and the maxillary sinus, or antrum of Highmore.

The **orbital fascia** (Plates XCII; XCIII) resembles the deep fascia of other locations. It envelops and forms sheaths for the muscles, vessels, and nerves of the orbit, and sends partitions, or septa, into the orbital fat which separate it into lobules. Posteriorly, or at the apex of the orbit, the orbital fascia is continuous with the orbital periosteum around the origins of the muscles. It passes anteriorly as a single layer between the muscles, and where each of the muscles is lacated it exists as two layers which envelop the muscle. Near the apex of the orbit it is thin and lax, but as it passes anteriorly it becomes much stronger and more adherent to the muscles. At about opposite the equator of the eyeball it divides into two laminæ, the anterior and the posterior. The *anterior lamina of the orbital fascia* passes forward to blend with the orbital periosteum at the orbital margin, and to the deep surface of the palpebral fascia in the eyelids, thus forming a funnel-shaped partition which supports the fornix of the conjunctiva. The *posterior lamina of the orbital fascia* turns posteriorly behind the posterior third of the eyeball, and loosely envelops the optic nerve and its sheath.

The anterior lamina is a strong membrane throughout its extent, the portion beneath the eyeball being known as the *suspensory ligament of the eyeball,* because after excision of the superior maxilla (*maxilla*), the lower portion of the anterior lamina forms a hammock-like sling which supports the eyeball and prevents it from sinking downward. This ligament is attached, laterally, to the malar (*zygomatic*) bone and, medially, to the crest of the lacrimal bone. At the four rectus muscles the anterior lamina is stronger and forms *check ligaments,* the lateral and medial ones being stronger than the other two. The *lateral check ligament* passes laterally and anteriorly from the tendon of the lateral rectus muscle and under the lacrimal gland to be attached to the malar (*zygomatic*) bone just behind the lateral palpebral ligament. The *medial check ligament* passes medialward from the medial rectus muscle to be attached to the upper part of the crest of the lacrimal bone behind the tensor tarsi (*lacrimal part of orbicularis oculi*) muscle. These check ligaments of the rectus muscles prevent extreme action of these muscles, and after the rectus muscles are divided, they prevent the bellies of the muscles from retreating far back into the orbit.

The **capsule of Tenon** (**fascia bulbi**) is the membrane which envelops the posterior three-fourths of the eyeball. It is a thin, translucent, fibrous membrane formed by the posterior lamina and part of the anterior lamina of the orbital fascia, and extends from the insertions of the rectus muscles, posteriorly, over the

PLATE XCII.

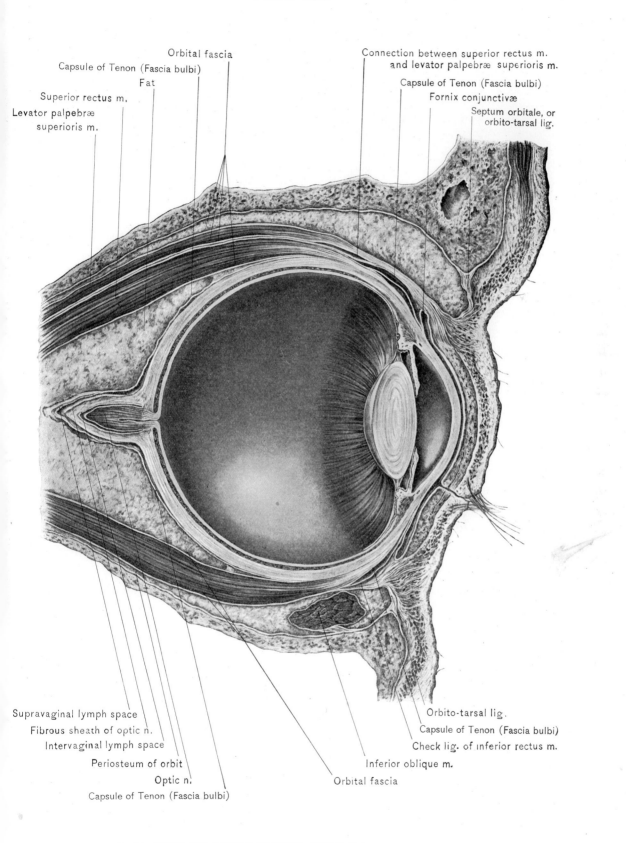

Orbital fascia

Capsule of Tenon (Fascia bulbi)

Fat

Superior rectus m.

Levator palpebræ
superioris m.

Connection between superior rectus m.
and levator palpebræ superioris m.

Capsule of Tenon (Fascia bulbi)

Fornix conjunctivæ

Septum orbitale, or
orbito-tarsal lig.

Supravaginal lymph space

Fibrous sheath of optic n.

Intervaginal lymph space

Periosteum of orbit

Optic n.

Capsule of Tenon (Fascia bulbi)

Orbito-tarsal lig.

Capsule of Tenon (Fascia bulbi)

Check lig. of inferior rectus m.

Inferior oblique m.

Orbital fascia

ORBITAL FASCIA AND CAPSULE OF TENON (FASCIA BULBI)—SAGITTAL SECTION.

PLATE XCIII.

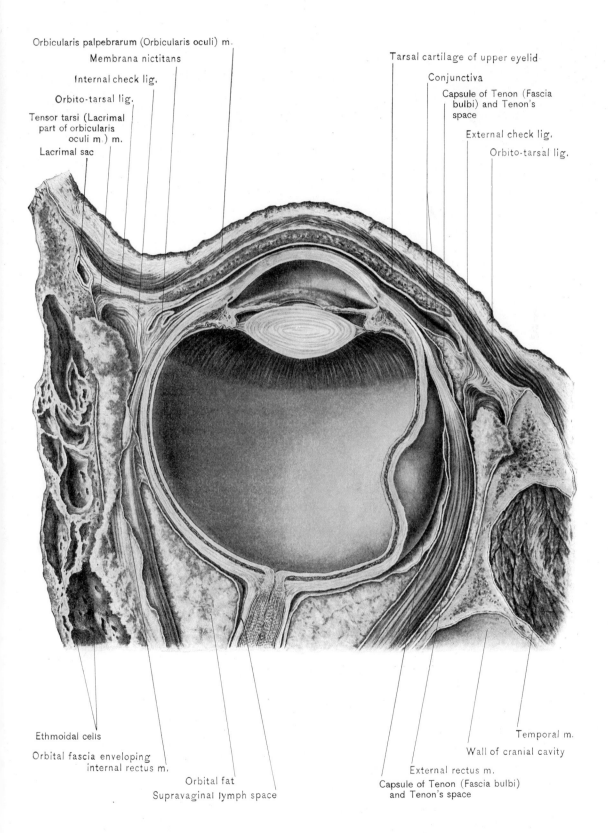

Orbicularis palpebrarum (Orbicularis oculi) m.

Membrana nictitans

Internal check lig.

Orbito-tarsal lig.

Tensor tarsi (Lacrimal part of orbicularis oculi m.) m.

Lacrimal sac

Tarsal cartilage of upper eyelid

Conjunctiva

Capsule of Tenon (Fascia bulbi) and Tenon's space

External check lig.

Orbito-tarsal lig.

Ethmoidal cells

Orbital fascia enveloping internal rectus m.

Orbital fat

Supravaginal lymph space

Temporal m.

Wall of cranial cavity

External rectus m.

Capsule of Tenon (Fascia bulbi) and Tenon's space

ORBITAL FASCIA AND CAPSULE OF TENON (FASCIA BULBI)—TRANSVERSE SECTION.

sclerotic coat of the eyeball almost to the point of entrance of the optic nerve, where it is reflected, posteriorly, over the sheath of the optic nerve to the apex of the orbit. In passing toward the apex of the orbit, the capsule approaches the sheath of the optic nerve but does not blend with it. The space between the sheath of the optic nerve and the capsule of Tenon (*fascia bulbi*) is the *supra-vaginal lymph space*, and that between the sclerotic coat and the capsule is *Tenon's (interfascial) space.* These two lymph spaces are in communication with each other. They also communicate with the subdural lymph spaces, thus establishing intracranial connections. The capsule of Tenon (*fascia bulbi*) is attached to the sclerotic coat and the sheath of the optic nerve by loose areolar tissue which permits free movement of the eyeball. The orbital surface of the capsule is in relation with the orbital fat. The capsule first comes in contact with the rectus muscles near the equator of the eyeball, where the capsule is pierced by the tendons of these muscles. The anterior margin of the capsule of Tenon (*fascia bulbi*) forms a circular line connecting the insertions of the rectus muscles.

The posterior two-thirds of the eyeball and the capsule of Tenon (*fascia bulbi*) may be said to form a ball-and-socket joint, permitting the various rotatory and gliding movements of the eyeball. The socket of the joint, or the capsule of Tenon (*fascia bulbi*), is held in position by the attachments of orbital fascia, and the globe is held in the socket chiefly by the rectus muscles.

After excision of the eyeball the muscles of the orbit are able to move the stump through their attachments to the capsule of Tenon (*fascia bulbi*).

The frontal nerve is the largest of the three branches of the ophthalmic division of the fifth nerve, the lacrimal, the nasal (*nasociliary*), and the frontal, and may be regarded as the continuation of the main trunk. It gains entrance to the orbit by way of the sphenoidal (*superior orbital*) fissure, lying lateral and on a plane slightly inferior to the fourth, or trochlear, nerve. It then passes forward with the supra-orbital artery between the levator palpebræ superioris muscle and the orbital periosteum. At a point about midway between the sphenoidal (*superior orbital*) fissure and the supra-orbital foramen, or notch, it divides into its terminal branches, the supra-orbital and the supratrochlear.

The **supra-orbital nerve** continues forward in the line of the frontal nerve, and with the supra-orbital artery leaves the orbit by way of the supra-orbital foramen, or notch. It then turns upward on the forehead and, dividing into a medial and a lateral branch, supplies the scalp as far back as the lambdoid suture. At the supra-orbital foramen it gives off a few filaments to the upper eyelid.

The **supratrochlear nerve** runs toward the medial side of the orbit, and, as its name implies, passes over the pulley of the superior oblique muscle. There it gives off a twig which communicates with the infratrochlear branch of the nasal (*nasociliary*) nerve.   It then passes out of the orbit accompanied by the frontal artery, gives a few twigs to the inner part of the upper eyelid, supplies the structures around the medial canthus of the eye and the root of the nose, and sends a few filaments to the lining membrane of the frontal sinus.

The **lacrimal nerve,** the smallest branch of the ophthalmic division, enters the orbit through the sphenoidal (*superior orbital*) fissure lateral and slightly inferior to the frontal nerve.   It then courses along the lateral wall of the orbit above the superior margin of the lateral rectus muscle, accompanied by the lacrimal artery.   Just behind the lacrimal gland it forms a loop of communication with the temporal branch of the orbital (*zygomatic*), or temporo-malar (*zygomatic*), nerve.   From this loop and the immediate portion of the nerve, twigs are given off which enter the lacrimal gland.   The remainder of the nerve continues forward, pierces the palpebral fascia, and supplies the skin and conjunctiva around the lateral canthus of the eyelids.   (Plate XCIV.)

The nasal (*nasociliary*) nerve is described with the nose at p. 391.

The **trochlear, or fourth, nerve** is the smallest of all the cranial nerves.   It enters the orbit through the medial end of the sphenoidal (*superior orbital*) fissure, occupying the highest position of all the structures which traverse it, and lying above and to the medial side of the frontal nerve.   It passes over the origin of the levator palpebræ superioris muscle, lies to the medial side of the frontal nerve, and enters the orbital surface of the superior oblique muscle, to which alone it is distributed.

The **lacrimal gland** is a distinctly lobulated structure, resembling an almond, which lies in the superolateral part of the orbit under the lateral angular (*zygomatic*) process of the frontal bone.   It is composed of two portions of unequal size, which are separated by the aponeurotic expansion of the levator palpebræ superioris muscle.   The separation is not perfect, there being gaps which allow communication between the portions of the gland.   Of the two portions, the upper is by far the larger, and is called the superior, or orbital, portion, or superior lacrimal gland; the lower is called the inferior, palpebral, or accessory portion, or inferior lacrimal gland.

The *superior,* or *orbital, lacrimal gland,* comprising the main part of the gland, is about the size of a small almond.   Its upper surface is convex and its lower surface concave.   It occupies the fossa lacrimalis of the frontal bone and is enclosed by a capsule, from which run fibrous trabeculæ to be inserted into the periosteum of the fossa.   These bands are called the *suspensory ligaments of the lacrimal gland.*   Below, it rests upon the fascial prolongation attached from the trochlea to the fronto-malar (*fronto-zygomatic*) suture.

PLATE XCIV.

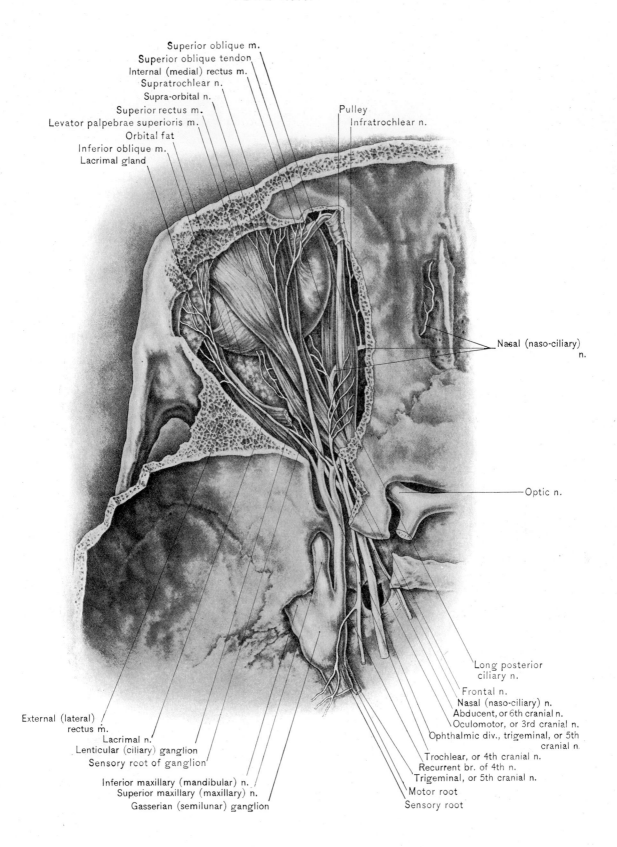

Superior oblique m.
Superior oblique tendon
Internal (medial) rectus m.
Supratrochlear n.
Supra-orbital n.
Superior rectus m.
Levator palpebrae superioris m.
Orbital fat
Inferior oblique m.
Lacrimal gland

Pulley
Infratrochlear n.

Nasal (naso-ciliary) n.

Optic n.

Long posterior ciliary n.
Frontal n.
Nasal (naso-ciliary) n.
Abducent, or 6th cranial n.
Oculomotor, or 3rd cranial n.
Ophthalmic div., trigeminal, or 5th cranial n.
Trochlear, or 4th cranial n.
Recurrent br. of 4th n.
Trigeminal, or 5th cranial n.
Motor root
Sensory root

External (lateral) rectus m.
Lacrimal n.
Lenticular (ciliary) ganglion
Sensory root of ganglion

Inferior maxillary (mandibular) n.
Superior maxillary (maxillary) n.
Gasserian (semilunar) ganglion

NERVES AND MUSCLES OF ORBIT.

PLATE XCV.

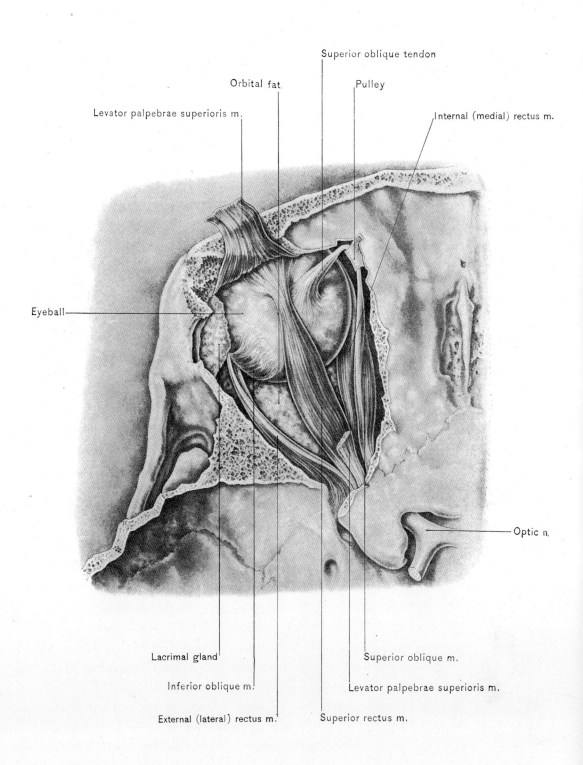

Superior oblique tendon

Orbital fat

Pulley

Levator palpebrae superioris m.

Internal (medial) rectus m.

Eyeball

Optic n.

Lacrimal gland

Superior oblique m.

Inferior oblique m.

Levator palpebrae superioris m.

External (lateral) rectus m.

Superior rectus m.

MUSCLES OF ORBIT.

The *inferior*, or *palpebral, lacrimal gland* is looser in texture than the orbital, and extends into the lateral third of the upper eyelid. It can be readily seen in this position when the eyelid is everted.

The lacrimal gland secretes the tears, which flow through from ten to fifteen very slender ducts into the lateral part of the superior conjunctival fornix about four millimeters above the superior margin of the tarsal cartilage, thence medial-ward over the ocular conjunctiva to the puncta lacrimalia, passing through the lacrimal canaliculi, lacrimal sac, and lacrimo-nasal duct into the inferior meatus of the nose.

The **Muscles of the Orbit** (Plate XCV) are: the levator palpebræ superioris, superior oblique, superior rectus, lateral and medial recti, inferior rectus, and inferior oblique. With one exception, the inferior oblique, they arise from the margin of the optic foramen and diverge as they pass forward to their insertions.

The **levator palpebræ superioris muscle** runs forward between the orbital periosteum and the superior rectus muscle, which lies immediately below it. It *arises* from the orbital roof, above and in front of the optic foramen, and passes forward. Gradually widening, it expands into a broad aponeurosis, passes between the two portions of the lacrimal gland, and splits into three lamellæ. The superficial lamella blends with the superior orbito-tarsal ligament; the middle lamella, the most easily demonstrable, is inserted into the anterior surface of the superior border of the tarsal cartilage; the deepest lamella is attached to the conjunctival fornix. The margins of the tendon are attached to the margin of the orbit, thus preventing excessive action of the muscle.

ACTION.—It raises the upper eyelid and retains it in that position.

NERVE SUPPLY.—From the superior division of the oculomotor nerve, a branch which pierces the superior rectus muscle.

The **superior oblique muscle** takes its *origin* from the orbital roof at the superior and medial margins of the optic foramen. It extends as a fleshy belly along the superomedial part of the orbital wall above the medial rectus muscle. It then narrows into a shining, slender tendon which enters the ring-like pulley attached to the frontal bone. Leaving the pulley, the tendon changes its course to a lateral and posterior direction. It then passes under the superior rectus muscle, and expands to be *inserted* into the sclera midway between the entrance of the optic nerve and the margin of the cornea, and between the superior rectus and lateral rectus muscles.

The *pulley*, or *trochlea, of the superior oblique muscle* is a fibrocartilaginous ring which is attached by a fibrous plate to the trochlear fossa in the under surface of the orbital plate of the frontal bone. The ring is lined by a synovial sheath which is continued over its contained tendon. Chronic serous effusion

27

into this synovial sheath sometimes develops in persons past middle life, and causes a cystic swelling at the upper and medial portion of the upper eyelid.

ACTION.—It rotates the eyeball medialward, and as the muscle is inserted into the posterior portion of the globe, it draws the cornea downward and slightly abducts it. It counteracts the tendency of the inferior rectus muscle to rotate the cornea lateralward, and the tendency of the superior and inferior recti muscles to adduct the cornea.

NERVE SUPPLY.—From the trochlear, or fourth cranial, nerve.

DISSECTION.—Divide the frontal nerve and the levator palpebræ superioris muscle, and dissect the latter free from the underlying structures. While dissecting up the levator palpebræ superioris muscle, a nerve filament should be observed which passes through the underlying muscle, the superior rectus, and enters the under surface of the posterior portion of the levator palpebræ superioris muscle. This filament is the branch of the oculomotor nerve, which supplies that muscle.

The **superior rectus muscle** is now fully exposed. It *arises* from the superior portion of the anterior margin of the optic foramen, and becomes broader as it passes forward between the levator palpebræ superioris muscle and the optic nerve. It is *inserted* by a thin, expanded tendon into the sclera, about six to eight millimeters (one-fourth to one-third of an inch) behind the superior margin of the sclero-corneal junction.

ACTION.—It rotates the eyeball upward, in addition to adducting and rotating the cornea medialward.

NERVE SUPPLY.—From the superior division of the oculomotor nerve.

DISSECTION.—This is a very important stage of the dissection, and requires great care in order not to destroy some of the important structures. Divide the superior rectus muscle and reflect it. While dissecting this muscle free from the underlying structures, observe the nerve filament, already mentioned, entering the under surface of the posterior portion of the divided muscle. This nerve is the superior division of the oculomotor nerve, and sends a perforating branch through the superior rectus muscle to supply the levator palpebræ superioris muscle. Remove a quantity of loose fat, and when working on the lateral side of the optic nerve, take especial care not to injure the lenticular (*ciliary*) ganglion or its connections. The optic nerve, as well as numerous structures above and upon each side of it, will now be exposed. These are the nasal (*nasociliary*) nerve, the ophthalmic artery and vein, and the long ciliary branches of the nasal (*nasociliary*) nerve, all of which cross the optic nerve. There may also be found the short ciliary nerves. These are more numerous than the long ciliary nerves, and one of the largest should be selected and followed backward until its source of origin, the lenticular (*ciliary*) ganglion, is reached. By careful work the roots of this ganglion can be worked out by tracing them backward from the ganglion. They will lead to the nasal (*nasociliary*) nerve, the inferior division of the oculomotor nerve, and the cavernous plexus of the cervical sympathetic.

In the posterior portion of the orbit the third, or oculomotor, nerve, the nasal branch of the ophthalmic nerve, the abducent, or sixth nerve, and the ophthalmic vein can be seen passing between the two heads of the lateral rectus muscle.

In the anterior portion of the orbit the reflected tendon of the superior oblique muscle can now be more readily seen, its terminal portion having been exposed by the reflection of the superior rectus muscle.

The **Nasal (Nasociliary) Nerve** (Plate XCIV) is a branch of the ophthalmic division of the fifth nerve. It is intermediate in size between the lacrimal and frontal nerves. Covered with dura mater, it gains access to the orbit through the sphenoidal (*superior orbital*) fissure, and passes between the two heads of the lateral rectus muscle and between the divisions of the oculomotor nerve. It then crosses to the medial wall of the orbit, passing over the optic nerve and immediately under the superior rectus muscle, taking a position between the superior oblique and the medial rectus muscles. After giving off the infratrochlear branch, it leaves the orbit through the anterior ethmoidal foramen. It then takes the following course: having passed through the anterior ethmoidal foramen, it again lies in the cranial cavity between the dura mater and the lateral part of the cribriform plate of the ethmoidal bone. Here it leaves the cranial cavity through the ethmoidal fissure, or nasal fissure, at the side of the crista galli, and becomes an occupant of the nasal fossa where it terminates in its internal, external, and anterior nasal branches. It thus has successively traversed the cranial cavity, the orbit, the cranial cavity again, and finally, the nasal cavity. It then gives off an internal and an external branch, and continues as the anterior, or terminal, branch.

The *internal*, or *septal*, *branch* supplies the anterior part of the septum.

The *external branch* supplies the anterior portion of the middle and inferior turbinate bones (*conchæ*) and the mucous membrane of the lateral nasal wall.

The *anterior*, or *terminal*, *branch* runs downward in the groove on the under surface of the nasal bone, passes between the lower edge of the nasal bone and the lateral nasal cartilage, and supplies the sides and tip of the nose.

The **branches of the nasal (nasociliary) nerve** in the orbit are four in number: the long root to the lenticular (*ciliary*) ganglion, the two long ciliary nerves, and the infratrochlear nerve.

The *ganglionic branch*, or *branch to the lenticular (ciliary) ganglion*, known as the long, upper, or sensory, root of that ganglion, arises from the nasal (*naso-*

ciliary) nerve as it passes between the two heads of the lateral rectus muscle. It is very slender, and measures about twelve millimeters (one-half inch) in length. It passes along the lateral side of the optic nerve and enters the posterior superior angle of the lenticular (*ciliary*) ganglion.

The *long ciliary nerves*, usually two in number, arise from the nasal (*nasociliary*) nerve as it crosses the optic nerve, and run medially along the optic nerve to enter the eyeball by piercing the sclera. One of these nerves usually unites with one of the short ciliary nerves. Their course between the sclera and choroid is described with the eyeball, at p. 462.

The *infratrochlear nerve* arises from the nasal (*nasociliary*) nerve just before it enters the anterior ethmoidal foramen. It traverses the medial orbital wall below the superior oblique muscle and its pulley, and forms a loop of communication with the supratrochlear nerve, sometimes behind, but usually in front of the pulley of the superior oblique muscle. It supplies the region around the medial canthus of the eyelids, including the lacrimal sac, the lacrimal caruncle, the skin of the upper eyelid, and the root of the nose.

The **Ophthalmic Artery** (Plate XCVI) is a branch of the cavernous portion of the internal carotid artery. It enters the orbit by passing through the optic foramen in company with the optic nerve, holding a position lateral, and a little inferior to the nerve. The ophthalmic artery, like arteries in other parts of the body in which the tissues must be freely movable, such as the facial and splenic, is very tortuous, to allow of its elongation. At first it lies lateral to the optic nerve, soon crossing over that nerve and running along and near the medial orbital wall, between the superior rectus and the medial rectus muscles. At the medial canthus of the eyelids it terminates by dividing into the nasal and frontal arteries.

The **branches of the ophthalmic artery** are: the retinal, ciliary, lacrimal, muscular, supra-orbital, ethmoidal, palpebral, nasal, and frontal.

The **central artery of the retina** arises from the ophthalmic artery just anterior to the optic foramen and while the vessel is still below the optic nerve. It enters the optic nerve obliquely, about fifteen millimeters behind the eyeball, and traverses the nerve to reach the interior of the eyeball and supply the retina.

The **ciliary arteries** consist of two sets, a posterior and an anterior set. The posterior set includes the short and the long ciliary arteries. These arteries being intermingled with the ciliary nerves are dissected with the nerves (see p. 418). They are distributed to the choroid, the ciliary processes, and the iris. They vary as to number and origin.

The **lacrimal artery** is given off from the ophthalmic artery between the superior rectus and the lateral rectus muscles, as the ophthalmic artery passes

PLATE XCVI.

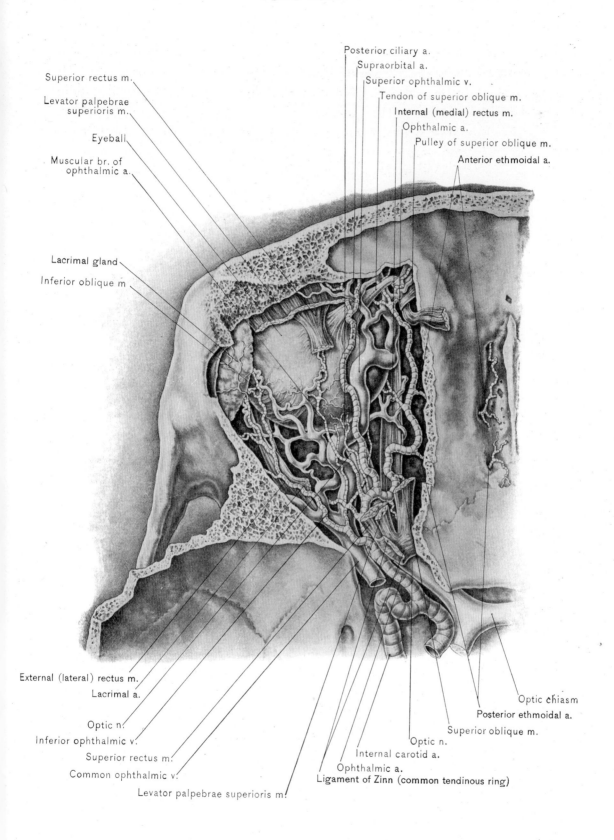

Posterior ciliary a.

Supraorbital a.

Superior ophthalmic v.

Tendon of superior oblique m.

Internal (medial) rectus m.

Ophthalmic a.

Pulley of superior oblique m.

Anterior ethmoidal a.

Superior rectus m.

Levator palpebrae
superioris m.

Eyeball

Muscular br. of
ophthalmic a.

Lacrimal gland

Inferior oblique m

External (lateral) rectus m.

Lacrimal a.

Optic n.

Inferior ophthalmic v.

Superior rectus m.

Common ophthalmic v.

Levator palpebrae superioris m.

Ligament of Zinn (common tendinous ring)

Ophthalmic a.

Internal carotid a.

Optic n.

Superior oblique m.

Posterior ethmoidal a.

Optic chiasm

ARTERIES AND VEINS OF ORBIT.

upward over the lateral surface of the optic nerve just after the artery enters the orbit.   It passes forward and lateralward, in company with the lacrimal nerve, to the lacrimal gland, which it supplies, finally terminating in the conjunctiva and eyelids.   It sends off twigs as follows: (1) a *recurrent branch*, which passes backward through the sphenoidal (*superior orbital*) fissure to anastomose with the middle meningeal artery; (2) *muscular branches* to the lateral rectus muscle; (3) *malar (zygomatic) branches*, which traverse the malar (*zygomatic*) bone to enter the temporal fossa, one anastomosing with the deep temporal arteries and the middle temporal artery, and the other with the transverse facial artery; (4) *palpebral branches*, which form an arch in each eyelid with the palpebral branches of the ophthalmic artery; (5) some *anterior ciliary branches*.

The **muscular branches of the ophthalmic artery** are variable in number and origin, and are distributed to the muscles of the orbit.   They give off most of the anterior ciliary arteries.

The **supra-orbital artery** arises from the ophthalmic artery as that vessel crosses the optic nerve.   It accompanies the frontal nerve upon the levator palpebræ superioris muscle, and runs between this muscle and the periosteum of the roof of the orbit, emerging upon the forehead through the supra-orbital notch, or foramen.   Having reached the forehead, it divides into a superficial and a deep branch, the former ramifying in the superficial fascia, and the latter in the areolar tissue layer of the scalp.   It anastomoses with the superficial temporal artery, the angular artery, and the supra-orbital artery of the opposite side.   Its branches are: (1) *periosteal*, to the roof of the orbit; (2) *muscular*, to the adjacent muscles; (3) *diploic*, to the diploë and frontal sinus; (4) *trochlear*, to the pulley of the superior oblique muscle; (5) *palpebral*, to the upper eyelid.

The **ethmoidal arteries** are two in number, posterior and anterior.

The *posterior ethmoidal artery*, the smaller and less constant of the two, passes lateralward between the medial rectus and the superior oblique muscles, and enters the posterior ethmoidal foramen.   Having reached the posterior ethmoidal cells, it gives off branches which nourish their walls and their lining mucous membrane.   It then enters the cranial cavity, and gives off branches to a small area of dura mater and nasal branches which pass downward through the cribriform plate (*lamina cribrosa*) of the ethmoidal bone, to supply the mucous membrane of the roof of the nose, especially the upper posterior part of the septum.

The *anterior ethmoidal artery* is larger than the posterior, and traverses the anterior ethmoidal foramen, in company with the nasal (*nasociliary*) nerve.   It accompanies the nerve within the cranial cavity and out of that cavity through the ethmoidal fissure into the nose.   Its branches are: *ethmoidal*, to the walls and mucous membrane of the anterior and middle ethmoidal cells; *meningeal*, to the dura mater in the anterior cranial fossa; *nasal*, to the latero-anterior part of the mucous membrane of the nose; *frontal*, to the frontal sinus; *terminal*, accompanying the terminal branch of the nasal nerve to the skin of the nose.

The **medial palpebral arteries** are two in number, superior and inferior. They arise from the ophthalmic artery, either separately or by a common trunk, almost opposite the pulley of the superior oblique muscle. They pass, one above and the other below the tendo oculi (*medial palpebral ligament*), run between the tarsal cartilage and the orbicularis palpebrarum (*orbicularis oculi*) muscle, near the edge of the eyelid, and anastomose with the lateral palpebral branches of the lacrimal artery, thus forming a vascular arch in each eyelid (arcus tarseus superior et inferior). They also supply the lacrimal duct and caruncle and the adjacent conjunctiva.

The **nasal artery** (**dorsal nasal**) is the lower terminal branch of the ophthalmic artery. It leaves the orbit by piercing the orbito-tarsal ligament, or palpebral fascia, above the tendo oculi (*medial palpebral ligament*). It then passes down the side of the nose, and anastomoses with the angular, or lateral nasal, branches of the facial (*external maxillary*) artery, giving off branches to the walls of the lacrimal sac and to the skin of the root of the nose.

The **frontal artery** is the upper, terminal branch of the ophthalmic artery. It leaves the orbit at the medial canthus of the eyelids by piercing the palpebral fascia, and passes upward on the forehead, anastomosing with the supra-orbital, the anterior temporal, and the frontal artery of the opposite side.

The **Ophthalmic Veins** are two in number, the superior and the inferior.

Neither these veins nor their tributaries have valves. They communicate freely with veins corresponding to the arteries with which the branches of the ophthalmic artery anastomose. They thus form important emissaries connecting the cavernous sinus with the facial (*anterior facial*) vein.

The **superior ophthalmic vein,** the larger of the two ophthalmic veins, arises at the medial portion of the upper eyelid by a free anastomosis with the frontal, supra-orbital, and angular veins, and following a straighter course than the ophthalmic artery, crosses over the optic nerve to reach the medial end of the sphenoidal (*superior orbital*) fissure, where it joins the inferior ophthalmic vein.

The **inferior ophthalmic vein** is formed by the union of the inferior muscular, and posterior ciliary veins in the lower lateral portion of the orbit. It lies below the plane of the optic nerve, and communicates with the pterygoid plexus of veins by a twig which passes through the spheno-maxillary (*inferior orbital*)

PLATE XCVII.

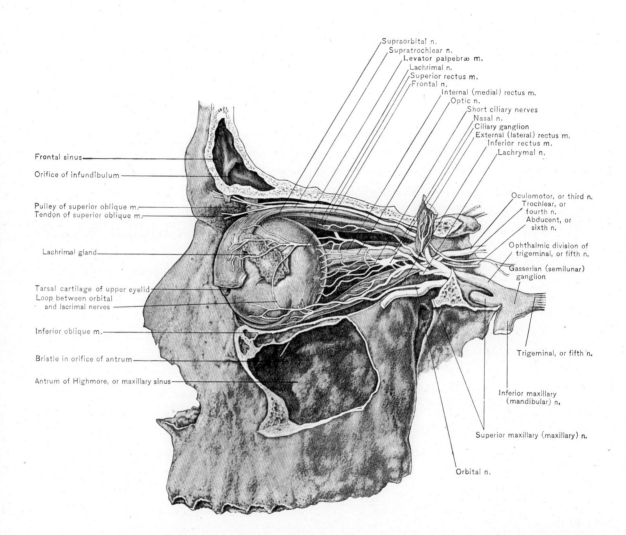

Supraorbital n.
Supratrochlear n.
Levator palpebræ m.
Lachrimal n.
Superior rectus m.
Frontal n.
Internal (medial) rectus m.
Optic n.
Short ciliary nerves
Nasal n.
Ciliary ganglion
External (lateral) rectus m.
Inferior rectus m.
Lachrymal n.

Frontal sinus

Orifice of infundibulum

Pulley of superior oblique m.
Tendon of superior oblique m.

Lachrimal gland

Tarsal cartilage of upper eyelid
Loop between orbital
and lacrimal nerves

Inferior oblique m.

Bristle in orifice of antrum

Antrum of Highmore, or maxillary sinus

Oculomotor, or third n.
Trochlear, or
fourth n.
Abducent, or
sixth n.

Ophthalmic division of
trigeminal, or fifth n.

Gasserian (semilunar)
ganglion

Trigeminal, or fifth n.

Inferior maxillary
(mandibular) n.

Superior maxillary (maxillary) n.

Orbital n.

NERVES OF ORBIT.
426

fissure. It then runs to the posterior portion of the orbit, and either joins the superior ophthalmic vein or empties directly into the cavernous sinus.

Phlebitis of the ophthalmic veins may extend to the cavernous sinus and cause fatal thrombosis. The communication between the facial (*anterior facial*) and the superior ophthalmic veins makes infections along the course of the facial (*anterior facial*) vein exceedingly dangerous, since intracranial complications may result from a lesion in this area.

Pulsation of the ophthalmic vein and of the orbit may be produced by an arterio-venous aneurysm between the internal carotid artery and the cavernous sinus. This pulsation may be transmitted to the dilated palpebral and frontal veins. Pulsation of the orbit may also be caused by traumatic aneurysm of one of the arteries of the orbit, or by pulsation transmitted to the terminal portion of the ophthalmic vein from an aneurysm of the internal carotid artery.

The **ciliary, lenticular, or ophthalmic, ganglion** (Plate XCVII) is a small, reddish, quadrilateral body, slightly larger than the head of an ordinary pin; both its surfaces are slightly convex. It lies about six millimeters (one-fourth of an inch) in front of the sphenoidal (*superior orbital*) fissure, between the optic nerve on the medial side and the lateral rectus muscle on the lateral side. It is usually situated at the lateral side of the ophthalmic artery, to which, at times, it is closely adherent. Like all the sporadic ganglia connected with the trigeminal nerve, it has afferent and efferent filaments. The afferent filaments are three in number, and are termed its roots; the efferent filaments are the branches of distribution.

The **roots** of the ciliary ganglion are motor, sensory, and sympathetic. The *motor*, or *short*, *root* is a visceral motor root derived from that branch of the oculomotor nerve which runs to the inferior oblique muscle. It enters the postero-inferior angle of the ganglion. The *sensory*, or *long*, *root* springs from the nasal (*nasociliary*) branch of the ophthalmic division of the trigeminal nerve. It passes along the lateral side of the optic nerve, and enters the posterosuperior angle of the ganglion to pass through it. The *sympathetic root* has its origin in the cavernous plexus, and is somewhat difficult to dissect satisfactorily. It enters the posterior portion of the ganglion, either in company with the sensory root, or sometimes alone in the form of a bunch of fine filaments, or occasionally, in company with the motor root.

BRANCHES.—From the anterior border of the ganglion from three to six delicate filaments, the short ciliary nerves, are given off; they run forward to the eyeball and, by subdividing, they number twenty when they reach the globe; they are arranged in an upper and lower group. They surround the optic nerve and pierce the sclerotic coat in a circle around the entrance of that nerve. After penetrating the sclerotic coat, they are joined by the long ciliary nerves. They are sensory and trophic nerves to the eyeball, and motor nerves to the radial fibers of the iris, the ciliary muscle, and the cornea. The motor oculi filaments supply the circular muscle fibers of the iris, and the sympathetic fibers supply the radial muscle fibers of the iris. These motor filaments, which come from the oculomotor nerve, are cerebral sympathetic fibers, probably having their origin in the nucleus of Edinger and Westphal. They are concerned with contraction of the pupil. The dilator fibers of the pupil have their origin in the upper thoracic sympathetic fibers, and reach the cranium by way of the cervical sympathetics. Although a few of these fibers course through the ciliary ganglion, the major portion of them form the long ciliary nerves.

The **oculomotor, or third, nerve** lies in the lateral wall of the cavernous sinus, holding the highest position of all the nerves in this location. It is the principal motor nerve of the intrinsic and extrinsic muscles of the eyeball. It passes to the sphenoidal (*superior orbital*) fissure, where it divides into a superior and an inferior division, each of which then passes through the sphenoidal (*superior orbital*) fissure between the heads of the lateral rectus muscle, separated from each other by the nasal branch of the ophthalmic nerve.

The *superior division*, the smaller of the two, has already been traced. It supplies the superior rectus muscle and the levator palpebræ superioris muscle.

The *inferior division* very soon breaks up into three branches. Two of these are comparatively short, and enter the ocular surface of the inferior and medial recti muscles, to which they are distributed; the branch to the medial rectus muscle passes under the optic nerve. The third branch, pursuing a longer course, runs along the floor of the orbit to supply the inferior oblique muscle. It occupies the interval between the inferior and lateral rectus muscles, and enters the inferior oblique muscle at its posterior border. Near its origin it gives off the motor root to the ciliary ganglion.

The oculomotor nerve supplies the ciliary ganglion and the muscles of the orbit, with the exception of the lateral rectus and superior oblique muscles. Through the ciliary ganglion it supplies the ciliary muscle and the sphincter pupillæ.

The **abducent, or sixth, nerve** passes forward in the medial wall of the cavernous sinus, lying on the lateral side of, and slightly posterior to the internal carotid artery. It enters the orbit through the medial part of the sphenoidal (*superior orbital*) fissure, between the inferior division of the oculomotor nerve and the ophthalmic vein. It then passes between the heads of the lateral rectus muscle, to terminate in the ocular surface of that muscle and supply it. It is entirely motor.

PLATE XCVIII.

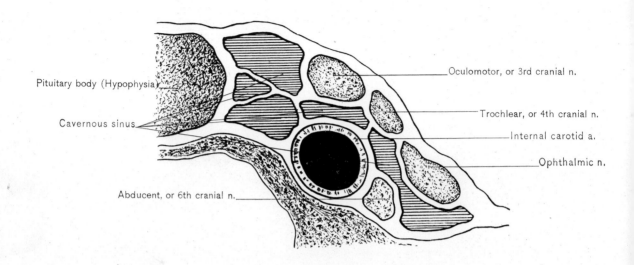

Pituitary body (Hypophysis)

Cavernous sinus

Oculomotor, or 3rd cranial n.

Trochlear, or 4th cranial n.

Internal carotid a.

Ophthalmic n.

Abducent, or 6th cranial n.

SECTION OF CAVERNOUS SINUS.

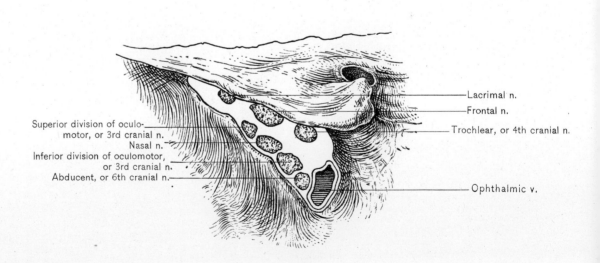

Superior division of oculomotor, or 3rd cranial n.

Nasal n.

Inferior division of oculomotor,
or 3rd cranial n.

Abducent, or 6th cranial n.

Lacrimal n.

Frontal n.

Trochlear, or 4th cranial n.

Ophthalmic v.

STRUCTURES TRAVERSING THE SPHENOIDAL FISSURE.

PLATE XCIX.

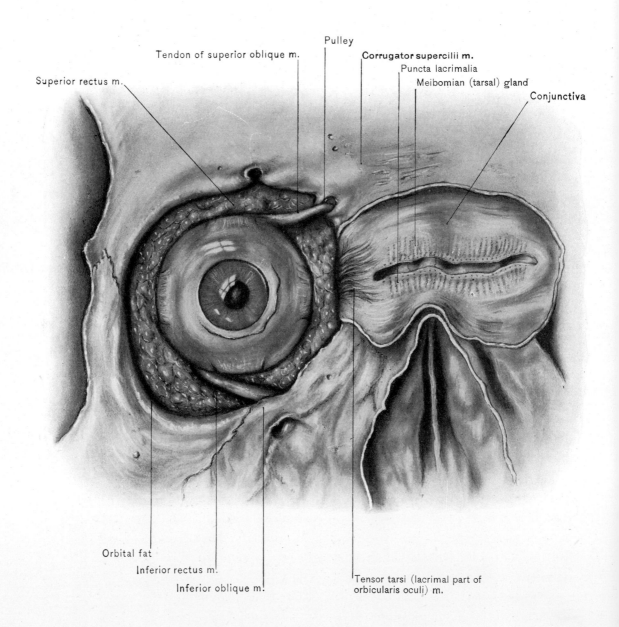

Pulley

Tendon of superior oblique m.

Corrugator supercilii m.

Puncta lacrimalia

Superior rectus m.

Meibomian (tarsal) gland

Conjunctiva

Orbital fat

Inferior rectus m.

Inferior oblique m.

Tensor tarsi (lacrimal part of orbicularis oculi) m.

TENSOR TARSI (LACRIMAL PART OF ORBICULARIS OCULI) AND CORRUGATOR SUPERCILII MUSCLES.

The **arrangement of the nerves of the orbit** (Plate XCVIII) in the walls of the cavernous sinus and in the sphenoidal (*superior orbital*) fissure is as follows: in the *lateral wall of the cavernous sinus*, from above downward, are the oculomotor nerve, the trochlear nerve, and the ophthalmic division of the trigeminal nerve; in the medial wall is the abducent nerve, in relation with the lateral side of the internal carotid artery. These nerves are separated from the cavity of the sinus by its endothelial lining. In the *sphenoidal (superior orbital) fissure*, in the order named from without medialward, are the lacrimal, the frontal, and the trochlear, or fourth, nerve. They pass above the origin of the muscles, while the other nerves and the ophthalmic vein are lower down, and enter the orbit between the two heads of the lateral rectus muscle. The nerves lying on a lower plane in the sphenoidal (*superior orbital*) fissure are, from without medialward: the superior division of the oculomotor nerve, the nasal (*nasociliary*) nerve, the inferior division of the oculomotor nerve, and the abducent, or sixth, nerve. The ophthalmic vein lies medial to the abducent nerve.

The **optic nerve** enters the orbit through the optic foramen, in company with the ophthalmic artery, and passes into the eyeball about two millimeters (one-tenth of an inch) medial to the posterior pole of that organ. It is invested by a sheath of dura mater, arachnoid, and pia mater, and is surrounded by an extension of the capsule of Tenon (*fascia bulbi*), the orbital fat and vessels, and the recti muscles. The lateral fibers of the dura blend with those of the lateral third of the sclera, those of the arachnoid end on the medial wall of the intervaginal space, while the pia mater assists in forming the medial third of the sclera. It is pierced and traversed by the vena and the arteria centralis retinæ.

The **lateral rectus muscle** is seen along the lateral wall of the orbit. It has two heads of origin: its upper head *arises* from the lateral margin of the optic foramen, beneath the superior rectus muscle, and its lower head, partly from the superolateral part of the ligament, or annulus, of Zinn and partly from a small spine of bone situated on the lower margin of the sphenoidal (*superior orbital*) fissure. Between these two heads pass the oculomotor nerve, the nasal (*nasociliary*) nerve, the abducent nerve, and the ophthalmic vein. The lateral rectus muscle is *inserted*, by an expanded tendon, into the sclerotic coat of the eyeball about six to eight millimeters (one-fourth to one-third of an inch) behind the lateral margin of the cornea. (Plate XCIX.)

NERVE SUPPLY.—From the abducent, or sixth cranial, nerve.

ACTION.—It abducts the cornea.

The **medial rectus muscle** lies along the medial wall of the orbit, below the superior oblique muscle, the ophthalmic artery, and the nasal (*nasociliary*) nerve. It *arises* through the ligament, or annulus, of Zinn from the medial

28

margin of the optic foramen, and is *inserted* into the sclerotic coat of the eyeball about six to eight millimeters (one-fourth to one-third of an inch) posterior to the medial margin of the cornea.

NERVE SUPPLY.—From the inferior division of the oculomotor nerve.

ACTION.—It abducts the cornea.

The **inferior rectus muscle** *arises* from the lower margin of the optic foramen through the ligament, or annulus, of Zinn. It passes forward along the floor of the orbit and below the optic nerve, and is *inserted* into the sclerotic coat of the eyeball about six to eight millimeters (one-fourth to one-third of an inch) from the lower margin of the cornea.

NERVE SUPPLY.—From the inferior division of the oculomotor nerve.

ACTION.—It depresses the cornea, adducts it, and rotates it laterally.

The inferior rectus muscle can be better studied after the dissection of the vessels, the nerves, and the other muscles has been completed, and those structures have been removed.

Ligament, or annulus, of Zinn (common tendinous ring).—At the ocular surfaces of the origin of the *four recti muscles*, these muscles will be seen to *arise* from a common tendinous ring, the ligament, or annulus, of Zinn, attached around the optic foramen, and which may be divided into a superior and an inferior common tendon. The *superior common tendon* is attached to the superior margin and the superolateral part of the margin of the optic foramen, and gives origin to the superior rectus muscle, part of the medial rectus, and the superior head of the lateral rectus muscle. The *inferior common tendon* is attached to the inferior part of the medial margin, the inferior margin, and the inferior part of the lateral margin of the optic foramen, and gives origin to the inferior rectus and part of the medial rectus muscle, and to the inferior head of the lateral rectus muscle.

DISSECTION.—The inferior oblique muscle is next exposed. Its position and relations differ greatly from those of the other orbital muscles, and can best be seen after the following dissection: release the eyeball from any position in which it may be held, evert the lower eyelid, and remove the conjunctiva at the inferior fornix; also remove the fat lying in the floor of the anterior portion of the orbit and clean the exposed muscle. In doing this be careful not to cut the nerve which enters the posterior border of the inferior oblique muscle.

The **inferior oblique muscle** *arises* by a flat tendon from the orbital plate of the superior maxilla (*maxilla*) to the lateral side of the orbital orifice of the lacrimal duct. It passes upward, lateralward, and backward under the inferior rectus muscle, and then upward between the globe and the lateral rectus muscle. It ends in a membranous tendon which is *inserted* into the sclera on the superior and lateral side of the globe, behind the orbital equator and under cover of the external oblique, below and lateral to the insertion of the superior oblique muscle.

NERVE SUPPLY.—From the longest branch of the inferior division of the oculomotor nerve, which enters the muscle at its posterior margin.

ACTION.—It rotates the eyeball laterally, and elevates and abducts the cornea. In abducting the cornea it counteracts the tendency of the superior rectus and inferior rectus muscles to adduct the cornea.

DISSECTION.—The ocular conjunctiva should now be removed from the sclerotic coat of the eyeball as far forward as the margin of the cornea, so that the positions of the attachments of the four recti muscles can be observed.

The recti muscles are *inserted* by thin, flat, slightly expanded tendons into the sclerotic coat of the eyeball, six to eight millimeters (one-fourth to one-third of an inch) from the margin of the cornea.

ACTION.—The actions of the recti and oblique muscles of the orbit are somewhat complex, as almost every movement of the eyeball is performed by two or more muscles. It should be noted that the movements of the eyeball are bilateral, the medial rotation of one eye being accompanied by the lateral rotation of the other. It must also be noted that the globe cannot be moved away from its position, in which it is closely retained by the capsule of Tenon (*fascia bulbi*) and the attachments of the orbital fascia, forward movement being prevented by the recti muscles. The only movements of the eyeball are rotation around any axis of the globe, limited by the attachments of the orbital fascia lying between the muscles and the adjacent structures, such as the orbital periosteum and the palpebral fascia. These movements are more easily understood if only the motion of the cornea is considered.

Adduction of the cornea, as already indicated, is performed by the medial rectus muscle, and abduction of the cornea by the lateral rectus muscle and the two oblique muscles.

Elevation of the cornea, as in looking directly upward, is performed by the superior rectus muscle, the inferior oblique muscle preventing adduction of the cornea and its rotation medialward. Rotation of the cornea medialward is the movement of the uppermost portion of the cornea medialward and downward.

Depression of the cornea is performed by the inferior rectus muscle, the superior oblique muscle preventing adduction of the cornea and its rotation lateralward.

Rotation of the cornea medialward is performed by the superior rectus and the superior oblique muscles, and rotation of the cornea lateralward, by the inferior rectus and the inferior oblique muscles.

Movement of the cornea in an oblique direction such as, upward and lateralward, is performed chiefly by the superior rectus and lateral rectus muscles.

Excessive action of the various muscles is prevented by the attachments of the anterior lamella of the orbital fascia.

Strabismus, or deviation of the sagittal axis of one eyeball from its normal position, occurs either from hyperactivity of one or more muscles or from hypo-activity of the opposing muscles. This condition is more commonly caused by defective refraction in the affected eye or unequal refraction in the two eyes. The first requisite is to correct the error in refraction, and as a last resort the tendon or tendons of the hyperactive muscle or muscles may be divided or the tendon of the hypo-active muscle may be advanced to a new position. After division of the tendon, extreme retraction of the muscle is prevented by the anterior lamella of the orbital fascia; or the muscle may be sutured in its new position. The usual deformity is an internal, or convergent, strabismus. Paralysis of one or more ocular muscles may occur. If a single muscle is affected it is apt to be the superior oblique or the lateral rectus, since these have separate innervations.

DISSECTION.—The temporo-malar (*zygomatic*) nerve is the last structure to be dissected. The orbital contents must be removed completely, and the nerve will be found in a pad of fat in the retiring angle between the inferior and lateral orbital walls.

The **temporo-malar, or orbital (zygomatic), nerve** arises from the superior maxillary (*maxillary*) nerve in the spheno-maxillary (*pterygo-palatine*) fossa, and reaches the orbit by passing through the spheno-maxillary (*inferior orbital*) fissure. It then divides into two branches, temporal (*zygomatico-temporal*) and malar (*zygomatico-facial*).

The **temporal branch (zygomatico-temporal)** forms a loop of communication with the lacrimal nerve, and then runs beneath the orbital periosteum to reach the spheno-malar (*zygomatic*) foramen. Having traversed this foramen and entered the temporal fossa, it pierces the deep layer of the temporal fascia. It takes a short course upward between the two layers of the temporal fascia, and pierces its superficial layer. It communicates with the temporal branch of the facial nerve, and is distributed to the skin of the anterior temporal region.

The **malar (zygomatico-facial) branch** runs forward in the orbital fat, and leaves the orbit by passing through the malar (*zygomatic*) foramen. It communicates with the malar (*zygomatic*) branch of the facial nerve and supplies the skin of the cheek.

PLATE C.

Tendo oculi

Lacrimal sac

Lacrimal canaliculus

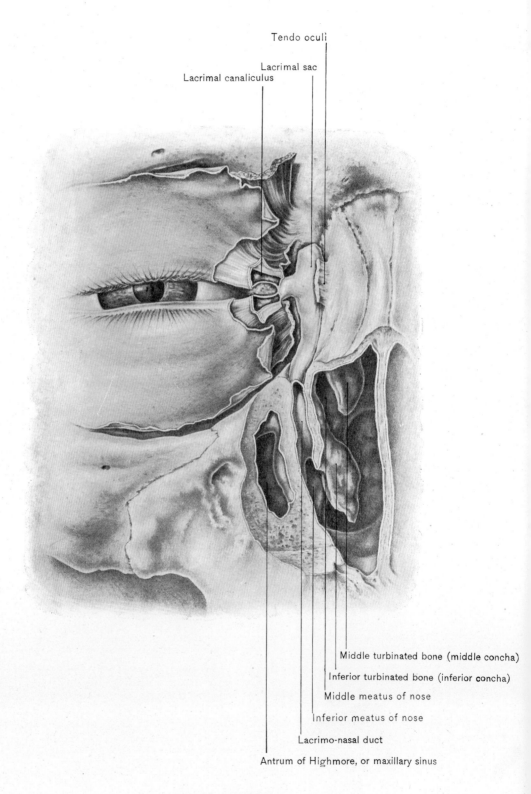

Middle turbinated bone (middle concha)

Inferior turbinated bone (inferior concha)

Middle meatus of nose

Inferior meatus of nose

Lacrimo-nasal duct

Antrum of Highmore, or maxillary sinus

LACRIMAL APPARATUS.

PLATE CI.

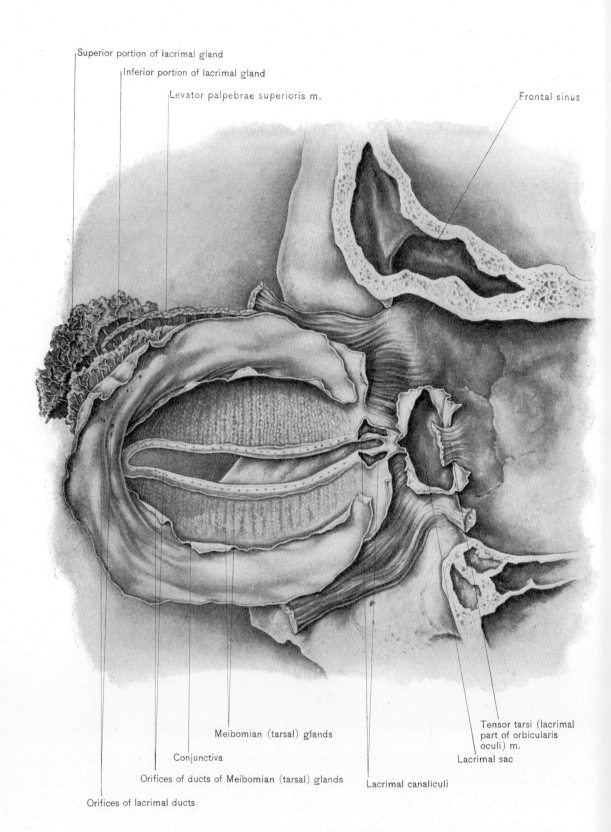

Superior portion of lacrimal gland

Inferior portion of lacrimal gland

Levator palpebrae superioris m.

Frontal sinus

Tensor tarsi (lacrimal
part of orbicularis
oculi) m.

Meibomian (tarsal) glands

Lacrimal sac

Conjunctiva

Lacrimal canaliculi

Orifices of ducts of Meibomian (tarsal) glands

Orifices of lacrimal ducts

MEIBOMIAN (TARSAL) GLANDS AND LACRIMAL APPARATUS.

PLATE CII.

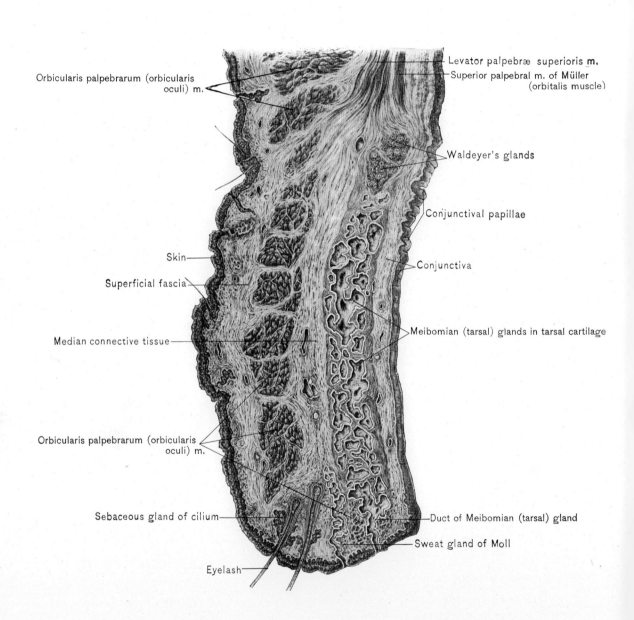

Levator palpebræ superioris **m.**

Superior palpebral m. of Müller (orbitalis muscle)

Orbicularis palpebrarum (orbicularis oculi) m.

Waldeyer's glands

Conjunctival papillae

Skin

Superficial fascia

Conjunctiva

Median connective tissue

Meibomian (tarsal) glands in tarsal cartilage

Orbicularis palpebrarum (orbicularis oculi) m.

Sebaceous gland of cilium

Duct of Meibomian (tarsal) gland

Sweat gland of Moll

Eyelash

SAGITTAL SECTION OF UPPER EYELID.

The **lymphatics of the orbit** pass through the spheno-maxillary (*inferior orbital*) fissure to the internal maxillary (*deep facial*) and deep parotid lymph glands.

THE LACRIMAL APPARATUS (Plates C; CI)

DISSECTION.—Insert slender probes into the puncta lacrimalia and lacrimal canaliculi, and open the latter as far as the lacrimal sacs.

The **lacrimal punctum** occupies the margin of the eyelid near the medial extremity.

The **lacrimal canaliculi** are two narrow canals, one in each eyelid, extending from the lacrimal punctum to the lacrimal sac. For a short distance from the lacrimal punctum the course of each canaliculus is vertically away from the margin of the lid, then turning abruptly, it forms a right angle, passes medially, and pierces the medial division of the tendo oculi (*medial palpebral ligament*) to reach the lacrimal sac. Before entering the lacrimal sac the lacrimal canaliculi of the upper and lower lids frequently join and open into the sac by a common orifice. In passing a probe into the lacrimal canaliculi their angular course should be remembered. Occasionally, the canaliculi do not unite but separately enter a diverticulum of the sac, known as the *sinus of Maier*.

DISSECTION.—Next make a vertical section through the upper and the lower eyelids to demonstrate their several layers of tissue.

The **eyelids** (Plate CII) are composed of: skin, superficial fascia, the orbicularis palpebrarum (*orbicularis oculi*) muscle, areolar tissue, palpebral ligaments, the orbito-tarsal ligament, or palpebral fascia, tarsal cartilage, Meibomian (*tarsal*) glands, conjunctiva, vessels, nerves, and lymph vessels. The upper eyelid also contains the aponeurosis of the levator palpebræ superioris muscle. The most superficial layer is the skin; the second layer is the superficial fascia, which contains no fat in this location; the third layer is composed of delicate areolar tissue; in the fourth layer are the tarsal cartilage, the palpebral fascia, or orbito-tarsal ligament, the palpebral ligaments, the Meibomian (*tarsal*) glands, and in the upper lid the aponeurosis of the levator palpebræ superioris muscle; the fifth layer is composed of conjunctiva and subconjunctival tissue. The eyelids are described on p. 239.

DISSECTION.—Open the lacrimal sac, and, after passing a probe through the lacrimo-nasal duct, saw away the anterior wall of that duct.

The **lacrimal sac** is the upper, dilated end of the lacrimo-nasal duct, and rests in the lacrimal groove, a depression in the lower anterior portion of the medial wall of the orbit. The lacrimal sac is invested by a fibrous capsule, which is attached to the margins of the lacrimal groove, and is continuous with the orbital periosteum. It is lined with mucous membrane, which is continuous with that of the lacrimal canaliculi and the lacrimo-nasal duct. The mucous membrane is, in turn, attached by loose, submucous tissue to the fibrous capsule.

The **lacrimo-nasal, nasal,** or **lacrimal (naso-lacrimal) duct,** which is the lower portion of the tear passage, extends from the lacrimal sac to the uppermost part of the anterior portion of the inferior meatus of the nose. It varies from twelve to twenty-four millimeters in length. It is directed downward and slightly backward and laterally. Its course is indicated by a line drawn from the anterior edge of the first upper molar tooth to the medial canthus of the eye. Its walls are formed by the superior maxillary (*maxillary*), lacrimal, and inferior turbinated bones (*inferior conchæ*), and are lined by mucous membrane continuous with that of the nose and lacrimal sac, the sac and the duct forming the **lacrimal (naso-lacrimal) canal.** The nasal orifice of the duct is guarded by a valvular flap of mucous membrane, the *valves of Hasner (plica lacrimalis).*

THE EYEBALL

The **eyeball** is a globular body, so situated in the anterior portion of the orbital fossa as to be protected by the orbital margins from injury by large objects. It is situated nearer the lateral than the nasal wall and nearer the superior than the inferior wall. It is freely movable around its axes, so that objects may be seen without appreciable muscular effort. These axes are practically parallel when both eyes are fixed on a distant object. When looked at in cross section it will be seen that the eyeball is composed of the parts of two spheres: a smaller anterior, or corneal, portion, and a larger posterior, or scleral, portion.

The **mobility of the eyeball** is permitted by the relation existing between the globe and the capsule of Tenon (*fascia bulbi*) (described with the orbit, at p. 406). The eyeball and capsule of Tenon (*fascia bulbi*) form a ball-and-socket joint. Backward, lateral, vertical, and oblique movements of the eyeball *en masse* are prevented by the attachments of the orbital fascia to the orbital margins and the palpebral fascia, and forward movement of the organ is checked by the recti muscles; therefore, the only movements of the eyeball are those of rotation around its axes. Excessive rotation, as already stated, is prevented by the attachments of the anterior lamella of the orbital fascia and its thickened portions, designated check ligaments.

Exophthalmos, or protrusion of the eyeball from the orbit, may be caused by tumors or foreign bodies in the orbit, myopia, orbital abscess, cavernous sinus thrombosis, or enlargement of the eyeball by disease. It sometimes exists slightly after tenotomy of one of the recti muscles; it is one of the symptoms of exophthalmic goiter.

Enophthalmos, or sinking of the eyeball, occurs after partial absorption of the orbital fat in wasting disease, and is associated with general emaciation. Here it is more apparent than real, but a true enophthalmos may result from a paralysis of the orbitalis (Müller's) muscle or from an injury to Tenon's capsule (*fascia bulbi*) and the check ligaments.

Being a globular body, the eyeball has an **anterior pole,** located at the center of the cornea, and a **posterior pole,** at the center of the posterior segment of the eye, which is the portion covered by the sclera. It also has an **equator,** midway between the two poles; an **axis,** or **sagittal diameter,** connecting the poles; a **vertical** and a **transverse diameter** at the equator. It is not quite spherical, because the cornea is a segment of a smaller sphere, and projects forward like a watch-glass, increasing the sagittal diameter, or axis; the transverse is slightly greater than the vertical diameter. The axis, or sagittal diameter, of the adult eye measures about twenty-four and a half millimeters; the transverse equatorial diameter, about twenty-four millimeters, and the vertical equatorial diameter, about twenty-three and a half millimeters. From these measurements it will be seen that the eyeball is slightly elongated from behind forward, and compressed from above downward. The axes of the two eyeballs are parallel with each other, although the axes of the two orbits are divergent anteriorly.

DISSECTION.—By the time the orbit has been dissected, the human eyeball will be so far decomposed that it cannot be easily or profitably dissected. Fortunately, an adequate substitute is found in the eye of the pig, the sheep, or the bullock. Of these, the pig's eye corresponds more nearly in size to the human eye; but the bullock's eye, on account of its greater size, is more easily dissected. At least a half dozen bullocks' eyes should be procured before the dissection is begun. The globe must be thoroughly cleaned down to the sclera. The best way to accomplish this is as follows: with scissors and forceps make a circular incision through the conjunctiva close to, and parallel with the margin of the cornea. The conjunctiva, the capsule of Tenon (*fascia bulbi*), the fat, the fascia, and the muscles are then gradually worked free from the sclera from before backward, as far as the point of entrance of the optic nerve. When about half way back, the *venæ vorticosæ* will be seen emerging; and when near the optic nerve, the circle around it, formed by the *posterior ciliary arteries* and the *ciliary nerves,* will be noticed.

The **Conjunctiva** is a mucous membrane covering the anterior surface of the eyeball and the posterior surface of the eyelids. It consists of a parietal layer, the palpebral portion, which lines the eyelids, and of a visceral layer, the ocular portion, which covers the anterior third of the eyeball. The visceral layer is subdivided into a sclerotic and a corneal portion.

The **palpebral portion of the conjunctiva** has been described with the eyelids under the Dissection of the Face, at p. 446.

The **sclerotic portion of the conjunctiva** is loosely adherent, except at the margin of the cornea. It contains small blood-vessels, which are derived from the palpebral vessels, branches of the lacrimal, infra-orbital, supra-orbital, and frontal vessels, which are not perceptible under normal conditions, but when congested the conjunctival vessels are distinguished from the anterior ciliary vessels by the fact that the former move with the conjunctiva, while the latter are fixed in the sclera and remain stationary. The lax submucous tissue which connects the conjunctiva with the sclera permits the surgeon to slide flaps of conjunctiva. Its laxity accounts for the occurrence of subconjunctival hemorrhages after sudden, severe, muscular effort, as in paroxysms of whooping cough. Hemorrhages, if associated with traumatism about the head, should arouse suspicion, as they may result from fracture of the anterior fossa of the skull with leakage of blood into the orbit.

The **corneal portion of the conjunctiva** consists of layers of epithelial cells, and forms the anterior layer of the cornea. It is closely adherent, perfectly transparent, and gives the cornea its mirror-like characteristics. It contains no blood-vessels.

Extensive destruction of the conjunctiva may be produced by caustics accidentally introduced between the eyelids and the eyeball. This more frequently occurs under the lower eyelid, on account of its position. The lid may adhere to the globe, causing **symblepharon**; or cicatricial contraction from chronic conjunctivitis or other causes may produce **entropion,** or inversion of the eyelid and eyelashes. Adherence of the two raw surfaces may be prevented by sliding a bridge of conjunctiva from above the cornea and placing it upon the raw surface below. In **purulent ophthalmia,** or purulent conjunctivitis, which is usually due to gonococcic infection of the conjunctiva, involvement of the cornea may lead to permanent blindness. *Ophthalmia neonatorum* is the most common form of this infection.

Coats and Refracting Media of the Eye.—The eyeball contains three superimposed coats, inclosing three refracting media, or so-called humors. The coats, named from without inward are: a fibrous, a vascular, and a nervous coat. The refracting media, enumerated from before backward are: the aqueous humor, the crystalline lens, and the vitreous humor.

The **Fibrous Coat** is composed of two portions: a posterior opaque portion, the sclera, and an anterior, transparent portion, the cornea. (Plate CIII.)

PLATE CIII.

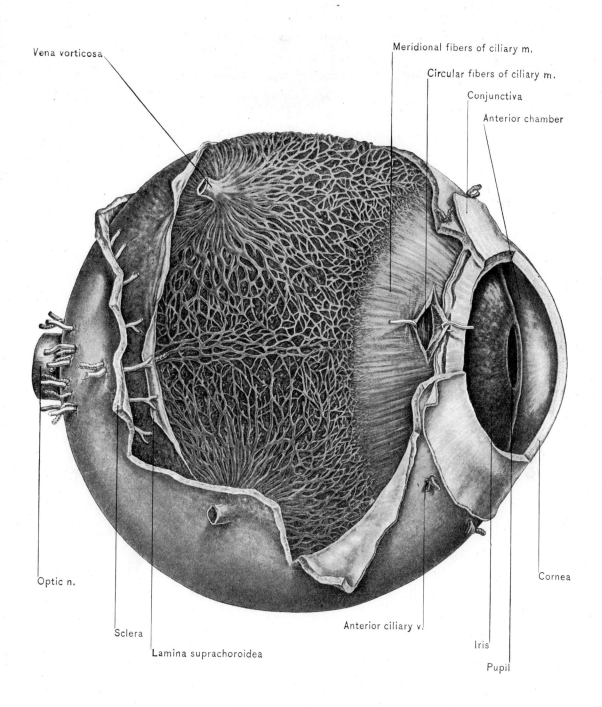

Vena vorticosa

Meridional fibers of ciliary m.

Circular fibers of ciliary m.

Conjunctiva

Anterior chamber

Optic n.

Sclera

Lamina suprachoroidea

Anterior ciliary v.

Iris

Pupil

Cornea

EXTERNAL AND MIDDLE COATS OF THE EYEBALL.

PLATE CIV.

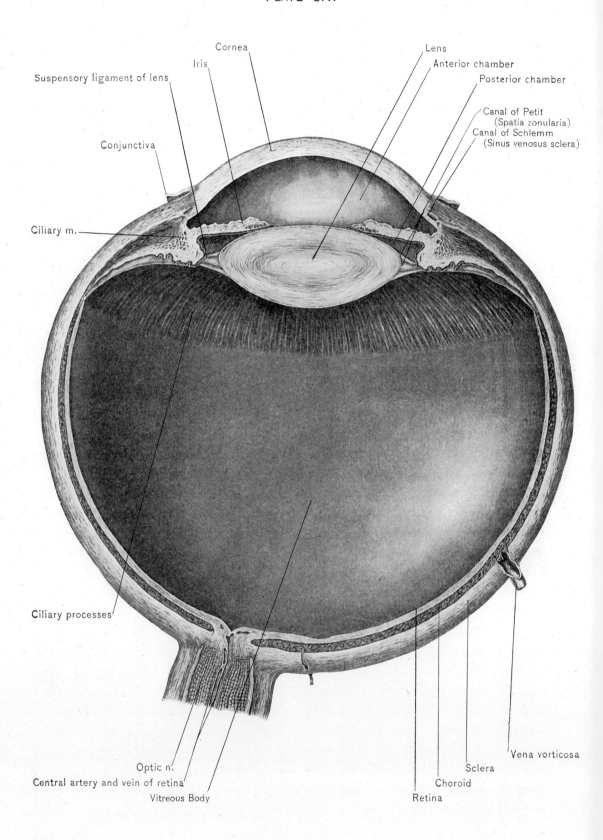

Cornea

Lens

Iris

Anterior chamber

Suspensory ligament of lens

Posterior chamber

Canal of Petit
(Spatia zonularia)

Canal of Schlemm
(Sinus venosus sclera)

Conjunctiva

Ciliary m.

Ciliary processes

Optic n.

Central artery and vein of retina

Vitreous Body

Vena vorticosa

Sclera

Choroid

Retina

MERIDIONAL SECTION OF EYE.

DISSECTION.—In order to observe all parts of the sclerotic coat clearly, detach it from the underlying tissues and remove it. To do this make an incision midway between the center of the cornea (the anterior pole) and the corresponding posterior point (the posterior pole). With a sharp knife make a short cut just deep enough to expose the black, underlying choroid; a pair of scissors with delicate blades and sharp points should then be used to complete the equatorial incision. With the handle of the scalpel the halves of the sclerotic coat should be separated from the subjacent tissues, as one removes the skin of an orange. At only two points will any difficulty be met. One is at the entrance of the optic nerve, where it is necessary to cut off the optic nerve close to the choroid; the other point is anteriorly, where the ciliary body is attached to the sclera. By the use of slight force this attachment can be torn with the forceps, and the anterior half, composed of the sclera and the cornea, removed entire. This results in escape of the aqueous humor. The remainder of the globe should be laid aside in diluted alcohol until required for further study.

The **sclera**, or **sclerotic coat** (Plate CIV), incloses the posterior five-sixths of the eyeball, the remaining anterior one-sixth of its wall being completed by the cornea. It is incomplete posteriorly at the entrance of the optic nerve, the opening, the *optic foramen*, being partially filled by a layer of sclerotic tissue, the *lamina cribrosa sclerae*. The sclera is white, opaque, and tough, and maintains the normal conformation of the globe. It consists of interlacing bundles of white, fibrous connective tissue. It is thickest posteriorly, and thinnest just behind the insertions of the recti muscles, about six to eight millimeters (one-fourth to one-third of an inch) from the cornea, where it is sometimes ruptured in cases of injury to the eyeball. Between the cornea and the insertions of the tendons of the recti muscles it again becomes thicker, on account of its reinforcement by fibers from those tendons. In disease of the eye, such as glaucoma, in which there is increased intra-ocular tension, compression of the ciliary nerves against the unyielding sclerotic coat causes intense pain.

At its anterior margin the sclerotic coat is directly continuous with the cornea, and the slight groove at this point is called the *scleral sulcus*. About six millimeters (one-fourth of an inch) behind the sclero-corneal junction the sclerotic coat receives the insertions of the rectus muscles. At this point it also receives and transmits the anterior ciliary vessels, which form a ring around the cornea; congestion of these vessels is evident in iritis. In the sclera, just behind the sclero-corneal junction, is the *sinus venosus sclerae*, or the *canal of Schlemm*, a circular blood channel surrounding the margin of the cornea. This canal transmits venous blood, and is in close relation with certain lymph spaces, the *spaces of Fontana (spatia anguli iridis)*, in the pectinate ligament of the iris. In conjunction with the spaces of Fontana (*spatia anguli iridis*) the canal of Schlemm (*sinus venosus scleræ*), by absorbing the excess of aqueous humor, is supposed to maintain the normal intra-ocular tension.

The *lamina cribrosa* is in the posterior portion of the sclera, and is the point of entrance of the optic nerve, whose dural and pial investments blend with the sclera. Minute openings which form a circle around the lamina cribrosa transmit the posterior ciliary vessels and ciliary nerves. The point of entrance of the optic nerve is not at the posterior pole or in the visual axis of the eye, but lies about two and a half millimeters (one-tenth of an inch) to its nasal side and slightly below it. As this nerve passes through the sclera it is constricted, and instead of passing as a compact bundle, it is broken up into fasciculi which separately pierce the fibrous lamina cribrosa. The lamina has an opening in the center larger than the perforations produced by the individual nerve bundles; this is called the *porus opticus*, and transmits the central artery of the retina.

Except at the entrance of the optic nerve and at the sclero-corneal junction, the sclerotic is but feebly attached to the subjacent vascular coat. Its innermost layer which, on account of its deep color, is called the *lamina fusca*, is in relation with the vascular coat, to which it is attached by a layer of loose connective tissue, the *lamina suprachoroidea*.

The **cornea** is the circular anterior window of the eyeball, and comprises about one-sixth of the circumference of the globe. It is perfectly transparent, and is somewhat thinner at its center than at its periphery. Its transparency is lost in certain diseases, such as interstitial keratitis, which is frequently caused by syphilis. It is more convex than the remainder of the eyeball, and consequently forms part of a sphere smaller than the sclera, and hence projects further than the latter. The dissector can readily prove this fact by closing his own eye and moving the loose skin of the upper lid over the globe with his finger. The cornea is part of the fibrous coat of the eye, and at its periphery is continuous with the sclera. Owing to the fact that the transition of the sclera into the cornea occurs first on the inner aspect of the former, the sclera seems to overlap the cornea; thus the margin of the cornea becomes beveled on its external aspect and the sclera on its internal aspect. The fact that this apparent overlapping is greater above and below than at the sides, accounts for the fact that the transverse diameter of the cornea is slightly greater than the vertical.

The cornea being convex, assists in bringing rays of light to a focus upon the retina. If the convexity of the cornea is excessive, the rays are brought to a focus before reaching the retina, producing **myopia,** or **near-sightedness.** If the cornea is insufficiently convex, the rays reach the retina before being collected to a focus, producing **hypermetropia,** or **far-sightedness.** When the curvature of the cornea is irregular, the rays of light are not regularly brought to a focus, the resulting error of refraction being known as **astigmatism,** which may also be produced by irregular refraction in the lens.

The cornea consists of five layers which from without inward are: the anterior epithelium, the anterior limiting membrane (*anterior elastic lamina*), the substantia propria, the posterior limiting membrane (*posterior elastic lamina*), and the posterior endothelium.

The *anterior epithelium* is continuous with the epithelial covering of the adjacent conjunctival sclera.

The *anterior limiting membrane,* situated immediately below the epithelium, may be considered as a differentiation of the anterior part of the substantia propria.

The *substantia propria* constitutes the main portion of the sclera, and is composed of numerous laminæ of modified connective tissue with a few elastic fibers, between which are freely anastomosing lymph channels, through which it is nourished. Like the other layers of the cornea, it contains no blood-vessels. The lymph vessels, or channels, end in loops at its periphery. In interstitial keratitis the laminæ are affected, and effusion into the lymph channels causes haziness and loss of transparency of the cornea.

The *posterior limiting membrane* is not so firmly united to the substantia propria as the anterior limiting membrane. At the sclero-corneal junction it splits into fibers which interlace and form the pectinate ligament of the iris. The spaces between these interlacing fibers are the spaces of Fontana (*spatia anguli iridis*). The *posterior endothelium* covers the inner surface of the posterior limiting membrane. This layer is reflected onto the anterior surface of the iris.

Ulcers and wounds of the cornea, as a rule, heal readily, notwithstanding the absence of blood-vessels. But ulcers may perforate the cornea and allow the aqueous humor to escape, and with the stream of the escaping aqueous humor the pupillary margin of the iris may be prolapsed through the opening in the cornea. Scars resulting from ulcers or wounds of the cornea may produce an opacity resembling a small puff of smoke, *nebula,* or a pearly white opacity, known as *leukoma.* These opacities, if situated at the center of the cornea, interfere with the passage of light to the most sensitive portion of the retina, making it necessary to form an artificial pupil, or if the leukoma is excessively large, the sight of the eye may be lost.

In elderly persons there is frequently seen an opacity of the corneal tissue near the margin of the cornea; this opacity usually begins at the upper part of the cornea, and extends to its lower part; subsequently, the extremities of the two hazy crescents meet, and a complete **arcus senilis** results. This condition is due to fatty or hyaline degeneration of the corneal tissue, probably the result of defective vascular supply.

In **pannus** the cornea appears to contain blood-vessels. Through irritation from granular lids, trachoma, or inverted eyelashes, blood-vessels grow into the corneal conjunctiva, and later may enter the corneal tissue.

Staphyloma of the cornea is a bulging forward of a corneal scar and adherent iris. It is produced by increased intra-ocular tension pushing forward the iris and even the lens against a weakened cornea, and causing repulsive disfigurement.

A **conical cornea** is thin, protrudes further forward than normally, and retains its transparency. As a result, vision is imperfect.

Blood Supply.—The blood supply of the cornea is indirectly derived from the anterior ciliary and the long posterior ciliary arteries. No blood-vessels are found in the cornea, nutrition being supplied by imbibition of lymph into the lymph channels of the cornea.

Nerve Supply.—The cornea receives a rich nerve supply from the ciliary nerves. Its nerves are merely axis cylinders, and, therefore, do not affect its transparency.

The pectinate ligament of the iris.—At the corneal margin the fourth layer, the posterior limiting membrane of the cornea, breaks up into fibrillæ, some of which form the attachment of the ciliary muscles, others run into the base of the iris. These fibrillæ comprise the pectinate ligament of the iris, and bridge over the angle between the cornea and the base of the iris. This ligament contains lymph spaces, the *spaces of Fontana* (*spatia anguli iridis*), which communicate, on the one hand, with the anterior chamber of the eye and, on the other, with the canal of Schlemm (*sinus venosus scleræ*).

The **Vascular Coat,** or the uveal tract, the middle coat of the eye, has been exposed throughout by the previous dissection. It consists of three portions: the iris anteriorly, next the ciliary body, which lies behind the iris, and posteriorly, the choroid.

The **iris,** the anterior portion of the middle tunic, is a perforated circular curtain interposed between the lens and the cornea. It is attached only at its margin, where it is joined to the cornea, anteriorly, by means of the pectinate ligament of the iris, and posteriorly, by the ciliary body. These attachments are not very strong; consequently, injuries to the eye may cause the iris to be torn away from the cornea and the ciliary body without damage to either of these two structures. It is contractile and expansile, and floats in the clear aqueous humor, separating the anterior chamber of the eyeball from the posterior chamber; the two chambers communicate with each other through the central opening of the iris, called the **pupil.** In the fetus the pupil is closed by the pupillary membrane, which disappears before birth. By change in size of the pupil the iris regulates the amount of light admitted to the interior of the eye. Both contraction and dilatation of the pupil are active processes, the presence of circular and radiating muscle fibers having been demonstrated. Near the pupil the posterior surface of the iris is in contact with the lens, hence in iritis the iris may adhere to the lens, producing **posterior synechia**; or the iris may adhere to the cornea, resulting in **anterior synechia**.

The iris receives much support from contact with the lens; consequently, when the lens is dislocated posteriorly, or after cataract operations, the iris may be tremulous through lack of support.

The **Argyll Robertson pupil** is one which does not react directly or indirectly to stimulation by light, but retains its power of accommodation for distance. It is a diagnostic sign in locomotor ataxia, and has been observed in cerebral syphilis, general paralysis of the insane, and poisoning by carbon bisulphid.

The **color** of the iris varies in different individuals, and is largely dependent on the amount and position of its pigment. In blue eyes the stroma of the iris is entirely free from pigment, the latter being confined to the posterior pigment layer, from which position it is seen through the superimposed strata of the iris. In darker eyes the stroma cells of the iris also acquire pigment; this is small in amount in light gray eyes, greater in brown eyes, while in very dark eyes the colored particles are very numerous, and sometimes appear as almost continuous pigmented areas; in the albino, on the other hand, even the retinal portion of the iris is devoid of pigment. The color of the iris may be greatly altered during inflammation of that structure, through effusion into the tissues of the iris. The swelling thus produced causes sluggish movement of the iris and encroachment upon the pupil.

Blood Supply.—From the ciliary vessels; consequently, iritis is usually associated with choroiditis.

Nerve Supply.—The nerve supply of the iris is derived from two sources: the sphincter of the pupil is innervated by the oculomotor, or third, nerve through the short ciliary nerves, while the dilator muscle fibers are innervated by the cervical sympathetic through the long ciliary branches.

The path for the iris reflex (that is, the contraction and dilatation of the pupil induced by variations in the amount of light falling into the eye) is along the optic nerve and tract to the geniculate body, or perhaps the anterior pair of corpora quadrigemina, thence to the nucleus of the oculomotor, along the latter nerve to the ciliary ganglion, and then through the ciliary nerves to the iris. Interference with this path by lesions in the optic nerves or tracts or in the central nervous system leads to disturbances which the clinician utilizes for diagnostic purposes.

Coloboma, or a fissure of the iris, is a common congenital defect; it is usually situated below the pupil, and is due to persistence of the choroid cleft of the embryo.

Aniridia (Irideremia), or congenital absence of the iris, is a rare defect; it is usually bilateral.

The **ciliary body,** the intermediate portion of the vasular tunic, or uveal tract, is composed of three portions: the ciliary muscle, the choroid portion, or ciliary processes, and the ciliary ring, or orbicularis ciliaris. The ciliary body extends from the posterior, or ciliary, margin of the iris to a point opposite the ora serrata, or the anterior limit of the visual part of the retina. In meridional sections of the eyeball it is triangular. Laterally, the triangle is formed by the ciliary muscle, and is in contact with the sclera; the posteromedial side is directed toward the vitreous chamber of the eyeball, and contains the ciliary processes; the anterior side is directed toward the aqueous chamber, and gives attachment to the margin of the iris at about its middle. The ciliary body is well supplied with branches from the ciliary vessels and nerves. For branches of the ciliary ganglion see the the nerve-supply of the iris at p. 455. Inflammation spreads rapidly from the ciliary body to the iris, the choroid, the retina, and the cornea. It is called the dangerous area of the eye, because traumatic inflammation of the ciliary body in one eye may be followed by sympathetic ophthalmia beginning in the ciliary body of the other eye. This is supposed to be due to the rich nerve supply of that region.

The **ciliary muscle** (Plates CV; CVI) forms a conspicuous white band between the choroid and the iris, and behind the sclero-corneal junction. It bears on its inner surface the ciliary processes. In cross section of the ciliary body or in longitudinal section of the eyeball, it appears as a triangular band of muscle fibers. The shorter anterior side of the triangle extends from the sclero-corneal junction toward the ciliary processes, and at the angle of junction of the other two sides it joins the anterior margin of the choroid. It consists of fasciculi of muscle tissue, the interstices of which are filled with similar strands of connective tissue. The muscle tissue, like all similar structures in the eyeball, is composed of involuntary muscle fibers arranged in two sets, meridional and circular. The *meridional,* or *longitudinal, fibers (tensor choroidea), arise* from the sclera and the sclero-corneal junction, pass backward, and are *inserted* into the choroid opposite the ciliary processes. The *circular fibers,* or ring muscle of Müller, are placed internal to the meridional fibers in the ciliary body, and encircle the outer, or attached, margin of the iris.

BLOOD SUPPLY.—The ciliary muscle and ciliary body are supplied with blood from the long posterior ciliary and the anterior ciliary anteries.

PLATE CV.

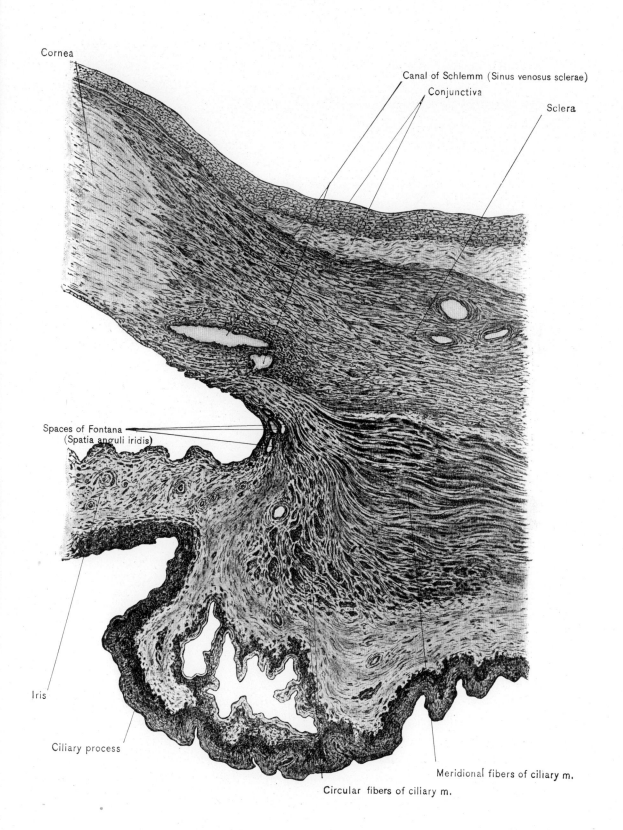

Cornea

Canal of Schlemm (Sinus venosus sclerae)

Conjunctiva

Sclera

Spaces of Fontana
(Spatia anguli iridis)

Iris

Ciliary process

Meridional fibers of ciliary m.

Circular fibers of ciliary m.

MERIDIONAL SECTION OF CILIARY REGION OF EYEBALL.

PLATE CVI.

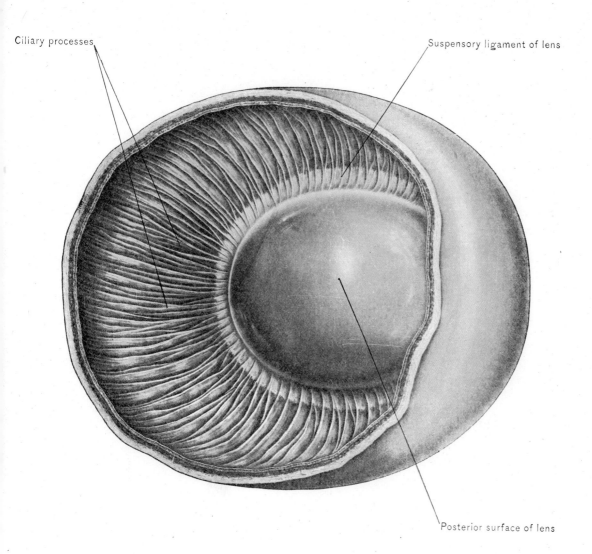

Ciliary processes

Suspensory ligament of lens

Posterior surface of lens

CILIARY REGION (FROM LION'S EYE IN MUSEUM OF UNIVERSITY OF PENNSYLVANIA).

Nerve Supply.—From the long and short ciliary nerves.

Action.—The ciliary muscle possesses the function of accommodation, and permits variation in the degree of convexity of the lens to enable the rays of light to reach a focus on the retina. As the ciliary muscle contracts it pulls the ciliary processes forward and relaxes the suspensory ligament of the lens; lessened tension upon this ligament relaxes the capsule of the lens, and allows the anterior surface of the lens to bulge forward. In the hyperopic, or far-sighted, eye, in which the anteroposterior axis of the eyeball is too long, the ciliary muscle is overworked in endeavoring to bring the rays of light from near objects to a focus upon the retina; consequently, in hypermetropia the ciliary muscle, and especially the ring muscle of Müller, is hypertrophied. After a severe illness, or after frequent and long-continued periods of reading, this muscle is unable to perform the required amount of work, and the hypermetropic state ensues, which should be relieved by a convex lens. As the oculomotor nerve supplies the medial rectus as well as the ciliary muscle, and does not supply the lateral rectus muscle, convergent squint is frequently associated with hypermetropia. A properly selected convex lens removes the cause of the spasm of the medial rectus muscle, and the strabismus disappears.

Dissection.—Secure a fresh eye, and with a sharp, thin-bladed knife or a pair of scissors cut the globe in half slightly anterior to the equator. Scoop out the jelly-like vitreous, leaving intact the lens and its attachments. Place the bowl-like preparation thus produced in a shallow tray containing dilute alcohol, and wash out the pigment with a small camel's-hair brush. A clear posterior view of the ciliary processes will then be secured, another dissection being necessary in order to obtain an anterior view of the processes. The cornea may be removed by making a circular incision just anterior to the sclero-corneal junction. Four meridional incisions should be made through the sclera and carried backward to about six millimeters (one-quarter of an inch) from the posterior pole of the eye. The flaps thus formed should be pinned back, and the whole preparation placed in dilute alcohol held in a wax- or cork-lined tray. With delicate forceps and scissors the iris is then removed, when an anterior view of the ciliary processes may be had.

The **ciliary processes** are some seventy or eighty irregular projections from the internal surface of the ciliary body. They are longitudinal folds of the forward continuation of the choroid. Their broader extremities are directed forward and form a circle, the *corona ciliaris*, which gives attachment to the suspensory ligament of the lens. Toward the posterior part of the ciliary body they become less prominent and subdivide, the inner surface of the ciliary body here being almost smooth and forming the *orbicularis ciliaris*, or ciliary ring.

The ciliary processes are the most vascular portion of the eyeball; like the choroid, they are composed of connective-tissue stroma, pigment, and numerous blood-vessels. It is by osmosis from the blood-vessels of the eyeball that the aqueous humor is supposed to be replenished. As the iris and the anterior portion of the ciliary body are continuous and their blood-vessels are in free communication, iritis seldom exists without cyclitis; hence the resultant disease is called irido-cyclitis.

The **choroid proper** extends from the posterior termination of the ciliary body to the optic nerve, by which it is pierced. Like the sclera, it is found in the posterior portion of the globe, and consists mainly of blood-vessels, areolar tissue, and pigment. Externally, it is in relation with the sclerotic coat, to which it is connected by the lamina suprachoroidea; internally, it is adherent to the pigment layer of the retina.

It is composed of four layers: the lamina suprachoroidea, the choroid proper, which contains the larger vessels, the chorio-capillaris, and the membrana, or lamina, vitrea. Its outer layer, the *lamina suprachoroidea*, is in immediate contact with the sclera, and is composed of loose areolar, non-vascular tissue, containing pigment. This layer is so loosely connected with the lamina fusca of the sclera that after traumatism of the eye extensive hemorrhages may occur between the sclera and the choroid. The next layer is the *choroid stroma*, or *proper* tissue of the choroid, and contains large blood-vessels, the most conspicuous of which are the four *venæ vorticosæ*, each of which is formed by a number of veins converging at one point and forming a whorl. They are located at equidistant points along the equator of the eyeball, and to them the small veins converge, returning the blood from the whole uveal tract. The larger vessels are in the outer part of this layer, which is known as the lamina vasculosa. The *choriocapillaris* is the inner vascular layer, and is composed of capillary blood-vessels. Between this lamina and the lamina vasculosa is a network of fine elastic fibers, the intermediate stratum. The *membrana*, or *lamina*, *vitrea* (*lamina basalis*), the fourth, or internal, layer, is transparent and nearly structureless. It supports the retinal pigment, which usually adheres to it when the retina is removed.

The choroid contains so much pigment that it is one of the few structures affected by primary **melanotic sarcoma.**

The **ciliary nerves** (Plate CVII) have two sources of origin: the *long ciliary nerves* arise from the nasal branch of the ophthalmic nerve, and the *short ciliary nerves* spring from the lenticular (*ciliary*) ganglion. They pierce the sclera around the optic nerve, and pass forward between the sclera and the choroid; at the posterior part of the globe they groove the inner surface of the sclera and are intimately attached to it. They pass forward to the ciliary body,

PLATE CVII.

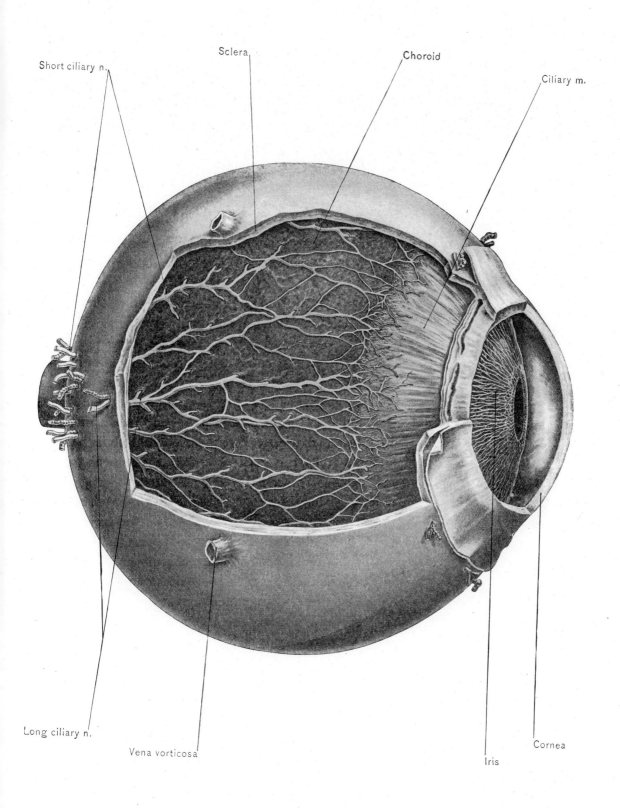

Short ciliary n.

Sclera

Choroid

Ciliary m.

Long ciliary n.

Vena vorticosa

Iris

Cornea

CILIARY NERVES.

PLATE CVIII.

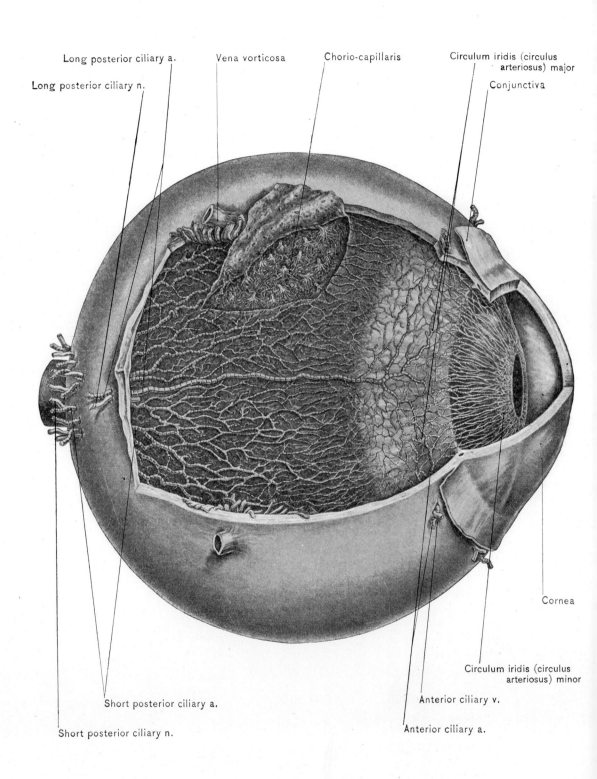

Long posterior ciliary a.

Long posterior ciliary n.

Vena vorticosa

Chorio-capillaris

Circulum iridis (circulus arteriosus) major

Conjunctiva

Cornea

Circulum iridis (circulus arteriosus) minor

Anterior ciliary v.

Anterior ciliary a.

Short posterior ciliary a.

Short posterior ciliary n.

CILIARY ARTERIES.

PLATE CIX.

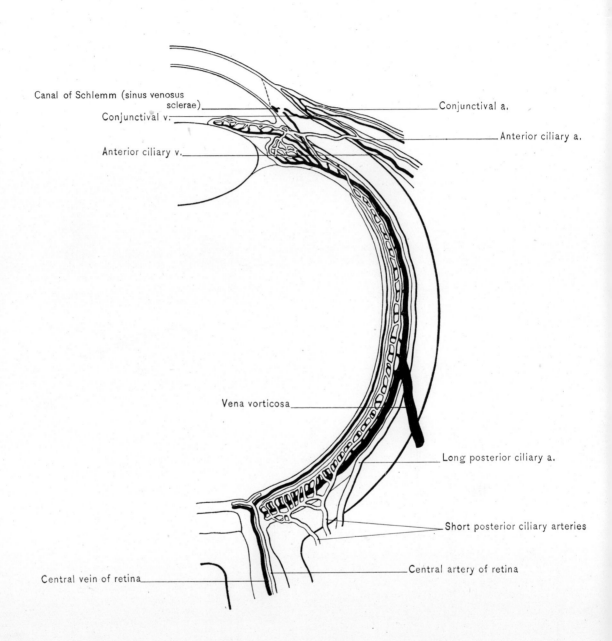

Canal of Schlemm (sinus venosus sclerae)

Conjunctival v.

Anterior ciliary v.

Conjunctival a.

Anterior ciliary a.

Vena vorticosa

Long posterior ciliary a.

Short posterior ciliary arteries

Central artery of retina

Central vein of retina

BLOOD-VESSELS OF EYEBALL (AFTER LEBER).

PLATE CX.

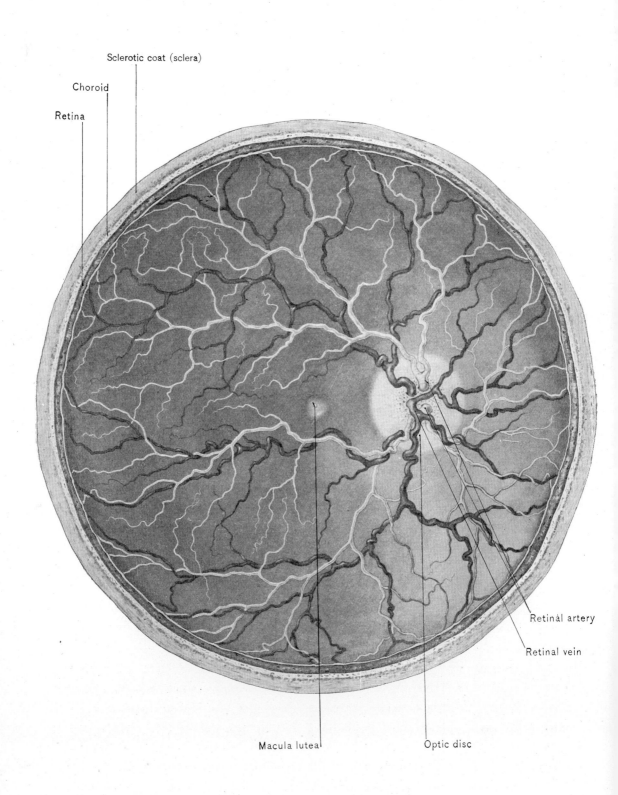

Sclerotic coat (sclera)

Choroid

Retina

Retinal artery

Retinal vein

Macula lutea

Optic disc

RETINA OF POSTERIOR HALF OF RIGHT EYEBALL (ENLARGED).

where they break up to form a plexus, from which fibers are distributed to the ciliary muscle, the iris, and the cornea. Compression of these nerves against the resisting sclera in increased intra-ocular tension, as in glaucoma, causes intense pain in the eyeball and anesthesia of the cornea.

The **ciliary arteries** consist of the short posterior, the long posterior, and the anterior. The *short posterior ciliary arteries*, twelve to twenty in number, pierce the sclera aronud the optic nerve, and are distributed to the choroid. The *long posterior ciliary arteries* pierce the sclera just external to the circle formed by the perforations for the short ciliary arteries, and run forward in the choroid. In the ciliary body around the attached margin of the iris they anastomose with the anterior ciliary arteries, to form the *circulum iridis major (circulus arteriosus major);* branches from this circle enter the iris, and at the outer margin of the sphincter muscle of the iris anastomose and form the *circulum iridis minor (circulus arteriosus minor)*. (Plate CVIII.)

The *anterior ciliary arteries* are usually eight in number, two arising from each of the arteries which supply the rectus muscles. They pierce the sclera near the sclero-corneal junction, and enter into the circulum iridis major (*circulus arteriosus major*).

The **ciliary veins** (Plate CIX) which have their origin in the middle coat of the eyeball are the venæ vorticosæ and the anterior ciliary veins. The *venæ vorticosæ* have already been described (p. 462). The *anterior ciliary veins* arise from small veins in the ciliary muscle, and pierce the sclera near the margin of the cornea, receiving veins connected with the canal of Schlemm (*sinus venosus sclerae*). They also receive conjunctival and episcleral veins, and empty into the veins which accompany the arteries to the rectus muscle.

DISSECTION.—The choroid, the ciliary body, and the iris should be carefully stripped from the eyeball in which they were exposed. This should be done under diluted alcohol. When completed, the retina will be seen. If a portion of the detached choroid is inspected, on its inner surface irregular black patches will be observed. These are fragments of the pigment layer of the retina, which have become detached on account of their firm adhesion to the lamina vitrea of the choroid.

The **Retina** (Plate CX), the third and innermost coat of the eye, is the nervous tunic. It is the end organ of the optic nerve specialized for the function of vision. Morphologically, it extends from the point of entrance of the optic nerve at the foramen sclerae to the free margin of the iris. It consists of three parts: the posterior portion is situated between the choroid and the vitreous body, and extends from the optic nerve entrance to the ciliary body, where the retina suddenly becomes thin along an irregular line, thus forming the **ora**

serrata. This posterior portion is the optic part, or **pars optica retinæ,** and terminates at the ora serrata. The next portion, the ciliary part, or the **pars ciliaris retinæ,** lines the inner surface of the ciliary body, extending as far forward as the insertion of the iris. The anterior portion lines the internal surface of the iris, and is called the **pars iridica retinæ.** The pars optica retinæ is the only part which has a visual function, the pars ciliaris and pars iridica retinæ being mainly continuations of the pigment layer beyond the ora serrata, at which the highly specialized layers of the retina suddenly diminish in thickness. (Plate CXI.)

When viewed from the interior, a circle, the *optic disc,* is seen at the point of entrance of the optic nerve. The optic disc is sometimes called the porus opticus, but this name should be applied only to the foramen in the lamina cribrosa traversed by the central artery of the retina. This disc lies two and a half millimeters (one-tenth of an inch) to the nasal side of the posterior pole of the eye. As this is the *blind spot* of the retina, it is placed outside of the direct line of vision. Exactly in the center of the retina, at the posterior pole, and in the direct line of vision, a small yellow spot, the *macula lutea,* is seen in a fresh eye; the depression in the center of the macula lutea is termed the *fovea centralis.* The macula lutea is the point at which vision is most acute. For that reason it is situated in a line with the centers of the lens, pupil, and cornea, so that it receives the rays of light brought to a focus by the lens. Rays from other points, passing through the lens, strike other portions of the pars optica retinæ and produce collateral vision, which is less distinct.

The retina is derived from the two layers of the optic cup, which is an extension of the anterior cerebral vesicle and is, therefore, ectodermic in origin. The outer layer of the cup remains as the pigment layer of the retina, while the inner layer gives rise to the remaining and more specialized portion of it. During life the inner layer is pink and transparent; but after death it becomes hazy and opaque.

BLOOD SUPPLY.—Partly from the arteria centralis retinæ, which can be seen entering the eye at the optic disc. It gives off an ascending and a descending branch, each of which bifurcates into a nasal and a temporal branch. Like the vessels of the brain, the lungs, etc., its branches are end arteries, not anastomosing in the substance of the retina, either with each other or with the ciliary arteries. A portion of the nourishment of the retina is derived from the posterior ciliary vessels, through the chorio-capillaris of the choroid.

The **retinal veins** converge to form two vessels which enter the optic nerve at the optic disc, and soon join to form one *vena centralis retinæ,* which pursues a course in the nerve corresponding to that of the artery.

DISSECTION.—The following method will be found the most satisfactory for studying the vitreous body and lens. The eyeball should be kept from one to three

PLATE CXI.

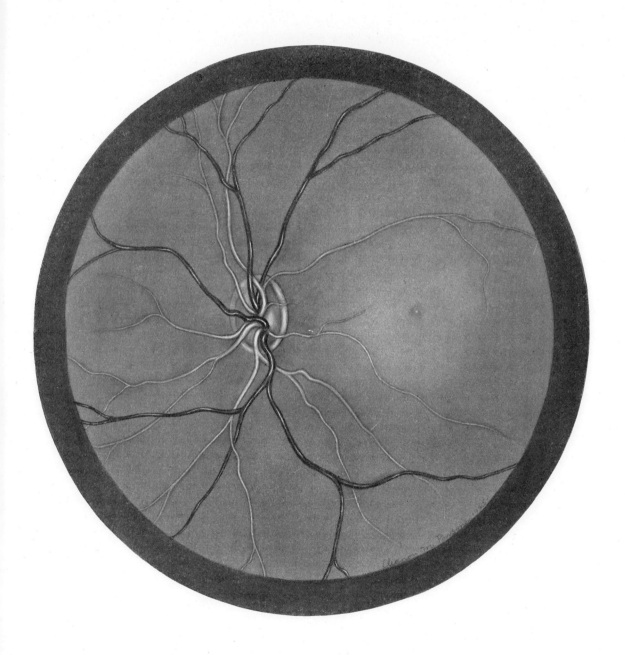

NORMAL FUNDUS OF LEFT EYE

days before being used.   Divide and turn back the three tunics at the equator. This should be carefully done over a vessel of diluted alcohol, into which the so-called "eye kernel," composed of the vitreous body and the lens, is allowed to fall.   The "eye kernel" is then placed in a strong picrocarmin solution for a few minutes, and when removed, it should be well washed.   By this method the hyaloid membrane, the lens capsule, and the zonule of Zinn (*zonula ciliaris*) are stained red.   By gently shaking the solution, the coloring matter will enter the hyaloid canal, which can thus be recognized.

The **vitreous body** is a soft, gelatinous, perfectly transparent substance, composed of semi-solid connective tissue.   It occupies the posterior cavity, or vitreous chamber, of the globe.   The *vitreous chamber* is bounded, posteriorly and laterally, by the retina, and anteriorly, by the lens and the zonule of Zinn (*zonula ciliaris*).   The vitreous body consists of the vitreous substance, inclosed by the **hyaloid membrane,** except anteriorly, where the vitreous substance comes into direct contact with the lens capsule, receiving the lens into a depression, the **patellar fossa** (*hyaloid fossa*) of the vitreous body.   It has an indistinctly reticulated structure, and may contain small corpuscular bodies which occasionally produce shadows upon the retina, the so-called **muscæ volitantes.** Running from the optic disc to the center of the posterior surface of the lens is a narrow canal, lined by a prolongation of the hyaloid membrane, and called the **hyaloid canal, canal of Stilling,** or **canal of Cloquet.**   During fetal life this canal transmits an artery, the hyaloid artery, to the lens, and in the adult it contains the remains of the supporting connective tissue or, rarely, an atrophied vessel.

The **zonule of Zinn** (**zonula ciliaris**), or **suspensory ligament of the lens,** is the thickened portion of the hyaloid membrane extending from the ciliary body to the lens.   At the ora serrata the hyaloid membrane becomes attached to the ciliary body and remains attached as far as the peripheral, or anterior, ends of the ciliary processes.   From the apices of the ciliary processes thick bands of the hyaloid membrane pass over to the lens, to its periphery and to its anterior surface.   The hyaloid membrane, in this region, is thrown into numerous folds, caused by the plications of the choroid portion of the ciliary body, to which it is so closely apposed.   At the ciliary margin of the ligament these folds become converted into two series of stiff fibers: one consisting of the fibers which spring from the apices of the ciliary processes; the other, of those which spring from the depressions between the processes.   The former are inserted into the periphery and the adjacent parts of the posterior portion of the capsule of the lens, and the latter go to the anterior surface of the lens, blending with the superficial layers of the anterior portion of the lens capsule   The lens is thus maintained in position.   The tension of the zonule of Zinn (*zonula ciliaris*) is modified by contraction of the ciliary muscle, by which the suspensory ligament is relaxed; the lens is then less firmly compressed, and by its own elasticity becomes more convex, and its focal distance is decreased. This function is known as **accommodation**.

The **canal of Petit** (**spatia zonularia**), a narrow lymph channel which encircles the margin of the lens, is triangular on section, and is bounded, anteriorly, by the anterior lamina of the suspensory ligament of the lens; posteriorly, by the hyaloid membrane, and medially, by the capsule of the lens. It is subdivided into two portions by the fibers of the posterior lamina of the suspensory ligament of the lens. The lymph in the canal of Petit (*spatia zonularia*) is derived from the ciliary vessels, and is supposed to supply nutrition to the lens.

DISSECTION.—By carefully inserting a fine blowpipe into the canal of Petit (*spatia zonularia*) it may be distended with air or with a colored fluid. When so dilated, it presents a series of sacculations, due to the undulations in the zonule of Zinn (*zonula ciliaris*) produced by the ciliary processes. Remove the lens by cutting through the zonule of Zinn (*zonula ciliaris*) with a pair of scissors.

The **crystalline lens** is a biconvex, transparent body, lying behind the iris and the aqueous humor, and in front of the vitreous body. Its rounded margin is a short distance from, and parallel to the corona ciliaris of the ciliary body, to which it is firmly attached by the suspensory ligament of the lens. The center of the anterior surface of the lens is the anterior pole, and the center of the posterior surface is the posterior pole. The convexity of the anterior surface of the lens is not so great as that of the posterior surface. The central portion of the anterior surface is opposite the pupil, and in contact with the aqueous humor of the anterior chamber. At the margin of this central portion the lens is in contact with the posterior surface of the pupillary margin of the iris; external to this margin the curvature of the lens carries it away from the iris; this interval between the lens and the iris is the posterior chamber of the eye, and is filled with part of the aqueous humor. Posteriorly, the lens is received into the patellar fossa (*hyaloid*) of the vitreous body. Peripherally, it is in relation with the zonule of Zinn (*zonula ciliaris*) and the canal of Petit (*spatia zonularia*).

The lens is composed of the lens capsule and the substantia lentis. The **capsule of the lens** is a strong, elastic, transparent membrane which surrounds the **substantia lentis,** or **lens substance,** a transparent, gelatinous material, translucent in the cadaver, and composed of transparent fibers joined by a transparent cement. The **cortex** (*cortical substance*), or peripheral portion, is soft, and the **nucleus** (*nucleus lentis*), or central portion, is firm.

DISSECTION.—With a sharp knife divide the anterior part of the capsule of the lens, and then express the lens substance through the opening as the pulp of a grape is squeezed from its skin; the capsule and lens substance can now be examined.

The capsule of the lens, or the suspensory ligament, may be ruptured by traumatism, and the lens escape into the vitreous or the aqueous humor. If the anterior portion of the capsule is torn, the aqueous humor will enter and produce opacity of the lens. This is done purposely in the treatment of soft cataract, so that the lens substance may be absorbed by the aqueous humor.

The **Chambers of the Eyeball** (Plate CIV) are situated in front of the lens; they are lymph spaces containing the aqueous humor, and are incompletely separated from each other by the iris.

The **anterior chamber** of the eye is bounded, anteriorly, by the cornea and posteriorly, by the iris and by that portion of the lens which presents at the pupil. It communicates with the posterior chamber through the pupil. At its lateral angle it is bounded by the pectinate ligament of the iris. This angle, which is formed by the peripheral portions of the cornea and iris, is called the *angle of the iris*, or the *filtration angle*. The anatomy of the structures at this angle is most important, for it is here that the excess of the aqueous humor escapes into the spaces of Fontana (*spatia anguli iridis*) and thence by way of the canal of Schlemn (*sinus venosus sclerae*) into the anterior ciliary veins, thus reducing intra-ocular tension.

A collection of pus in the anterior chamber of the eye is known as **hypopyon.** It arises from suppurative inflammation of the cornea, iris, ciliary body, or choroid. The pus passes from the ciliary body through the pectinate ligament of the iris or the attached margin of the iris to reach the anterior chamber, causing cloudiness of the aqueous humor, and its solid portion gravitates to the most dependent part of the anterior chamber, varying its position with movements of the head.

The **posterior chamber** of the eye is a circular space, triangular on cross-section, and situated posterior to the iris. It is bounded anteriorly by the iris; posteriorly by the lens and the zonule of Zinn (*zonula ciliaris*); laterally by the anterior portion of the ciliary body, and medially by the pupillary margin of the iris.

The **Lymphatic System of the Eyeball** is imperfect. Lymph vessels are present only in the conjunctiva, the lymph being contained in spaces and perivascular lymph channels. These spaces are divided into an anterior and a posterior set.

The **anterior lymph passages** of the eye include the lymph spaces of the cornea and the iris, and the anterior and posterior chambers of the eyeball.

The *lymph spaces of the cornea* are situated between the lamellæ of the corneal substance. At the periphery of the cornea the lymph flows into the conjunctival lymph vessels.

The *lymph spaces of the iris* open into the aqueous humor of the anterior chamber of the eye at small indentations called the *crypts of the iris*, and at the periphery of the iris they communicate with the spaces of Fontana (*spatia anguli iridis*).

The *aqueous humor* is composed of about ninety-five per cent water, one per cent of salts and a minute quantity of albumen. It is situated in the anterior and posterior chambers of the eye. It is produced in the ciliary body by transudation from the plexus of vessels. The aqueous humor passes from the posterior chamber through the pupil into the anterior chamber of the eye, and escapes by way of the spaces of Fontana (*spatia anguli iridis*), the canal of Schlemm (*sinus venosus scleræ*), and the anterior ciliary veins, a part of it being absorbed and eliminated by the iris.

The **posterior lymph passages** of the eye include the hyaloid canal, the perichoroidal space, Tenon's space (*interfascial space*), the intervaginal (*subdural*) space of the optic nerve, and the supravaginal space.

The *hyaloid canal*, or central canal of the vitreous body, extends from the optic disc forward to the posterior pole of the lens. In the embryo it contains the hyaloid artery, which disappears later, although the canal remains as a lymph channel which is drained by the intervaginal (*subdural*) space of the optic nerve.

The *perichoroidal lymph space*, situated between the choroid and the sclera, is continued along the vessels of the choroid and especially along the venæ vorticosæ. Its lymph escapes into Tenon's space (*interfascial space*) by perforations in the sclera around the venæ vorticosæ.

Tenon's space (*interfascial space*), situated between the sclera and Tenon's capsule (*fascia bulbi*), drains the perichoroidal space, and opens into the supravaginal space.

The *intervaginal* (*subdural*) *lymph space* is situated between the dural and pial sheaths of the optic nerve. It opens into the subdural and subarachnoid spaces of the brain.

The *supravaginal lymph space* is situated between the dural sheath of the optic nerve and the posterior extension of Tenon's capsule (*fascia bulbi*).

The greater portion of the lymph of the eyeball escapes by way of the chambers of the aqueous humor, the spaces of Fontana (*spatia anguli iridis*), the canal of Schlemn (*sinus venosus scleræ*), and the anterior ciliary veins; consequently, any obstruction in the anterior lymph channels causes increased intra-

PLATE CXII.

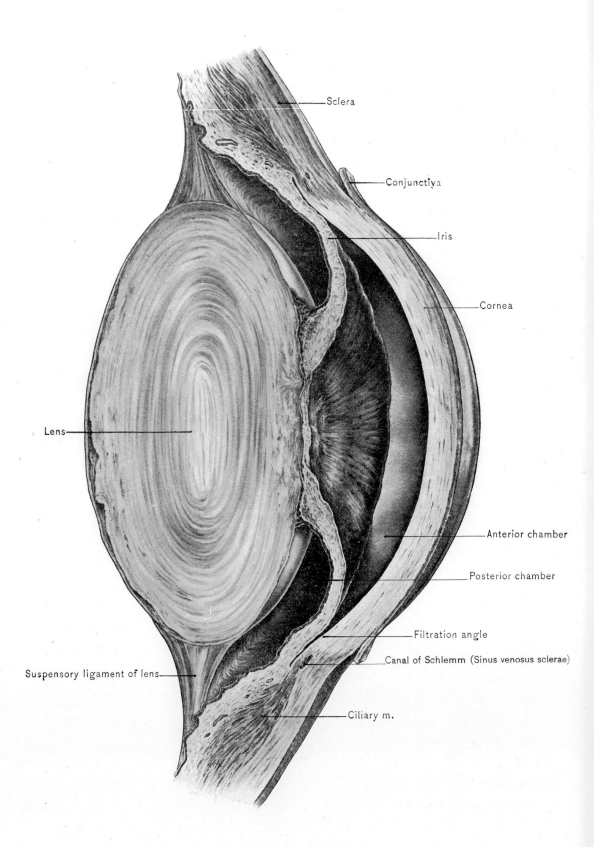

Sclera

Conjunctiva

Iris

Cornea

Anterior chamber

Posterior chamber

Filtration angle

Canal of Schlemm (Sinus venosus sclerae)

Ciliary m.

Suspensory ligament of lens

Lens

ANNULAR POSTERIOR SYNECHIA.

PLATE CXIII.

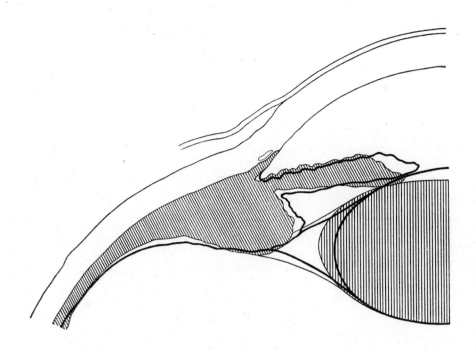

THE DARK AREAS REPRESENT THE LENS, IRIS, AND CILIARY BODY AT REST; AND THE BROAD OUTLINES INDICATE THE CHANGED POSITION OF THOSE STRUCTURES DURING ACCOMMODATION (AFTER FUCHS).

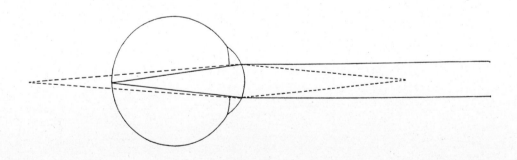

EMMETROPIC EYE.

PLATE CXIV.

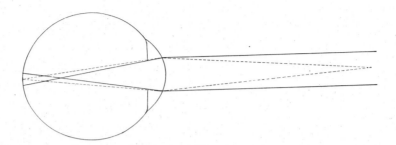

MYOPIC EYE.

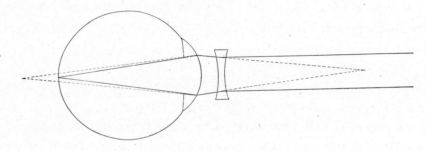

MYOPIC EYE WITH CONCAVE LENS.

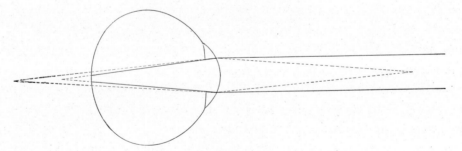

HYPEROPIC EYE.

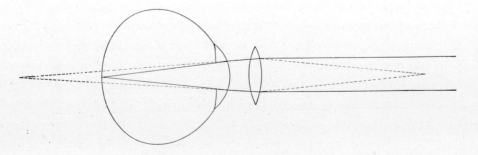

HYPEROPIC EYE WITH CONVEX LENS.

ocular tension. Such obstruction occurs in **annular posterior synechia,** (Plate CXII) in which the whole pupillary margin of the iris is adherent to the anterior surface of the capsule of the lens, and prevents the lymph of the posterior chamber, which is derived from the ciliary vessels, from entering the anterior chamber. The pressure in the posterior chamber causes the peripheral portion of the iris to project forward against the cornea, obliterating the filtration angle, and preventing the escape of lymph from the anterior chamber of the eyeball; the serious disease of the eye, *glaucoma,* which is characterized by increased intra-ocular tension, is thus produced. Glaucoma also develops from conditions not so readily demonstrable, such as hypersecretion of lymph, and other causes of retention of lymph, in the eyeball.

In **emmetropia,** (Plate CXIII) or normal vision, parallel rays of light, or those from distant objects, are brought to a focus on the retina when the eye is at rest, and divergent rays, or those from near objects, do not reach a focus on the retina without some exercise of the function of accommodation. Normal vision occurs in an eye whose axis, or sagittal diameter, is of the normal length, and whose media possess the proper refractive index.

In **hyperopia, hypermetropia,** (Plate CXIV) or far-sightedness, the axis, or sagittal diameter of the eye, is usually too short, although hyperopia may be due to absence of the lens, decreased convexity of the refracting surfaces of the eye, or diminished power of refraction in the refractive media of the eye. The result is that when the ciliary muscle is at rest, parallel rays of light, or those from distant objects, and divergent rays, or those from near objects, come in contact with the retina before being brought to a focus, forming circular diffusion of the light and a blurred image. The ciliary muscle attempts to compensate for the defect by contracting and allowing increased convexity of the lens, but the severe strain causes local and remote disorders, and, on account of failure of the muscle to perform the work required, reading becomes difficult. The defect is corrected by converging the rays with convex glasses.

In **myopia,** or near-sightedness, the anteroposterior, or sagittal, diameter is too long, and parallel rays of light are brought to a focus in front of the retina, so that distant objects are indistinct because the image is blurred. Divergent rays, or those from near objects at a certain distance, are brought to a focus upon the retina. Myopia occasionally results from increased refractive power of the lens; when this occurs in an old person, *second sight* is produced and convex glasses may be discarded. As there is no mechanism in the eye which can compensate for the defect, and the patient can see near objects, continued eye strain may cause serious disease of the myopic eye. The defect is corrected by concave glasses which cause the rays to diverge.

Exenteration of the orbital contents is performed for malignant disease. The lateral canthus is split, and the orbital contents, including the periosteum, are all removed except at the apex of the orbit.

Evisceration of the eyeball is performed in staphyloma of the cornea, disfiguring leukoma, and in some infective conditions. The cornea is circumcised at the sclero-corneal margin, and all the contents of the globe and the middle and internal coats of the eyeball are carefully removed, leaving the sclera intact. The sclera is stitched vertically and the conjunctiva transversely. After the wound heals, an artificial shell may be inserted over the stump. If there has been no infection in the eye before operation, a glass ball may be inserted into the cavity of the eye and the sclera and conjunctiva closed, as above.

Enucleation, or excision, of the eyeball.—The eyelids are separated with a speculum, and the ocular conjunctiva is divided close to, and entirely around the cornea. The conjunctiva and capsule of Tenon (*fascia bulbi*) are pushed backward over the eye. The recti muscles are grasped with forceps at their insertions and divided back of the forceps. The globe is drawn forward and medialward, and the optic nerve and adjoining structures are divided with scissors along the lateral side of the eyeball. The eye is then drawn out of its socket, and the remaining adherent tendons and other structures are severed. The cavity is irrigated with sterile water, and the stumps of the recti muscles are sutured together. The wound is cleansed, and a sterile dressing applied.

THE ORGAN OF HEARING (Plate CXV)

The organ of hearing consists of three portions: the external, the middle, and the internal ear. The **external ear** comprises the auricle, or pinna, and the external auditory meatus; the former is of no great importance physiologically; the latter is the canal which leads inward to the tympanic membrane. The **middle ear** is composed of the tympanum, the mastoid (*tympanic*) antrum, and the mastoid cells. The tympanum, is an air chamber which communicates with the naso-pharynx by means of the Eustachian (*auditory*) tube, and contains a chain of movable bones, the auditory ossicles. The mastoid (*tympanic*) antrum and mastoid cells are air chambers accessory to the tympanum. The **internal ear,** or **labyrinth,** is made up of a complex arrangement of cavities, the osseous labyrinth. It contains a fluid, the perilymph, together with a membranous cast of the bony structures known as the membranous labyrinth; the latter contains the endolymph, and within it are the specialized neuro-epithelial cells and the terminations of the auditory nerve.

PLATE CXV.

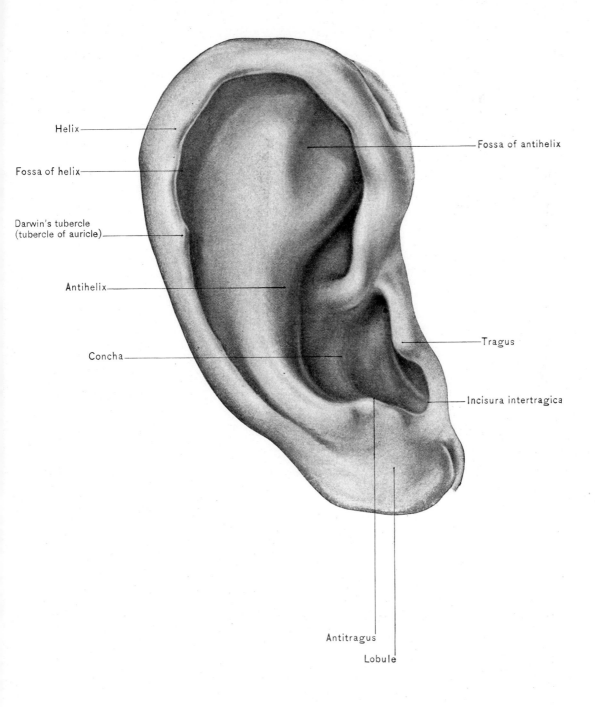

Helix

Fossa of helix

Darwin's tubercle
(tubercle of auricle)

Antihelix

Concha

Fossa of antihelix

Tragus

Incisura intertragica

Antitragus

Lobule

AURICLE.
487

PLATE CXVI.

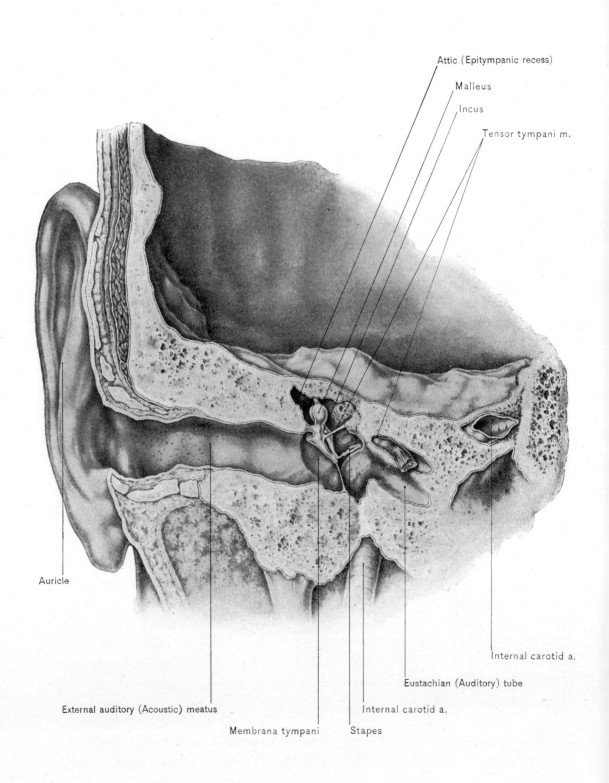

Attic (Epitympanic recess)

Malleus

Incus

Tensor tympani m.

Auricle

External auditory (Acoustic) meatus

Membrana tympani

Stapes

Internal carotid a.

Eustachian (Auditory) tube

Internal carotid a.

EXTERNAL AND MIDDLE EAR.

THE EXTERNAL EAR

The **Auricle** consists of a pliable framework of yellow, elastic cartilage covered with integument.   The external surface is concave, and conducts the sound waves to the external auditory meatus, although accidental or intentional amputation of the auricle causes but slight diminution in acuteness of hearing. The outer concave surface presents a number of elevations and depressions described at p. 250.

The auricle is developed in the embryo from six small tubercles which form at the external extremity of the first branchial cleft.   As a result of imperfect fusion of these tubules **supernumerary auricles,** or **auricular fistulæ,** may occur near the external auditory meatus.   If the orifice of one of these fistulæ is closed, a **dermoid cyst** of the auricle is formed.   Supernumerary auricles may also develop at the external extremity of the other branchial clefts.   Congenital absence of the auricle is very rare.

The **integument of the auricle,** which is continuous with that lining the external auditory meatus, is thin, and contains sebaceous glands and, in certain situations, hairs and sudoriferous glands.   The sebaceous glands are most abundant in the concha, where their orifices can often be seen filled with foreign material, in persons who are careless as to cleanliness.   *Sebaceous cysts* not infrequently develop in the skin of the auricle.   The integument is more firmly attached over the concave surface of the auricle than on the convex, or cranial, surface.

The **subcutaneous tissue of the auricle** forms a thin lamina almost devoid of fat.   This lack of subcutaneous fat, which affords protection from cold to the blood-vessels, and the exposed position of the auricle account for the frequency of **frost-bite** in this location, which occasionally causes gangrene of the auricle.

The yellow elastic **cartilage of the auricle,** which gives form to that structure, presents several fissures and processes (see p. 256).

The **intrinsic muscles of the auricle** are small, rudimentary, and unimportant.   They have been described with the face, at p. 255.

The **External Auditory Canal, or Meatus** (**External Acoustic Meatus**), (Plate CXVI) is a slightly curved passage, convex upward, which leads inward and a little forward for a distance of about twenty-five millimeters (one inch), to the membrana tympani.   Its general direction is downward, inward and slightly forward. The highest portion of the canal is about at its middle.   Drawing the auricle upward and backward has a tendency to straighten the canal; this is done when inspecting the canal or introducing an instrument.   Owing to the obliquity of the tympanic membrane, the anterior and inferior walls of the external auditory meatus are longer than the other walls, and the internal extremity of the canal is wedge-shaped, terminating in a narrow recess, the **sinus** of the external auditory meatus. Small foreign bodies which have lodged in the sinus of the canal must be removed carefully, as the instrument closely approaches the membrana tympani. The meatus is elliptical at the external orifice, the vertical diameter of the canal being the greater; near the membrana tympani the transverse diameter is the greater. Although the orifice of the external meatus is elliptical, ear specula which are round are more desirable than the elliptical instruments, because they can be rotated while being introduced. The lateral third of the wall of the external auditory meatus is cartilaginous and continuous with the cartilage of the auricle; this portion is about eight millimeters (three-eighths of an inch) in length, and the cartilage presents one or two fissures, known as the incisuræ, or fissures of Santorini (*incisuræ cartilagines*), which are filled with fibrous tissue. Parotid abscesses opening into the canal usually pass through these deficiencies in the cartilage. The inner, or osseous, portion is somewhat longer, and measures less in diameter than the cartilaginous portion, its average length being about sixteen millimeters (five-eighths of an inch). At birth the osseous portion is represented merely by an incomplete bony ring, the **annulus tympanicus,** and a mass of epithelial cells and cerumen fills the canal. The upper end of the mandible is in close relation with the cartilaginous and bony portions of the meatus. Opening of the mouth draws the cartilage forward. This may account for the open mouth of the listener.

The **integument** lining the meatus is thin, and firmly attached to the underlying parts; consequently, inflammatory processes, such as furuncles, are accompanied by considerable pain; the cutaneous lining is continued over the tympanic membrane as a delicate covering, forming the outer layer of that structure. Hairs and sebaceous glands, as well as slightly modified sweat glands which secrete the cerumen, or ear wax, are found in the cartilaginous portion of the meatus. When the cerumen, or wax, is secreted too rapidly, the meatus becomes occluded, and deafness and tinnitus aurium result. No hairs or glands are found in the osseous portion of the external auditory meatus.

In **otitis externa** the skin of the external auditory meatus is inflamed, and there may be a purulent discharge from that canal.

Occlusion of the external auditory meatus may occur as a congenital defect or from the presence of polypoid growths arising from granulations projecting through a perforation in the membrana tympani in chronic otitis media, from exostoses from the bony wall, from foreign bodies, or from an excessive quantity of cerumen.

Foreign bodies may remain in the external auditory meatus for many years without causing injury or inconvenience, and they may remain undiscovered until otoscopic examination for some condition in no way connected with the presence of a foreign body. Unskilful attempts at removal have inflicted nearly all the injuries following the presence of these foreign bodies. No attempt should be made to remove a foreign body until it is seen in the meatus. Insects or other foreign bodies may be removed by syringing gently with a slender stream of warm water, or a small hook may be inserted and kept in view, while the canal is being well illuminated. If the walls of the canal are swollen, removal of the foreign body should be deferred until the swelling has subsided.

RELATIONS.—A portion of the parotid gland is in relation with the lower and anterior wall of the external auditory meatus. This explains why parotid tumors cause narrowing of that canal, and why abscesses of the parotid gland may open into it, since the fissures in the cartilage afford a favorable site for perforation. The anterior wall of the meatus is also in relation with the condyle of the mandible, so that firm closure of the mouth has a tendency to narrow the lumen of the meatus. When the condyle is driven forcibly backward, as by a blow or a fall on the chin, the bony wall of the meatus may be fractured. The posterior and upper walls of the canal are formed by parts of the mastoid and of the squamous portion of the temporal bone, and often only a thin, osseous partition separates it from the mastoid cells, so that caries of the osseous wall of the external auditory meatus may be followed by mastoid disease.

BLOOD SUPPLY.—The blood supply of the external auditory meatus is derived from branches of the internal maxillary, posterior auricular, and superficial temporal arteries.

The *veins* accompany the corresponding arteries and empty into the temporal, internal maxillary, and posterior auricular veins.

NERVE SUPPLY.—From branches of the auriculo-temporal, the great auricular, and the auricular branch of the vagus nerve. Interesting reflex disturbances are at times caused by the presence of foreign bodies, wax, or specula, through irritation reflected along the auricular branch of the vagus nerve and referred to the parts supplied by the parent trunk; coughing, faintness, and nausea and vomiting may thus be induced. Sneezing is also produced by the presence of foreign bodies or specula in the external auditory meatus. The irritation is probably reflected along the auriculo-temporal nerve to the Gasserian (*semilunar*) ganglion or other centers of the trigeminal nerve, and thence referred to the nose through branches of the superior maxillary (*maxillary*) nerve. **Earache** associated with toothache in the upper teeth may be explained in the same manner. Earache frequently is associated with toothache in the lower teeth and disease of the tongue; the pain in the ear is probably due to irritation reflected along the inferior dental (*inferior alveolar*) nerve and the lingual nerve, and referred to the ear through the auriculo-temporal, the other sensory branch of the inferior maxillary (*mandibular*) nerve.

The **lymphatics of the external auditory meatus** follow the veins and terminate in the parotid and posterior auricular lymph glands.

DISSECTION.—Open the tympanum with a chisel by removing its bony roof (*tegmen tympani*); the opening is made to the lateral side of the elevation produced by the superior semicircular canal, and is enlarged carefully, uncovering also the mastoid (*tympanic*) antrum and the internal auditory meatus.

THE MIDDLE EAR (Plate CXVI)

The **Tympanum,** or **Middle Ear,** includes the tympanum, or tympanic cavity, the Eustachian (*auditory*) tube, and the mastoid cells. The tympanic cavity is a small, irregular air chamber, situated in the petrous portion of the temporal bone, lined with mucous membrane; it is interposed between the external auditory meatus and the internal ear. Its anteroposterior length measures about fifteen millimeters (three-fifths of an inch); its width is from two to six millimeters (one-twelfth to one-sixth of an inch); it is narrowest opposite the center, or umbilicus, of the tympanic membrane which is opposite the promontory; vertically, including the recesses epitympanicus, or attic, it is about sixteen millimeters (somewhat more than half an inch). (Plate CXVII.)

The **recessus epitympanicus,** or **attic,** is the highest portion of the tympanic cavity. It is situated above the level of the tympanic membrane, and contains the head of the malleus and part of the incus, and leads into the mastoid (*tympanic*) antrum.

The **roof of the tympanum (paries tegmentalis)** consists of a thin plate of bone, *tegmen tympani*, which separates the tympanum from the cranial cavity; it forms part of the anterosuperior surface of the petrous portion of the temporal bone. Destruction of this osseous lamina or extension through it of the inflammatory process in chronic otitis media may lead to meningeal or cerebral complications, such as extradural abscess, meningitis, abscess of the temporal lobe of the cerebrum, and cerebellar abscess. In children under one year of age the presence of the petro-squamous suture in the tegmen tympani favors this complication.

The **floor (paries jugularis)** is formed by a thin, bony plate situated between the tympanum and the jugular fossa. Destruction of this plate of bone by caries in otitis media may cause fatal hemorrhage or septic thrombosis of the internal jugular vein, embolism, and metastatic abscess.

The **anterior wall (paries carotica)** is quite narrow, and is deficient superiorly, inasmuch as the Eustachian (*auditory*) tube opens into the tympanum in

PLATE CXVII.

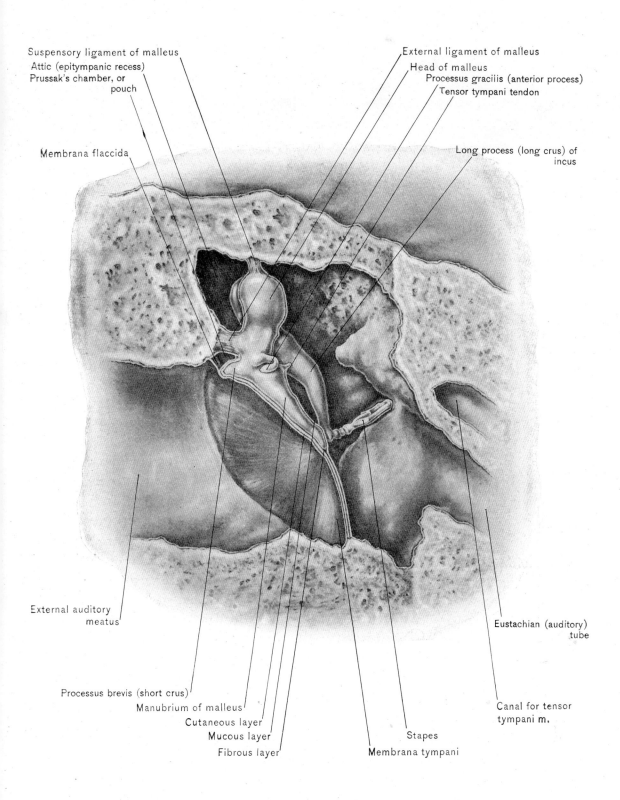

Suspensory ligament of malleus
Attic (epitympanic recess)
Prussak's chamber, or
pouch

External ligament of malleus
Head of malleus
Processus graciiis (anterior process)
Tensor tympani tendon

Membrana flaccida

Long process (long crus) of
incus

External auditory
meatus

Eustachian (auditory)
tube

Processus brevis (short crus)
Manubrium of malleus
Cutaneous layer
Mucous layer
Fibrous layer

Stapes
Membrana tympani

Canal for tensor
tympani m.

ANTERIOR VIEW OF RIGHT TYMPANUM.

this situation about four millimeters (one-sixth of an inch) above the floor. Just above the entrance of the tube is the opening of the canal which lodges the tensor tympani muscle. Owing to the position of the tympanic orifice of the Eustachian (*auditory*) tube above the level of the floor of the tympanum, fluid which has entered the tympanum by way of the Eustachian (*auditory*) tube, as in snuffling water in surf-bathing or in using a nasal douche, cannot all escape through the tube, and otitis media may result. Below the orifice of the Eustachian (*auditory*) tube the anterior wall is composed of a thin, bony lamina, situated between the tympanum and the carotid canal. Caries of this thin plate of bone may occur in otitis media, leading to ulceration into the internal carotid artery, resulting in fatal hemorrhage.

The **Eustachian** (**Auditory**) **Tube** (Plate CXVI) is the anterior extension of the tympanic cavity which connects the middle ear with the naso-pharynx. It passes inward, downward, and forward from the tympanum, is about thirty-five millimeters (one and a half inches) in length, and in its several portions varies from two to five millimeters (one-twelfth to one-fifth of an inch) in diameter. It consists of a bony portion about twelve millimeters (one-half inch) long, and a cartilaginous portion about twenty-five millimeters (one inch) in length. The *cartilaginous portion* is somewhat trumpet-shaped, being widest at the *pharyngeal* orifice. It is formed by a cartilaginous plate which is triangular in shape and folded upon itself, thus leaving on the inferior and lateral aspect of the tube an interval which is filled with fibrous tissue, the fascia salpingo-pharyngea, and by a part of the tensor palati (*tensor veli palatini*) muscle, called the *dilator tubæ*. (See also description of pharynx at p. 323.) The *bony portion*, which is smaller than the cartilaginous portion of the tube, is situated at the junction of the squamous and petrous portions of the temporal bone; the *isthmus tubæ*, its narrowest portion, is situated at the junction of the bony and cartilaginous parts. The Eustachian (*auditory*) tube is lined with mucous membrane which is continuous with that of the naso-pharynx and of the middle ear. Consequently, inflammatory processes of the naso-pharynx, by direct continuity of the tissues, may lead to involvement of the middle ear. The tympanic orifice of the Eustachian (*auditory*) tube is situated in the anterior wall of the tympanum, about four millimeters (one-sixth of an inch) above the floor of that cavity, and the pharyngeal orifice is in the lateral wall of the naso-pharynx, behind the posterior naris, at the level of the posterior extremity of the inferior turbinated bone (*inferior concha*). Normally, the canal is closed, except during swallowing, when it is opened by the tensor palati (*tensor veli palatini*) muscle, levator palati (*levator veli palatini*) muscle, and the salpingo-pharyngeus, which is the portion of the pharyngo-palatinus muscle attached to the Eustachian

32

(*auditory*) tube. The action of these muscles during swallowing affords an opportunity to inflate the middle ear, for diagnostic and therapeutic purposes, by way of the nose, the naso-pharynx, and the Eustachian (*auditory*) tube. Several methods are employed.

In the **Politzer method of inflation of the middle ear** the patient takes some water in his mouth; the nozzle of a rubber bag which contains air is inserted into one nostril; the nostrils are closed with the fingers of one hand, and as the patient swallows the water the bag is suddenly and forcibly compressed with the other hand. In the **method of Valsalva** the patient closes the mouth and nose firmly and puffs out the cheeks. Air is driven through the Eustachian (*auditory*) tube, and a sense of pressure and fullness is felt in the middle ear. This method is not altogether safe, on account of the increased tension produced in the blood-vessels, and the danger of hemorrhage and apoplexy. The middle ear may also be inflated by a rubber bag and an Eustachian catheter; the method for introducing the catheter is described at p. 323.

The Eustachian (*auditory*) tube may be closed by the extension of hypertrophic nasal and naso-pharyngeal catarrh into the tube, or the pharyngeal orifice of the tube may be obstructed mechanically by growths in the nose or in the naso-pharynx, or by adenoids. Occlusion of this tube causes autophony, or loud but muffled sound of the individual's voice, tinnitus aurium, or false sounds in the ears, a sensation of tension or distention in the ears, and more or less deafness.

In the mucous membrane of the Eustachian (*auditory*) tube and near the pharyngeal end of the tube, there are a few *mucous glands* and a quantity of lymphoid tissue; the latter is sometimes referred to as the *tubal tonsil*.

RELATIONS.—On the lateral side of the Eustachian (*auditory*) tube are the tensor palati (*tensor veli palatini*) and levator palati (*levator veli palatini*) muscles, the otic ganglion, the inferior maxillary (*mandibular*) nerve, and the middle meningeal artery; on the medial side is the wall of the pharynx.

BLOOD SUPPLY.—The blood supply of the Eustachian (*auditory*) tube is derived from the ascending pharyngeal, middle meningeal, and Vidian arteries (*arteries of the pterygoid canal*). Its veins form a plexus connecting with the cavernous sinus.

NERVE SUPPLY.—From the tympanic plexus and from the pharyngeal branch of the spheno-palatine ganglion.

The **posterior wall of the middle ear** (**paries mastoidea**) presents, at its upper portion, a large opening which leads into the mastoid (*tympanic*) antrum; through this opening the mucous membrane is continuous from one cavity to the other, so that inflammation in the middle ear may lead to involvement of the mastoid air cells. Below the opening into the antrum, near the inner wall of the tympanum and posterior to the fenestra ovalis (*fenestra vestibuli*), is a hollow, cone-shaped, bony projection, known as the *pyramid*, at the summit of which there is a perforation for the passage of the tendon of the stapedius muscle. External to the pyramid is the *iter chordæ posterius*, through which the chorda tympani nerve enters the middle ear.

As the **Mastoid (Tympanic) Antrum and Mastoid Cells** communicate with the middle ear, they are cavities accessory to the tympanic cavity.

The **mastoid portion of the temporal bone** contains numerous spaces which are filled with air; these communicate with the middle ear, and are called mastoid cells; other spaces which occupy the tip of the process are filled with marrow. Of the air cavities, the *mastoid (tympanic) antrum* is the largest and most important. Leidy described the mastoid (tympanic) antrum as a part of the tympanum.

The **mastoid, or tympanic, antrum** varies in size, being usually from four to six millimeters (one-sixth to one-fourth of an inch) in diameter, and is situated posterior to the tympanum, about on a level with the highest part of that cavity. It is lined with mucous membrane, or muco-periosteum, which is directly continuous with that of the attic of the tympanum and mastoid cells. The mastoid (*tympanic*) antrum is well developed at birth.

The **roof of the mastoid (tympanic) antrum (tegmen tympani)** is a thin plate of bone about one millimeter in thickness, situated lateral to the eminence produced by the superior semicircular canal; it separates the mastoid (*tympanic*) antrum from the cranial cavity, and is perforated by minute veins which empty into the superior petrosal sinus; at times, the tegmen is distinctly cribriform; it may be partly or wholly absorbed in old age.

The **floor of the antrum,** which frequently is on a lower level than the communication between the tympanum and the antrum, is formed by the substance of the mastoid portion of the temporal bone, and usually contains the orifices of some of the other mastoid cells.

The **anterior wall of the antrum** is thin, and at times perforated; it separates the mastoid (*tympanic*) antrum from the bony part of the external auditory meatus. Inflammatory processes may extend from the mastoid (*tympanic*) antrum through this wall to the external auditory meatus, or vice versa. Through this wall a mastoid abscess may be evacuated by way of the external auditory meatus.

The **posterior wall of the antrum** is a bony lamina of variable thickness, separating the antrum from the groove for the sigmoid sinus, a part of the lateral (*transverse*) sinus; through it small veins pass from the middle ear and mastoid (*tympanic*) antrum to the sigmoid sinus. By way of these veins the septic material of otitis media or of mastoid disease may reach the sigmoid portion of the lateral (*transverse*) sinus, and cause septic thrombosis and embolism. It is due to this intimate anatomic relation that this sinus is so frequently the seat of disease. In infants this infective inflammation is rare. This is due to the fact that in them the mastoid cells are not developed and that the squamous covering of the antrum is not closely united to the mastoid, so that purulent secretions are not kept under tension. The infantile internal ear, however, is more easily invaded by middle ear inflammation, and meningitis is apt to occur.

The **inner wall of the mastoid (tympanic) antrum** is from fourteen to eighteen millimeters (nine-sixteenths to three-fourths of an inch) distant from the base line of the suprameatal triangle (Macewen). The facial canal lies in the inner wall of the passage from the mastoid (*tympanic*) antrum to the tympanum. This canal, which is separated from the tympanum by a thin, osseous lamina, is situated above the fenestra ovalis (*fenestra vestibuli*) of the tympanum; on the inner side of the antro-tympanal passageway the canal curves and then descends to the stylo-mastoid foramen. The wall of the canal is thin in children, and may be defective in that portion which lies over the fenestra ovalis (*fenestra vestibuli*); the nerve within the canal is therefore more likely to be affected in otitis media in children than in the same disease in adults.

The **outer wall of the mastoid (tympanic) antrum** is formed by the descending plate of the squamous portion of the temporal bone; the antrum is from twelve to fifteen millimeters (one-half to three-fifths of an inch) distant from the surface of the bone. In the infant the outer wall of the mastoid (*tympanic*) antrum is about two millimeters in thickness; it increases rapidly in thickness during the second year, and in a child nine years of age it is ten millimeters thick. In infants the descending plate of the squamous bone is separated from the mastoid process by a suture, the masto-squamous suture, which at times persists wholly or partially. In children, on account of the tenuity of the external wall of the mastoid (*tympanic*) antrum and the presence of this suture, pus may find its way to the exterior through the middle ear and the mastoid (*tympanic*) antrum, and form a subperiosteal abscess over the mastoid portion of the temporal bone. This wall has been known to be perforated spontaneously by absorption of the bone. In such cases an air tumor, or **pneumatocele,** which can be inflated through the Eustachian (*auditory*) tube, may form over the mastoid process.

The **suprameatal triangle of Macewen** is bounded above by the posterior root of the zygoma, which runs nearly horizontally backward; the antero-inferior boundary is formed by the posterosuperior margin of the bony meatus; the posterior boundary is formed by a perpendicular line extending from the most posterior portion of the bony meatus to the posterior root of the zygoma. The

PLATE CXVIII.

Suspensory ligament
of malleus

Head of malleus

Incus

Roof of tympanic cavity

Mastoid (tympanic)
antrum

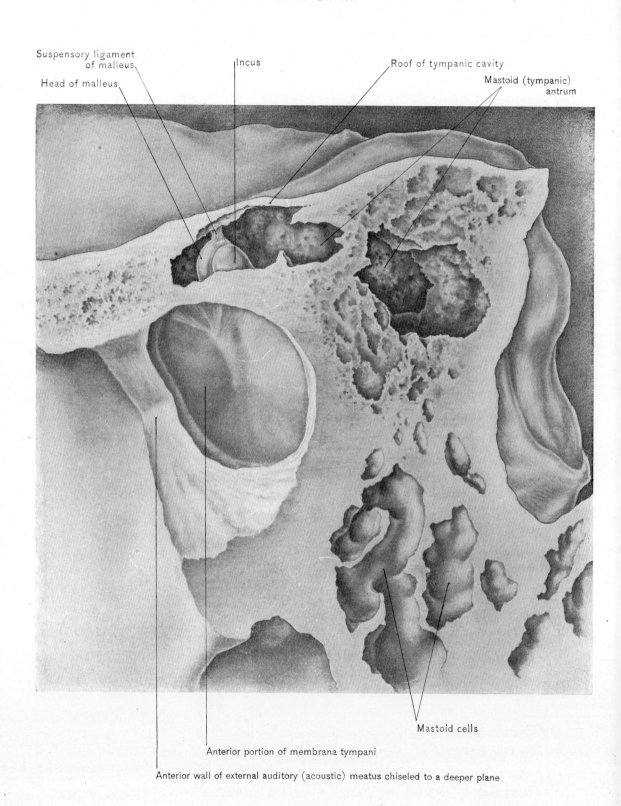

Mastoid cells

Anterior portion of membrana tympani

Anterior wall of external auditory (acoustic) meatus chiseled to a deeper plane

MEMBRANA TYMPANI AND ITS INCLINATION.

apex of this triangular area is directed forward, and the area itself is usually somewhat depressed. Through this triangle the mastoid (*tympanic*) antrum may be reached with safety, if the perforation is directed medialward and somewhat upward and forward, or parallel with the external auditory meatus. If the mastoid process is opened behind this triangle, the knee of the sigmoid portion of the lateral (*transverse*) sinus is in danger of being injured, particularly if the perforation is made directly medialward, as that sinus is only from three to six millimeters from the posterior extremity of the mastoid antrum. The posterior root of the zygoma indicates the level of the floor of the cranial cavity; should the operator pierce the bone above this line, the cranial cavity is likely to be opened. As previously stated, the mastoid antrum in the adult is usually from twelve to fifteen millimeters (one-half to three-fifths of an inch) from the surface of the bone; for this reason the chisel should enter the mastoid (*tympanic*) antrum at a depth not greater than fifteen millimeters. As the result of longstanding disease, the bone over the mastoid (*tympanic*) antrum may be thickened and sclerosed. If the inner wall of the antrum is encroached upon, the facial nerve may be injured by the instruments used by the operator. The facial nerve emerges from the petrous portion of the temporal bone and then passes backward along the upper margin of the medial wall of the tympanic cavity just above the oval window. From here it goes downward across the lower and medial wall of the aditus ad antrum just below the upper and deeper portion of the bony wall of the meatus; then downward, more deeply buried in the plate of bone which forms the posterior wall of the auditory meatus, it emerges posterior to the styloid process. The facial nerve is more liable to injury in the deep portion of the posterior meatal wall, just over the aditus ad antrum.

The **mastoid cells** vary greatly as to number and size. They are absent at birth, and prior to puberty they are few in number. They attain their full development in the young adult, and occupy the greater portion of the mastoid process, opening directly or indirectly into the mastoid (*tympanic*) antrum. They are lined with muco-periosteum which is continuous with that of the mastoid (*tympanic*) antrum. Posteriorly, they cease abruptly at the occipitotemporal suture. They are separated from the sigmoid portion of the lateral (*transverse*) sinus by a thin plate of bone, through which veins pass from these cells to the sinus, affording a ready means of infection and the formation of septic thrombosis of the sinus.

The **Outer Wall of the Middle Ear** is formed by the tympanic membrane and, to a slight extent, by bone.

The **tympanic membrane** (Plate CXVIII) is an elliptical, membranous disc, attached to a grooved ridge of bone at the bottom of the external auditory meatus. Its greatest diameter, measured from its posterosuperior portion forward and downward, is ten millimeters (two-fifths of an inch) in length; the vertical measurement is slightly less; it is one-tenth of a millimeter in thickness. The membrane is situated obliquely, its lateral surface being directed lateralward, downward, and forward. It is directed downward and lateralward, at an angle of about fifty-five degrees, and forward and lateralward, at an angle of about ten degrees. In the infant, at birth, this obliquity is greater and the membrane is almost horizontal. Its lateral surface is concave, the center being the deepest point of the concavity, for the extremity of the handle of the malleus is here attached, and, as it were, draws the membrane medially. The depressed center is known as the *umbo*. The bony ring to which the tympanic membrane is attached is incomplete above, leaving a notch, the *notch of Rivinus (tympanic notch)*, which is filled in by a thinner and looser portion of the membrane, known as the *membrana, or pars flaccida*, or *Shrapnell's membrane*. The circumference of the membrane which is fixed in the tympanic sulcus is thickened and is called the fibrocartilaginous ring. The tympanic membrane consists of three layers: a lateral, cuticular layer; an intermediate, fibrous stratum, or membrane propria, and a medial mucous membrane. (Plate CXIX.)

INSPECTION.—When viewed through a speculum during life, the tympanic membrane is of a pearly gray color, and appears smooth and polished. Extending downward and forward with its apex at the *umbo* is a *cone of light*, which is of value in the diagnosis of disease of the tympanum and tympanic membrane. The handle of the malleus and its short process and, posterior to the handle of the malleus, the long process of the incus, can frequently be seen through the membrane. From the short process of the malleus two folds extend to the margins of the notch of Rivinus *(tympanic notch);* these are known as the *anterior* and the *posterior folds* of the membrane, and between them is the *membrana flaccida*. The flaccid portion corresponds to the neck of the malleus. Owing to its laxity, perforations of the membrana flaccida cause only a slight loss of hearing. The remainder and major portion of the drum is known as the *membrana, or pars, tensa.*

Perforation, or rupture, of the tympanic membrane is frequently produced by traumatism, as by slender foreign bodies accidentally pushed far into the external auditory canal, or by the escape of pus from an otitis media. Perforation of the membrana flaccida occurs more commonly when the disease is confined to the attic; perforation of the posterior portion, when the disease is confined to the mastoid *(tympanic)* antrum. Perforation of the lower portion of the membrana tensa is most frequent on account of its low position, and, owing to the inelasticity of the membrane, these perforations do not gape much. Traumatic perforations

PLATE CXIX.

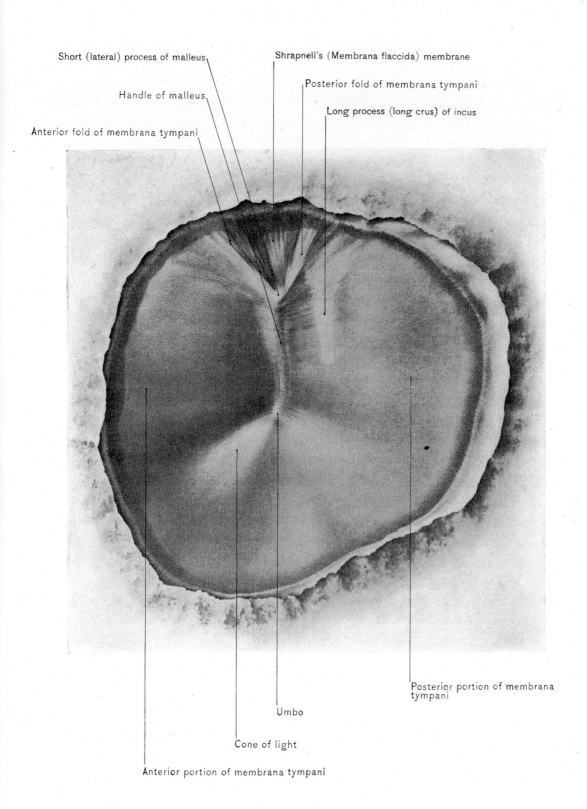

Short (lateral) process of malleus

Handle of malleus

Anterior fold of membrana tympani

Shrapnell's (Membrana flaccida) membrane

Posterior fold of membrana tympani

Long process (long crus) of incus

Posterior portion of membrana tympani

Umbo

Cone of light

Anterior portion of membrana tympani

LATERAL VIEW OF MEMBRANA TYMPANI OF LEFT EAR.

heal readily, whereas those associated with suppurative otitis media seldom close. Granulation tissue from the inflamed mucous membrane of the tympanum projecting through the perforation forms *polypoid growths* which conceal the opening and sometimes hide the tympanic membrane. These growths are associated with copious suppuration.

Paracentesis of the tympanum, or puncture of the tympanic membrane, is frequently practised by the surgeon to relieve tension and allow the discharge of pus.

The point selected is in the lower or subumbilical portion of the membrane, or wherever the bulging is greatest. Puncture of the upper portion of the membrane presents the danger of injuring the malleus, the incus, or the chorda tympani nerve, and puncture of the lower portion of the membrane requires caution owing to the medial wall of the tympanum being situated only from two to four millimeters (one-twelfth to one-sixth of an inch) medial to the tympanic membrane.

If the tympanic membrane has been destroyed by ulceration and the malleus and the incus have escaped with the pus, a plug of cotton inserted into the tympanum against the stapes will serve as an artificial tympanic membrane.

Blood Supply.—The blood supply of the tympanic membrane is derived mainly from the tympanic branches of the internal maxillary and the internal carotid arteries, the stylo-mastoid branch of the posterior auricular, the middle meningeal, and the ascending pharyngeal arteries.

Nerve Supply.—The chief nerve supplying the lateral surface of the tympanic membrane is the auriculo-temporal. According to Sappey, Arnold's nerve (*the auricular branch of the vagus*) supplies the lower portion of this surface of the membrane, and branches from the tympanic plexus supply the medial surface. The membrane is very sensitive.

The **medial wall of the tympanum (paries labyrinthica)** corresponds with the lateral wall of the internal ear It presents several points for examination: a conspicuous rounded elevation, the *promontory*, produced by part of the first turn of the cochlea, on which are faintly marked grooves for the tympanic plexus of nerves; above the posterior portion of the promontory is the *fenestra ovalis* (*fenestra vestibuli*), or oval window, a transverse oval foramen, which leads into the vestibule, and when the auditory ossicles are *in situ,* is closed by the base of the stapes; behind it, is the *pyramid*, at the summit of which is an opening for the tendon of the stapedius muscle; below the promontory is the *fenestra rotunda* (*fenestra cochleæ*), or round window, an opening which leads into the scala tympani of the cochlea, and in the recent state is closed by the *membrana tympani secundaria.* At the junction of the medial wall and the roof of the tympanum, above the oval window, is a rounded ridge of bone, passing antero-posteriorly, produced by the facial canal which lodges the facial nerve. The bony lamina separating this nerve from the cavity of the middle ear is very thin, especially in children, and in otitis media the facial nerve may become affected by neuritis, and may lead to paralysis of the muscles of expression upon the corresponding side of the face.   (Plate CXX.)

The **mucous membrane of the tympanum** lines the tympanic cavity, and is continuous with the mucous membrane of the Eustachian (*auditory*) tube and with that of the mastoid (*tympanic*) antrum.   It is a thin, transparent membrane closely adherent to the periosteum.   It forms the medial layer of the tympanic membrane, and is reflected over the ossicles and their ligaments, the tendons which enter the tympanic cavity, and the nerves of the middle ear.

Acute otitis media, or **acute middle ear disease,** may be followed by various complications, the most common of which is inflammation of the mastoid (*tympanic*) antrum and mastoid air cells, resulting in mastoiditis.   As the mucous membrane of the middle ear is directly continuous with that of the mastoid (*tympanic*) antrum, it will readily be seen how the inflammatory process may extend from the nose to the naso-pharynx, the Eustachian (*auditory*) tube, the tympanum, the mastoid (*tympanic*) antrum, and the mastoid cells.

In acute otitis media the pus usually escapes by perforation of the tympanic membrane, or may it pass out through the Eustachian (*auditory*) tube into the pharynx or through the canal for the tensor tympani muscle.   In **mastoiditis** the pus usually escapes through the tympanum and tympanic membrane, and may, after destruction of the compact bone on the intracranial surface of the mastoid process, enter the cranial cavity and form an extradural abscess; or it may enter the neck over or under the prevertebral fascia, point on the lateral surface of the mastoid process, or escape directly into the external auditory meatus.

Through carious destruction of the tegmen antri, or tegmen tympani, or through the perivascular lymphatics and the veins which pierce the tegmen, **extradural abscess, meningitis, thrombosis of the superior petrosal sinus, and cerebral and cerebellar abscess** may result from otitis media and mastoiditis. **Thrombosis of the sigmoid sinus** and consequent septic embolism may occur by extension of the inflammation along the veins from the mastoid (*tympanic*) antrum, mastoid cells, and tympanum, which empty into the sigmoid sinus.

The Contents of the Tympanum.—Plate CXVII.

The **Auditory Ossicles** form a chain of three small bones, the malleus, the incus, and the stapes, which transmit the impulses of sound waves from the tympanic membrane to the perilymph and endolymph of the internal ear.   The

PLATE CXX.

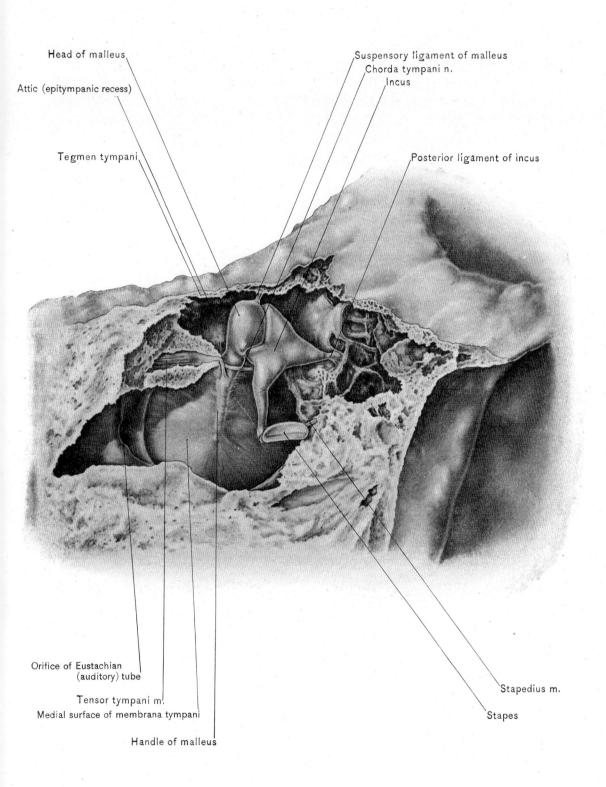

Head of malleus

Attic (epitympanic recess)

Tegmen tympani

Suspensory ligament of malleus
Chorda tympani n.
Incus

Posterior ligament of incus

Orifice of Eustachian
(auditory) tube

Tensor tympani m.
Medial surface of membrana tympani

Handle of malleus

Stapedius m.

Stapes

MEDIAL VIEW OF RIGHT TYMPANUM.

ossicles as well their ligaments and tendons are covered by the mucous membrane of the tympanum.

The **malleus,** or **hammer,** consists of a head, a neck, and three processes: the handle, the short (*lateral*) process, and the processus gracilis (*anterior process*). The rounded *head* is situated in the attic, the highest portion of the tympanic cavity, and above the level of the tympanic membrane; it is connected with the roof of the cavity by fibrous tissue which forms the so-called *superior ligament of the malleus.* On the posterior aspect of the head of the malleus is a cartilage-covered surface which articulates with the body of the incus. The constricted portion just below the head of the malleus is the *neck.* The *handle,* or *manubrium,* is connected with the fibrous layer of the tympanic membrane, and is situated between this layer and the mucous lining. The short (*lateral*) process is a small prominence below the neck, and gives attachment to the tensor tympani muscle. The *processus gracilis* (*anterior process*) is a long and slender process which passes forward to the Glaserian (*petro-tympanic*) fissure. In the adult it is often largely represented by fibrous tissue.

The **incus,** or **anvil,** resembles a bicuspid tooth with diverging roots. It consists of a body and two processes. The *body* presents a concavo-convex articular surface for the head of the malleus; the joint between these bones is surrounded by a capsular ligament and lined by a synovial membrane. The *short process* (*short crus*) passes backward, and is connected to the posterior wall of the tympanum by fibrous tissue. The *long process* (*long crus*) passes downward and backward nearly parallel with the handle of the malleus, and forms almost a right angle with the short process (*short crus*). It terminates in a small, rounded projection, the so-called *processus orbicularis* (*lenticular process*) which articulates with the head of the stapes.

The **stapes,** or **stirrup,** consists of a head, a neck, two crura, or branches, and a foot-piece, or base. The *head* articulates with the processus orbicularis (*lenticular process*) of the incus. This joint has a capsular ligament, and is lined by a synovial membrane. Just below the head is the *neck* from which the *crura, anterior* and *posterior,* diverge; they are grooved on their concave sides, and are attached to the *foot-piece,* or *base,* which fits into the oval window. The *base* of the stapes is united to the margin of that opening by fibrous tissue.

In otitis media the ligaments associated with the ossicles become indurated and stiffened; through loss of mobility the chain of bones cannot transmit impulses to the internal ear, and deafness ensues. In such cases hearing may be improved by removing the perforated tympanic membrane, the malleus, and incus, or by massage administered by means of sound. Caries of the malleus and incus frequently occurs in otitis media, and these bones are occasionally discharged with the pus in that disease.

The **Ligaments** situated in the tympanum attach the ossicles to the tympanic walls and limit their movements. They consist of the superior, the anterior, and lateral ligaments of the malleus, the posterior and superior ligaments of the incus, and the capsular ligaments.

The **superior,** or **suspensory, ligament of the malleus** is a slender, fibrous band which is attached to the lateral part of the roof of the tympanum and to the highest part of the head of the malleus. It limits downward and lateral movement of the head of the malleus and medial rotation of the handle of that bone.

The **anterior ligament of the malleus** is a strong, broad, fibrous band which surrounds the processus gracilis (*anterior process*) of the malleus. It is attached to the anterior wall of the tympanum around the Glaserian (*petro-tympanic*) fissure, some fibers passing through the fissure to become attached to the spine of the sphenoid, and to the anterior aspect of the head and neck of the malleus. It limits movement except in a forward direction. It occasionally contains muscle fibers, and has been described as the *laxator tympani muscle.*

The **lateral ligament of the malleus** is fan-shaped. Its apex is attached to the neck of the malleus, and its base to the margins of the notch of Rivinus (*tympanic notch*). It limits lateral rotation of the handle of the malleus. The posterior fibres of this ligament are known as the *posterior ligament* (Helmholtz); together with the anterior ligament it forms the "axis ligament" of the malleus, the axis around which the malleus rotates.

The **posterior ligament of the incus** is a short, thick band which attaches the extremity of the short process (*short crus*) of the incus to the posterior wall of the tympanum near the orifice of the mastoid (*tympanic*) antrum.

The **superior ligament of the incus** is inconstant. It appears chiefly as a fold of mucous membrane.

The **capsular ligaments** surround the articulations between the malleus and the incus, and the incus and the stapes.

The **Muscles of the Tympanum** are the stapedius and the tensor tympani.

The **stapedius muscle** *arises* from the triangular canal of the eminentia pyramidalis; its tendon passes through an aperture in the apex of the pyramid, and is *inserted* into the neck of the stapes, the lenticular process, and the capsular ligament.

NERVE SUPPLY.—From a branch of the facial nerve.

ACTION.—It draws the head of the stapes backward, thus pressing the posterior part of the base of that bone against the border of the oval window, and regulating the pressure in the vestibular contents, or the perilymph and endolymph.

The **tensor tympani muscle** is larger than the stapedius, and is situated in the bony canal which lies above, and parallel with the osseous portion of the Eustachian (*auditory*) tube. It *arises* from the cartilage of the Eustachian (*auditory*) tube, the adjacent surface of the greater wing of the sphenoidal bone, and the walls of the canal in which it lies. The tendon of the muscle winds around the end of the processus cochleariformis (*septum of musculo-tubal canal*), passes into the tympanum, and is *inserted* into the handle of the malleus near its root.

NERVE SUPPLY.—From the trigeminal, or fifth, nerve through the otic ganglion.

ACTION.—It draws the malleus toward the tympanic cavity, thus tightening and steadying the tympanic membrane and compressing the perilymph of the internal ear. Abnormal action of this muscle is one of the causes of snapping, buzzing, or ringing sounds in the ears.

BLOOD SUPPLY OF THE TYMPANUM.—The blood supply of the tympanum is derived from the tympanic branches of five vessels: the internal maxillary and internal carotid arteries; the stylo-mastoid branch of the posterior auricular artery; the petrosal branch of the middle meningeal artery, and a branch of the ascending pharyngeal artery which passes up the Eustachian (*auditory*) tube.

The *veins* empty into the temporo-maxillary (*posterior facial*) vein, the superior petrosal sinus, the lateral (*transverse*) sinus, the internal jugular vein, and the pharyngeal veins; numerous small venous channels pass through the tegmen tympani, communicating with the veins of the dura mater. These veins afford paths by which inflammatory processes may extend from the tympanum to the venous sinuses, the internal jugular vein, the meninges, and the brain.

The *lymphatics* arise from a network in the mucous membrane and terminate in the posterior auricular, parotid, and retropharyngeal lymph glands.

NERVE SUPPLY OF THE TYMPANUM.—The nerve supply of the tympanum is derived from numerous sources, for there are several nerves which enter the tympanic plexus of nerves.

The relation of *the facial nerve* to the tympanum has already been considered (p. 259).

The **chorda tympani nerve,** a branch of the facial nerve, through an opening in the posterior wall, the *iter chordæ posterius*, enters the tympanum near the upper part of the tympanic membrane, crosses the handle of the malleus, and then enters a small, bony canal, the *iter chordæ anterius*, near the Glaserian (*petro-tympanic*) fissure. In the tympanum it is covered by the tympanic mucous

33

membrane. Involvement of this nerve in otitis media may lead to abnormal sense of taste on one side of the anterior portion of the tongue. Although anatomically its relationship is important, it gives no branches to the structures of the tympanum.

The **tympanic plexus of nerves** ramifies in the grooves on the promontory and medial wall of the tympanum, and supplies its mucous membrane. It is formed by the tympanic branch of the glossopharyngeal nerve, a branch of the greater superficial petrosal nerve, a branch of the lesser superficial petrosal nerve, and the small deep petrosal (*carotico-tympanic*) nerve.

The *tympanic branch of the glossopharyngeal nerve* arises from the petrous ganglion of the glossopharyngeal nerve, and passes into the tympanum through a foramen in the floor near its medial wall.

The *branch of the greater superficial petrosal nerve*, is derived from the facial nerve, and passes into the tympanum through a foramen in the medial wall of that cavity just anterior to the oval window.

The *branch of the lesser superficial petrosal nerve*, which is also derived from the facial nerve, enters the tympanum near the canal for the tensor tympani muscle.

The *small deep petrosal (carotico-tympanic) nerve*, or tympanic branch of the carotid plexus of the cervical sympathetic, enters the tympanum through the carotico-tympanic canal.

The motor nerves to the tensor tympani and stapedius muscles have been described at p. 512. The former muscle receives its supply from the trigeminal while the latter is supplied by the facial.

THE INTERNAL EAR

The **Internal Ear,** or **Labyrinth.**—The most important portion of the organ of hearing is the labyrinth, situated in the substance of the petrous portion of the temporal bone. It consists of two sets of structures: the *bony* labyrinth and the *membranous labyrinth*, situated within the bony labyrinth.

The **Bony Labyrinth** (Plates CXXI; CXXII) is made up of three intercommunicating cavities: the vestibule, the cochlea, and the semicircular canals, which are lined by a delicate periosteum.

The **vestibule,** or middle portion of the bony labyrinth, situated between the cochlea and the semicircular canals, is an ovoid bony cavity, the antero-posterior diameter of which is about five millimeters (one-fifth of an inch). On the lateral wall is the *fenestra ovalis (fenestra vestibuli)* in communication with the tympanum. As previously stated, this is closed in the natural state by the base of the stapes and the periosteal lining of the vestibule. At the anterior

PLATE CXXI.

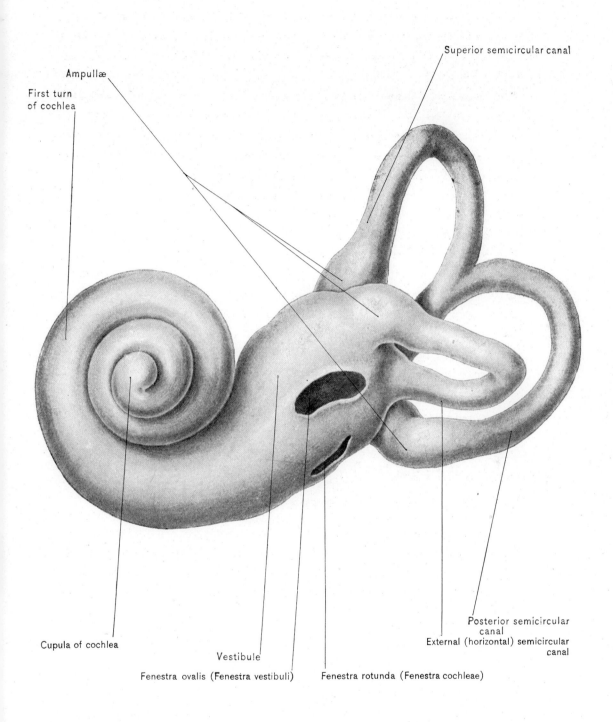

Superior semicircular canal

Ampullæ

First turn
of cochlea

Cupula of cochlea

Vestibule

Fenestra ovalis (Fenestra vestibuli)

Fenestra rotunda (Fenestra cochleae)

Posterior semicircular
canal
External (horizontal) semicircular
canal

LATERAL VIEW OF BONY LABYRINTH, OR COCHLEA, AND SEMICIRCULAR CANALS.

PLATE CXXII.

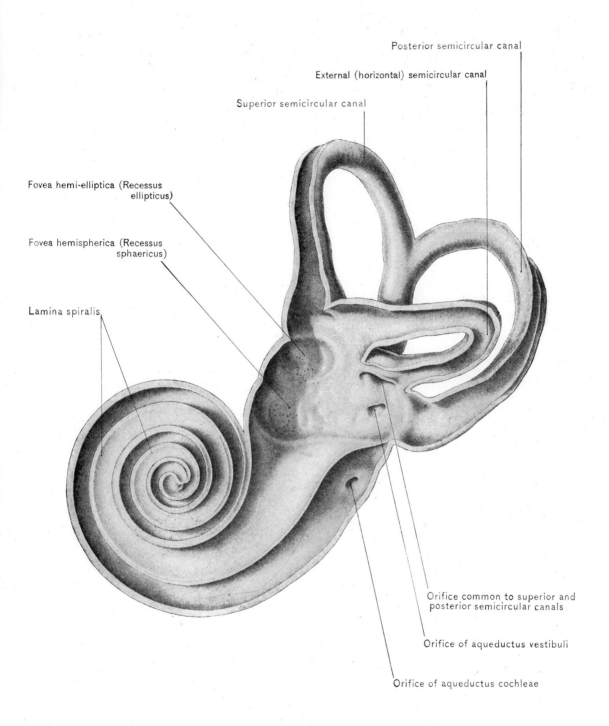

Posterior semicircular canal

External (horizontal) semicircular canal

Superior semicircular canal

Fovea hemi-elliptica (Recessus ellipticus)

Fovea hemispherica (Recessus sphaericus)

Lamina spiralis

Orifice common to superior and posterior semicircular canals

Orifice of aqueductus vestibuli

Orifice of aqueductus cochleae

INTERIOR OF OSSEOUS LABYRINTH OF LEFT INTERNAL EAR.

PLATE CXXIII.

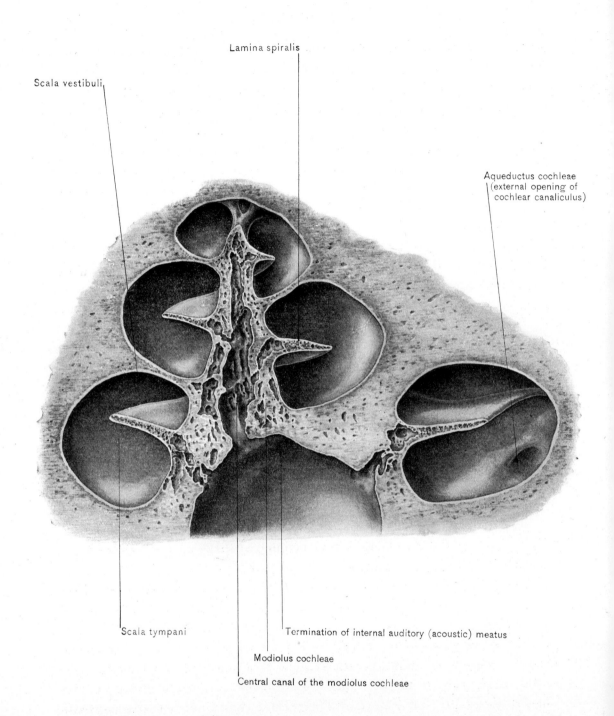

Lamina spiralis

Scala vestibuli

Aqueductus cochleae
(external opening of
cochlear canaliculus)

Scala tympani

Termination of internal auditory (acoustic) meatus

Modiolus cochleae

Central canal of the modiolus cochleae

SECTION OF OSSEOUS PORTION OF COCHLEA.

portion of the medial wall is a round depression, the *fovea hemispherica* (*recessus sphæricus*), the bottom of which is pierced by numerous small openings, *macula cribrosa media*, for the transmission of the vestibular branch of the auditory nerve. Posterior to the fovea hemispherica (*recessus sphæricus*) is a vertical crest, the *crista vestibuli*, the anterior end of which is known as the *pyramidalis vestibuli*. Posteriorly, the crista vestibuli divides into two limbs between which is a small depression, the *recessus cochlearis*, perforated by a number of small openings for the passage of nerve filaments of the ductus cochlearis the beginning of which is lodged in the cochlear recess. In the posterior portion of the medial wall is the small opening of the *aqueductus vestibuli*, a canal which extends to the posterior surface of the petrous portion of the temporal bone, and lodges the ductus endolymphaticus and a minute vein. At the infero-anterior portion of the vestibule is the comparatively large opening leading to the scala vestibuli of the cochlea. On the roof of the vestibule is the large oval fossa, the *fovea hemi-elliptica* (*recessus ellipticus*). Posteriorly, the vestibule communicates by five round openings with the semicircular canals.

The **semicircular canals,** three bony tubes about one and a quarter millimeters (one-twentieth of an inch) in diameter, are situated behind the vestibule. The *superior semicircular canal* lies nearly in the sagittal plane of the body, the *posterior*, in the coronal plane, and the *lateral*, or *horizontal*, in the transverse plane, thus occupying positions about at right angles to one another. Each semicircular canal forms more than a semicircle, and upon one extremity of each is an enlargement, the *ampulla*. They open by five orifices into the vestibule, since the non-ampullated extremities of the superior and posterior canals join, and have a common orifice. From the positions of these canals in the sagittal, coronal, and transverse planes, it may be inferred that they are associated with the maintenance of equilibrium.

The **cochlea** (Plate CXXIII) is situated anterior to the vestibule. When isolated from the investing bony substance it resembles a cone, the apex of which looks lateralward and somewhat downward and forward. The *base* is perforated by numerous foramina for branches of the auditory nerve, and is directed toward the internal auditory meatus. The base is nearly ten millimeters (two-fifths of an inch) in diameter, and the height of the cone is about six millimeters (one-fourth of an inch). The cochlea consists of a nearly horizontal central axis, the *modiolus*, or *columnella*, around which is wound a spiral bony tube, like the spirals in certain snail shells. The interior of the *modiolus* contains numerous canals for branches of the auditory nerve, the largest being the *canalis centralis modioli*. The **spiral canal** diminishes in diameter as it approaches the apex of the cochlea, makes two and a-half turns around the axis, and terminates in

a closed extremity, the *cupola*.   Projecting into the spiral canal from the modiolus is the bony *lamina spiralis*, which does not reach the outer wall of the cochlea.
From the free border of the lamina spiralis, or near it, two membranes extend,
in the natural state, the *basilar membrane* and the *membrane of Reissner (vestibular
membrane)*.   These two membranes are connected with the outer wall of the
cochlea, and inclose between them the *cochlear duct*, or *scala media;* they are, in
fact, two parts of the membranous cochlea.   The bony lamina spiralis and the
two membranes just mentioned divide the spiral canal into three parts: the
scala tympani, the *scala vestibuli*, and the *scala media (ductus cochlearis)* between
the two.

The *scala tympani* is on the basal side of the lamina spiralis, and opens into
the tympanum at the fenestra rotunda (*fenestra cochleæ*), although in the natural
state this opening is closed by the *membrana tympani secundaria*.   The *scala
vestibuli* is on the opposite side of the lamina spiralis, and opens into the vestibule.
These two scalæ communicate with each other by an opening at the summit of
the cochlea, known as the *helicotrema;* they contain the *perilymph* which communicates with the subarachnoid space of the brain along the sheath of the
auditory nerve.

The **Membranous Labyrinth** (Plate CXXIV), embryologically, is the earliest
formed and, therefore, the oldest part of the organ of hearing.   It is a cast (though
considerably smaller) of the bony labyrinth, except that the portion corresponding to the bony labyrinth has two compartments, the saccule and the utricle.
Between the outer surfaces of the membranous labyrinth and the walls of the
bony labyrinth is a space, the *perilymph space*, which contains the *perilymph*, or
liquor Contunii.   The space enclosed by the membranous labyrinth is the *endolymph* space and contains the *endolymph*.   It differs from the former space in that
it is lined with epithelium, the cells of which are highly specialized in certain
regions, to form the terminal portions of the cochlear and vestibular parts of
the auditory nerve.

The membranous labyrinth consists of the utricle, the saccule, the membranous semicircular canals (*semicircular ducts*) and the membranous cochlea.   The
utricle and the saccule are two vesicles found in the vestibule, the utricle
lying partly in the fovea hemi-elliptica (*recessus ellipticus*), and the saccule in
the fovea hemispherica (*recessus sphæricus*).   The **utricle** communicates with
the membranous semicircular canals (*semicircular ducts*) which open into the
utricle by five orifices.   Filaments of the vestibular branch of the auditory
nerve are distributed to a thickened portion of the walls of the utricle which
contains calcareous masses, the **otoliths**.   The **saccule**, which is smaller than
the utricle, receives branches of the auditory nerve through the perforations

PLATE CXXIV.

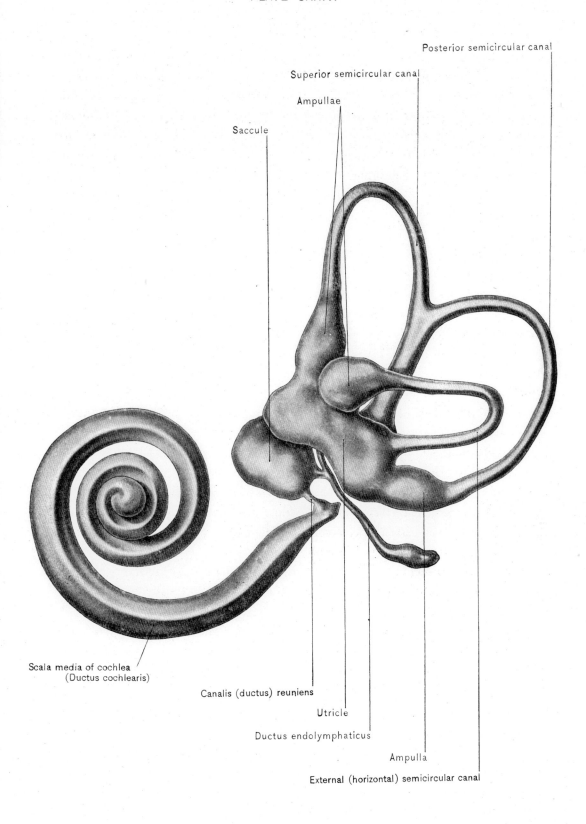

Posterior semicircular canal

Superior semicircular canal

Ampullae

Saccule

Scala media of cochlea
(Ductus cochlearis)

Canalis (ductus) reuniens

Utricle

Ductus endolymphaticus

Ampulla

External (horizontal) semicircular canal

DIAGRAM OF MEMBRANOUS LABYRINTH.

in the fovea hemispherica (*recessus sphæricus*); as in the utricle, these nerves are distributed to a thickened portion of the wall of the cavity, which is covered with otoliths. Passing from the saccule along the aqueductus vestibuli is a slender tube, the **ductus endolymphaticus,** which expands into the **saccus endolymphaticus,** a blind pouch which lies on the posterior surface of the petrous portion of the temporal bone beneath the dura mater; this canal is joined by a small tube from the utricle; the two portions of the membranous vestibule are thus brought into direct communication. The saccule communicates with the scala media (*ductus cochlearis*), or membranous labyrinth of the cochlea, by means of a short tube, the **canalis reuniens.**

The **membranous semicircular canals (semicircular ducts)** are about one-fourth the diameter of the osseous canals in which they lie; their extremities are ampullated.

The **membranous cochlea,** or **scala media (ductus cochlearis),** lies between the scala tympani and scala vestibuli. It follows the windings of the spiral tube of the cochlea, and ends blindly at both extremities, although near its basal end it communicates with the saccule by the canalis reuniens. Within the scala media (*ductus cochlearis*) is found the **spiral organ of Corti,** a complex arrangement of modified epithelial cells to which the final ramifications of the cochlear branch of the auditory nerve are distributed. For a detailed description of the more minute structure of the internal ear the reader is referred to works on systematic anatomy and histology.

Aural vertigo, also known as **Menière's symptom-complex,** is characterized by tinnitus, dizziness, reeling, and nausea and vomiting, in succession. It is due to abnormal increase of pressure in the membranous labyrinth. Cerumen or instillation of cold liquids into the external auditory meatus may produce this symptom, and it may also be due to abnormal conditions in the middle ear and to intermittent closure of the Eustachian (*auditory*) tubes.

Blood Supply.—The blood supply of the internal ear is derived from the auditory artery, a branch of the basilar, which enters the internal auditory meatus with the auditory nerve, and divides into branches for the cochlea and vestibule.

The *veins* which drain the internal ear are the vena aqueductus cochlea and vena aqueductus vestibuli. The *vena aqueductus cochlea* receives the veins of the cochlea, passes through the aqueductus cochleæ, and empties into the internal jugular vein. The *vena aqueductus vestibuli* receives the veins from the vestibule and semicircular canals, and empties into the superior petrosal sinus.

The *lymphatics of the internal ear* terminate in the tympanic and intra-cranial lymph vessels.

The **auditory (acoustic) nerve** is the nerve of the special sense of hearing. In the internal auditory meatus it divides into two branches, the cochlear and the vestibular; the former is distributed to the cochlea, and the latter to the walls of the membranous vestibule and ampullæ of the semicircular canals (see p. 100).

INDEX

In this Index the references in **heavy-face type** are to the pages containing plates illustrating the subject named. References in regular type are to the text.

Heavy-face type denotes plates illustrating the subject named

Heavy-face type denotes plates illustrating the subject named

Heavy-face type denotes plates illustrating the subject named

Heavy-face type denotes plates illustrating the subject named

Heavy-face type denotes plates illustrating the subject named

Heavy-face type denotes plates illustrating the subject named

Heavy-face type denotes plates illustrating the subject named

Heavy-face type denotes plates illustrating the subject named

Heavy-face type denotes plates illustrating the subject named

Heavy-face type denotes plates illustrating the subject named

Heavy-face type denotes plates illustrating the subject named

Heavy-face type denotes plates illustrating the subject named

Heavy-face type denotes plates illustrating the subject named

Heavy-face type denotes plates illustrating the subject named

Heavy-face type denotes plates illustrating the subject named

Heavy-face type denotes plates illustrating the subject named

Heavy-face type denotes plates illustrating the subject named

Heavy-face type denotes plates illustrating the subject named

Heavy-face type denotes plates illustrating the subject named

Heavy-face type denotes plates illustrating the subject named

Heavy-face type denotes plates illustrating the subject named

Heavy-face type denotes plates illustrating the subject named